T0400946

THE KNEE

CURRENT CONCEPTS IN KINEMATICS, INJURY TYPES, AND TREATMENT OPTIONS

MUSCULAR SYSTEM - ANATOMY, FUNCTIONS AND INJURIES

Additional books in this series can be found on Nova's website
under the Series tab.

Additional e-books in this series can be found on Nova's website
under the e-books tab.

THE KNEE

CURRENT CONCEPTS IN KINEMATICS, INJURY TYPES, AND TREATMENT OPTIONS

RANDY MASCARENHAS
EDITOR

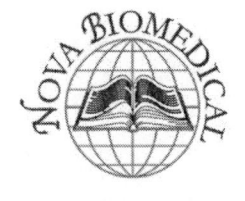

Nova Science Publishers, Inc.
New York

For permission to use material from this book please contact us:
Telephone 631-231-7269; Fax 631-231-8175
Web Site: http://www.novapublishers.com

NOTICE TO THE READER

The Publisher has taken reasonable care in the preparation of this book, but makes no expressed or implied warranty of any kind and assumes no responsibility for any errors or omissions. No liability is assumed for incidental or consequential damages in connection with or arising out of information contained in this book. The Publisher shall not be liable for any special, consequential, or exemplary damages resulting, in whole or in part, from the readers' use of, or reliance upon, this material. Any parts of this book based on government reports are so indicated and copyright is claimed for those parts to the extent applicable to compilations of such works.

Independent verification should be sought for any data, advice or recommendations contained in this book. In addition, no responsibility is assumed by the publisher for any injury and/or damage to persons or property arising from any methods, products, instructions, ideas or otherwise contained in this publication.

This publication is designed to provide accurate and authoritative information with regard to the subject matter covered herein. It is sold with the clear understanding that the Publisher is not engaged in rendering legal or any other professional services. If legal or any other expert assistance is required, the services of a competent person should be sought. FROM A DECLARATION OF PARTICIPANTS JOINTLY ADOPTED BY A COMMITTEE OF THE AMERICAN BAR ASSOCIATION AND A COMMITTEE OF PUBLISHERS.

Additional color graphics may be available in the e-book version of this book.

Library of Congress Cataloging-in-Publication Data

Library of Congress Control Number: 2012940514
ISBN: 978-1-61942-268-1

Published by Nova Science Publishers, Inc. † New York

CONTENTS

PREFACE

Knee injuries are common occurrences that affect the young active population and can lead to subsequent long term joint degeneration. This book provides an overview of current research examining knee injury mechanisms, prevention, and treatment options. Detailed discussions are included related to current treatment options for ACL injury, PCL injury, meniscal tears, patellofemoral instability, and combined knee pathology. Additionally, current advances in tissue engineering in ACL reconstruction and results following transphyseal ACL reconstruction in adolescents are examined. Furthermore, biomechanical studies and computerized modeling techniques are highlighted as methods for determining the mechanisms and sequelae of knee injuries, thus aiding in the development of injury prevention programs.

Chapter 1 - This chapter presents the results of cadaver simulation models to study non-contact sports injury mechanisms. The topics of interest include sports medicine injury mechanisms, biomechanics of injury, and post-traumatic osteoarthritis. Recently, numerous surveys have been conducted based on patient questionnaires and videos of ACL injuries to determine the loading mechanisms that cause this frequent and serious sports injury. The two most common scenarios were axial rotation of the tibia and valgus bending of the knee. But, as one of the studies pointed out; "whether the consistent valgus collapse observed in the videos was actually the cause of injury or simply a result of the ACL being torn is open for discussion". Therefore, the first objective was to measure the pre-failure and failure characteristics of the most common loading mechanisms in order to determine the cause-and-effect relationship between knee joint motion and potential ACL failure. A second objective is based on experiments showing that isolated ACL failure occurs due to anterior subluxation of the tibia caused by tibiofemoral (TF) compressive forces in the flexed knee.[154] The results support this loading mechanism in the extended knee as an important factor during non-contact, isolated ACL injuries. Finally, there is a large body of evidence for the association of ACL injury with long-term development of post-traumatic osteoarthritis. A final objective was to document the osteochondral microdamage that occurs at the time of acute ligamentous injury and which may play a role in chronic joint degeneration. Therefore, the contact pressure distributions in the TF joint were recorded during each injury mechanism. The regions in the tibial plateau where osteochondral microdamage occur were predicted in a finite element model and documented with imaging and histology. This was the first computer model to relate TF contact pressures with stress distributions in the cartilage and subchondral bone in order to validate the characteristic footprints of bone bruises and overlying cartilage degeneration that occur with specific injury mechanisms. These results are applicable to the clinical literature for comparison with the current mechanism-based classification of knee injuries and bone bruise patterns. This information may be used to develop new treatment regimens for dealing with post-traumatic osteoarthritis based on the injury mechanism and locations of osteochondral microdamage.

Chapter 2 - Although the knee is probably the most studied joint in the human body, the work carried out to date is still far from predicting true mechanical behavior and has not yet solved many of the doubts about the origin of several injuries. This is due mainly to the high cost involved with experimentation, technical difficulties in the measurement of stress and strain, and the inability to faithfully reproduce certain diseases and degenerative states in vivo. Faced with these difficulties, numerical simulation is an alternative fast, accurate and economical method capable of providing information that is often very difficult to otherwise obtain. The main objective of this study was to develop a knee three-dimensional computational model to analyze the role of joint ligaments and menisci in load transmission and joint stability. The authors present a computational model of a healthy adult male in full extension to other three different scenarios: flexion of 60 degrees on the femur (simplified model), static compression load of 1150 N on the tibia (full model) and flexion of 10 degrees to the tibia (full model). In the developed model, bones were considered to be rigid. Articular cartilage and menisci were considered to be linearly elastic, isotropic and homogeneous. Ligaments were considered hyperelastic and transversely isotropic. Initial strains on the ligaments and patellar tendon were also considered and the model was validated using experimental and numerical results obtained by other authors. The results obtained reproduce the complex, nonuniform stress and strain fields that occur in the soft tissue of the knee as a result of the kinematics of the human knee joint under a physiologic external load.

Chapter 3 - Objective: To determine the effect of a lower limb injury prevention program on athletes with greater knee valgus angles during landing at high risk for ACL injury, who have greater knee valgus angle during landing, and on players with a low risk for ACL injury. Methods: Forty-two female collegiate basketball athletes (84 limbs) participated in this study. Before and after the prevention program, which lasted four months, the peak knee valgus and peak knee flexion angles during the continuous jump test and the Star Excursion Balance Test (SEBT) scores were recorded. According to the average peak knee valgus angle of the continuous jump test, the subjects were divided into either a high- or a low-risk group. A 2-way ANOVA model (risk(2) × training(2)) was used to examine the main and interaction effects (risk/training/risk × training). Results: In the high-risk group, the post-training knee valgus angle decreased compared to the pre-training angle ($p < 0.01$). In the low-risk group, the post-training SEBT score was greater than the pre-training score ($p < 0.01$). Conclusions: The injury prevention program was effective in decreasing the risk of ACL injury in high-risk athletes with greater knee valgus angles during landing. Accordingly, screening for high-risk players and recommending a prevention program for them may allow for more effective prevention of ACL injuries. In low-risk players who did not have a valgus angle exceeding the cut-off value during landing, the prevention program resulted in improved balance ability, which may also lead to a decreased risk of lower limb injury. Based on these results, the authors conclude that enrolling all athletes in injury prevention programs may help reduce the risk of lower limb injury in sport.

Chapter 4 - Proprioception alterations induced by intense physical exercise may be associated with increased risk of injury. In this sense, the main purpose of the present chapter was to assess the effect of fatigue induced by a soccer match on knee joint position sense in elite soccer players. The second aim of this chapter was to identify possible gender differences in proprioceptive response to fatigue. Twenty soccer players (age: 18.4±1.1 years) were recruited. Knee joint position sense was evaluated using an open kinetic chain technique and active knee positioning, and was reported using absolute and relative angular errors. Knee angles were determined by computer analysis of videotape images of the knee joint using a two-dimensional automatic digitizing module. Joint position sense measures were obtained at rest and immediately after a soccer match. The perceived exertion or exercise intensity was assessed at the end of the match using Borg's rating of perceived exertion (RPE) scale. Of the 20 players, only 17 completed the soccer match reaching or exceeding the score of 15 on the RPE scale. This left 17 players (10 female) for the statistical analysis. After the soccer match a significant increase in absolute (2.1±1.1° to 4.0±2.3°, P=.001) and relative (0.7±2.0° to 3.5±3.1°, P<.001) angular errors was observed. When comparing genders, no differences at rest were observed in absolute (female, 1.8±1.0° vs. male, 2.5±1.2° P>.05) and relative (female, 0.5±1.7° vs. male, 0.8±2.6°, P>.05) errors. However, the absolute error after the match increased to 4.9±3.2°(P=.038) in males and to 3.3±1.2° (P=.014) in females. Additionally, the relative error post-match increased to 3.6±4.8° (P=.049) in males and to 3.3±1.2° (P=.004) in females. No gender differences were detected in the magnitude of the increase in both relative (male, 2.4±2.4° vs. female, 1.6±1.7°; P>.05) and absolute (male, 2.8±3.0° vs. female, 2.8±2.3°; P>.05) angular errors. In conclusion, the authors results indicate that fatigue induced by a soccer match has a marked deleterious effect on knee joint position sense in elite soccer players irrespective of gender.

Chapter 5 - Gait analysis is a broad term that can refer to many different methods of evaluating an individual's walking pattern. One of the main purposes of the rehabilitative process is to help patients achieve a high level of functional independence within the limits of their particular impairments. Human gait is one of the basic components of independent functioning that is commonly affected by either disease processes or injury.

Chapter 6 - Anterior cruciate ligament (ACL) injuries are increasingly common and ACL reconstruction, the gold standard of treatment, can result in relatively high rates of graft rupture in adolescent patients[1]. Additionally, up to 80% of patients undergoing ACL reconstruction may develop some degree of osteoarthritis in the long term[2]. Development of improved techniques in ACL reconstruction is thus of great clinical interest. The development of such techniques would be aided with the use of a large animal model to simulate ACL injury and treatment. While prior studies focusing on bio-enhanced primary ACL repair (where a suture repair was supplemented with a bioactive scaffold designed to stimulate ACL healing) have used an immature porcine model with promising results, study of this procedure in an adult animal model would be desirable. To study bio-enhanced ACL repair in adult animals, the authors selected an ovine model that has been previously used in studies focusing on ACL reconstruction and repair. The ovine model has anatomic and biomechanical similarities to the human knee. Prior studies have described the gross anatomy, histology, and biomechanics of the ACL in the healthy ovine knee. Additionally, there have been several studies investigating the biomechanical and histological outcomes of various ACL reconstruction techniques in an ovine model. The authors group recently completed a study in adult sheep evaluating the efficacy of this model in studying bio-enhanced ACL repair. In the authors experiment, eight skeletally mature sheep underwent unilateral ACL transection and bio-enhanced repair. Four animals each were euthanized after three and six months of healing, and AP laxity of the knee and structural properties of the repaired ACL were evaluated. Unpaired t-tests were used to compare the three and six month values. The average yield load, maximum load, and stiffness of the healing ligaments increased significantly from three to six months from 108 N to 320 N (p = 0.023), 121 N to 343 N (p = 0.034), and 28 N/mm to 58 N/mm (p = 0.035), respectively. All these values remained significantly lower than the contralateral control ACLs, but were comparable with results in the literature for ACL reconstruction in the ovine model. AP laxity was not significantly different between three and six months. In summary, the mature sheep has proven to be a reliable model for ACL reconstruction and bio-enhanced ACL repair. Bio-enhanced ACL repair in the mature sheep model resulted in progressively increasing yield load, maximum load and linear stiffness of the repair from three to six months of healing. Values obtained at six months validated the hypothesis that the functional outcomes of this new technique are comparable with those found in this model for ACL reconstruction. These promising results suggest that further work may result in a new and innovative strategy for the treatment of human ACL injuries, and that the mature ovine model is well-suited to development of new ACL treatment methods.

Chapter 7 - Anterior cruciate ligament (ACL) reconstruction ranks among the most commonly performed orthopaedic procedures worldwide. The concepts behind surgical management of ACL deficiency have continued to evolve over the past few decades. Historically, most ACL reconstruction methods have focused on single bundle (SB) reconstruction techniques that may not recreate native anatomy by ignoring the posterolateral (PL) bundle and its importance in rotatory stability. Recent data suggests that non-anatomic ACL reconstruction may lead to altered joint kinematics with concern for long-term joint health. A school of thought has emerged which suggests that a key to optimizing joint function and long term health may rest on an anatomic surgical approach to ACL injury. These approaches have focused on individualized surgery based on patient anatomy and anatomical restoration of the ACL, which consists of the anteromedial (AM) bundle (primary contributor to antero-posterior stability) and the PL bundle (allows rotatory stability). During the past several years, there has been an increasing trend towards double bundle (DB) ACL reconstruction in an attempt to restore anatomy and preserve the individual and synergistic functions of the AM and PL bundles. Recent biomechanical research suggests that anatomic DB ACL reconstruction can better reproduce native knee function when compared to conventional non-anatomic SB reconstruction. Further long-term clinical and biomechanical studies comparing anatomic DB ACL construction to non-anatomic SB reconstruction will more fully elucidate whether restoration of native knee joint kinematics and function have any bearing on future joint health.

Chapter 8 - Treatment of posterior cruciate ligament injuries may require different approaches ranging from conservative management to surgical reconstruction. With the varying success of surgical treatment, controversy exists as to which approach to use. PCL injuries occur at higher rates than previously believed (PCL injuries comprise 3% of all knee injuries and 37% of trauma cases with acute hemarthrosis[1]), and recent research has provided orthopedic surgeons with a better understanding of treatment algorithms and surgical techniques.

Chapter 9 - Meniscal injuries are common and can lead to significant morbidity. Historically, these injuries were managed with a total meniscectomy. However, knowledge of the anatomy and function of the meniscus has advanced considerably since the days when it was thought to be the functionless vestiges of a leg muscle. On the contrary, the meniscus is now known to be an integral component of the complex biomechanics of the knee. This is reflected in the various interventions and techniques employed to preserve the meniscus, and arthroscopic treatment of meniscal tears has become one of the most common procedures in the United States. It is the goal of this chapter to review the authors understanding of the meniscus and the associated treatment of meniscal injuries.

Chapter 10 - Patellar dislocation represents a common injury with a variety of causal factors. The incidence of patellofemoral instability is estimated to be approximately 5.8 per 100,000 with an increased incidence in adolescents of approximately twenty-nine per 100,000(1,2). It has been suggested that the recurrence rates after nonoperative treatment of an acute patellar dislocation range from 15-44% (2). However, once a second dislocation occurs, the rate of future instability events increases to nearly 50% (1). The extent of disability that occurs after an acute dislocation event should not be underestimated. Many patients experiencing patellar instability are young, active individuals that injure themselves during sporting activity. It has been shown that these individuals have definite limitations to return to their previous activity levels with a significant decrease in return to strenuous athletic activities even after six months of recovery (3). Because of the relatively low rate of re-dislocation after a primary event, a trial of conservative management with focus on regaining range of motion and strength should certainly be attempted. Once a second dislocation event occurs, more emphasis should be placed on causality and the possible benefit that can be gleaned from surgical treatment.

Chapter 11 - Patients presenting with knee pain may have multiple concurrent etiologies. With advancements in surgical techniques, implant designs, and imaging modalities, the ability to successfully perform complex procedures in even the most challenging patient is improving. However patients with multiple coexisting knee pathologies remain a difficult patient group, especially with regard to determining which (if any) of the lesions is the cause of symptoms. Cartilage lesions may be simply incidental in nature, and the decision to treat is based upon their confirmed contribution to patients' symptomatology.

Chapter 12 - Background: The surgical management of ACL rupture in the teenage athlete with open physes remains controversial. The purpose of this study was to evaluate the functional and radiographic outcome of transphyseal ACL reconstruction with medial hamstring autograft in skeletally immature patients with open physes. Hypothesis: Transphyseal ACL reconstruction with hamstring autograft can yield satisfactory clinical and functional outcomes with a low incidence of clinically significant leg length discrepancy or malalignment. Study Design: Case Series Methods: ACL reconstruction involved drilling tunnels through the tibial and femoral physes and placing a hamstring graft. Follow-up evaluation included objective clinical data (ROM and laxity testing), imaging (scanograms to assess for limb length discrepancies and MRI to assess for bony bar formation), and subjective patient-reported data (IKDC and ACL QOL forms). Results: Seventeen patients were reviewed at an average clinical follow-up of 8.2 years after surgery (range 5-9 years). No patients had significant leg-length discrepancies or bony bar formation. Subjective results showed an average ACL QOL score of 73.2 (range 37-100) and 88.2% of patients had normal or nearly normal knees as per the IKDC survey. Fifteen out of seventeen patients (88.2%)

returned to competitive sports after surgery. Conclusions: Transphyseal ACL reconstruction with semitendinosus/ gracilis autograft was performed successfully in seventeen skeletally immature adolescents with clearly open growth plates with little apparent risk for growth disturbance.

In: The Knee
Editor: Randy Mascarenhas

ISBN: 978-1-61942-268-1
© 2012 Nova Science Publishers, Inc.

Chapter I

BIOMECHANICAL RESPONSE OF THE KNEE IN SPORTS INJURY SCENARIOS

Eric G. Meyer[1] and Roger C. Haut[2]

[1] Experimental Biomechanics Laboratory, Biomedical Engineering Department, Lawrence Technological University, Southfield, MI, US
[2] Orthopaedic Biomechanics Laboratories, College of Osteopathic Medicine, Michigan State University, East Lansing, MI, US

ABSTRACT

This chapter presents the results of cadaver simulation models to study non-contact sports injury mechanisms. The topics of interest include sports medicine injury mechanisms, biomechanics of injury, and post-traumatic osteoarthritis. Recently, numerous surveys have been conducted based on patient questionnaires and videos of ACL injuries to determine the loading mechanisms that cause this frequent and serious sports injury. The two most common scenarios were axial rotation of the tibia and valgus bending of the knee. But, as one of the studies pointed out; "whether the consistent valgus collapse observed in the videos was actually the cause of injury or simply a result of the ACL being torn is open for discussion".[176] Therefore, the first objective was to measure the pre-failure and failure characteristics of the most common loading mechanisms in order to determine the cause-and-effect relationship between knee joint motion and potential ACL failure. A second objective is based on experiments showing that isolated ACL failure occurs due to anterior subluxation of the tibia caused by tibiofemoral (TF) compressive forces in the flexed knee.[154] The results support this loading mechanism in the extended knee as an important factor during non-contact, isolated ACL injuries. Finally, there is a large body of evidence for the association of ACL injury with long-term development of post-traumatic osteoarthritis. A final objective was to document the osteochondral microdamage that occurs at the time of acute ligamentous injury and which may play a role in chronic joint degeneration. Therefore, the contact pressure distributions in the TF joint were recorded during each injury mechanism. The regions in the tibial plateau where osteochondral microdamage occur were predicted in a finite element model and documented with imaging and histology. This was the first computer model to relate TF contact pressures with stress distributions in the cartilage and subchondral bone in order to validate the characteristic footprints of bone bruises and overlying cartilage degeneration that occur with specific injury mechanisms. These results are applicable to the clinical literature for comparison with the current mechanism-based classification of knee injuries and bone bruise patterns. [100] This information may be used to develop new treatment regimens for dealing with post-traumatic osteoarthritis based on the injury mechanism and locations of osteochondral microdamage.

1. INTRODUCTION

Injury in Sports

Sports Participation

Participation in sports, recreation, and exercise is increasingly popular and widespread in American culture. Approximately 50% of youths (aged 5-17 yrs.), accounting for more than 25 million people, regularly participate in vigorous physical activity. [49] The 1997 Centers for Disease Control and Prevention "Guidelines for schools and communities for promoting lifelong physical activity" states that the benefits of regular physical activity in childhood and adolescence include improvements in strength and endurance, help in building healthy bones and muscles, help in controlling weight, reduction of anxiety and stress, increasing self esteem and possibly improving blood pressure and cholesterol levels. [39]

There are also estimates of 25 million middle-aged people (15-20% of the U.S. population, depending on age and gender characteristics) participating in recreational sports. [220] The benefits of moderate and vigorous physical activities are also clear in adulthood. In a study of 50 to 70 year old Harvard alumni, greater energy expenditure was associated with increased longevity and was proportional to the intensity of the activities. [140] Benefits included decreased blood pressure, decreased risk of coronary heart disease, hypertension, colon cancer and diabetes and decreased obesity. [177] Along with a general emphasis on physical fitness, female participation in sports has seen a dramatic increase since the passage of Title IX in 1972.[169]

Injury Incidence

Each year 3-4.5 million children and adolescents are injured during sports participation with more than 775,000 of the injuries to young athletes requiring physician visits. [48,102] An estimated 800,000 lower extremity injuries are sustained nationally by American high school athletes. [74] Adult sports participants report musculoskeletal injuries at nearly twice the frequency of sedentary individuals (27-31% versus 15-17%, respectively). [107] In Scandinavia, sports injuries represent 10-19% of all acute injuries treated in emergency rooms. [20] Long-term participation in vigorous physical activities increases the risk of acute and chronic injuries such as ligament sprains or osteoarthritis (OA), respectively. [107]

Injuries to the lower extremity are among the most frequent injuries in all levels of sports and often account for more than 50% of reported injuries. [74] The knee is one of the most common sites of sports injury requiring an emergency room visit. [20] In particular, one in ten female athletes at the intercollegiate level suffers a season-ending knee injury annually.

[168] Additionally, female athletes participating in jumping and cutting sports have a three to six-fold higher incidence of serious knee injury than males. [75,104,181]

Risk Factors for Injury

A comprehensive model to describe the etiology of sports injuries would be very complex and include both intrinsic (age, sex and body composition) and extrinsic (shoe/surface traction, bracing and environmental factors) risk factors for a particular athlete, as well as an understanding of the inciting event (injury mechanism) that is associated with the onset of injury. [133] Each of these variables will have an effect on the load level in the lower extremity as well as the athlete's tolerance to that load before an injury occurs.

Intrinsic risk factors are generally difficult to control when attempting to reduce a particular athlete's likelihood of a lower extremity injury. Each athlete has a different set of these variables which can predispose them to more frequent injuries than an athlete with a different level of maturity, joint anatomy, or history of injury. Other intrinsic factors can be modified slightly with training. Physical fitness can be improved, skills in performing certain tasks such as landing can be taught, and psychological motivations like competitiveness can be monitored.

Exposures to extrinsic risk factors are easier to control, provided the variables linked with an increased susceptibility for injury can be identified in the first place. Therefore, knowledge about the types and magnitudes of force that produce injury is needed in order to implement policies that protect athletes from unnecessary risk. Examples of such policies to increase safety for the participants are rules that ban certain activities, mandated sports equipment, and the design of competition sites.

In some cases, however, tradeoffs and compromises make it difficult to control the extrinsic factors. While linear friction at the shoe-surface interface is necessary for athletic performance, [204] it is generally accepted that excessive rotational friction between the shoe and surface induces dangerous forces in vulnerable anatomic structures and may be a factor in lower extremity injury. A study of ACL injuries in high school football players documented a significant relationship between cleat design, the amount of torsional friction, and the risk of ACL injury. [138] In fact, the cleat design with the highest torsional moment was associated with an ACL injury rate two and a half times higher than of all other cleat designs combined. Although all injuries were sustained on natural grass, the authors also measured the frictional moments of each cleat on artificial turf and found these values to be even higher. Differences in injury frequency have also been documented for natural grass versus Astroturf surface types. These differences in injury frequency may be due to changes in the structure and materials, [96] the running speed of the players [210] or the coefficient of friction between the surface and shoe. [6] To complicate matters further, injury risk also depends on the player's position and the type of play at the time of injury, both of which influence the loading mechanisms on the lower extremity. Finally, the location of injury (ie. knee sprain vs. ankle sprain) may be dependent on the muscular activation and control present in the lower extremity at the time of injury. In uncontrolled movements, the knee may be the weakest link since ligamentous injury occurs at lower torques than in the ankle. [158] However, during controlled movements the musculature may have a greater ability to absorb torsional moments in the knee and therefore the ankle may have a lower failure torque.

Knee Biomechanics

Diarthrodial joints, such as the knee, allow movement by transferring forces between muscle and bone with very little friction while also providing cushioning and distributing the forces over large areas. The knee joint primarily functions as a hinge to produce flexion between the articular surfaces of the femoral condyles and tibial plateaus. [119] Contact between articular surfaces, muscle forces, and ligamentous restraint all play an important role in the stability of the knee by constraining joint motion.

Tissue Properties

The composition of ligaments is variable based on species and joint, depends on location within a particular ligament, and changes with age and activity as the tissue responds to the mechanical environment. [231] These changes in composition, especially of collagen fibers, affect the ligament's tensile properties. The ACL, in particular, loses 25-40% of its stiffness (200 N/mm to 125 N/mm) and 50-70% of its strength (1725 N to 730 N) as people age.

Defining the material properties of ligaments has been somewhat difficult, due to the complex anatomy and compositional organization of these tissues. The average elastic modulus of the ACL is 278 MPa, while the ultimate tensile strength is 40 MPa and occurs at approximately 12% strain. [35] The material properties of ligaments have a viscoelastic, non-linear stiffening response. There is little viscoelastic influence on the tissue's stiffness at relatively low strain rates (.66%/sec to 66%/sec), but the failure strain and energy absorbed before failure are significantly decreased when compared with higher strain rates. [173] In addition, at higher rates of loading, the failure mechanism is more commonly ligamentous rupture as compared to avulsions at lower rates of loading. Non-linear stiffening occurs due to progressive recruitment of crimped collagen fibrils and can be described in terms of four regions: clinical response, physiologic loading, microfailure and complete failure.[36] The physiological region is nearly linear and can range from approximately 169 N of force seen in the ACL during normal walking [163] to 630 N of force during jogging. [44] During the microfailure region and leading up to complete failure there are a series of unloadings that occur due to failure of individual collagen fibril bundles. [174]

The frictionless motion and cushioning properties of diarthrodial joints are provided by the articular cartilage (AC) layer on the contacting bone surfaces. Articular cartilage is characterized by a high degree of structural anisotropy. At birth and during development, however, the tissue is more isotropic in organization. The equilibrium tensile modulus of adult human knee cartilage is five to twenty times higher in the superficial zone than in the middle and deep zones. [3] By contrast, the confined compression modulus of bovine knee cartilage is significantly higher in the deep zone as compared to the superficial zone. [193] These differences are attributed to the orientation of collagen fibrils parallel to the surface of the superficial zone [227] and to the higher content of collagen and glycosaminoglycans in the deep zone. [130]

Age related changes in the mechanical properties of articular cartilage differ between locations within the body [124] and within the superficial, middle and deep zones. [123] The Young's modulus of cartilage increases until approximately 30 years of age at a value of 123 MPa. [63] Between 30 and 50 years of age, the material properties remain constant and then show a significant decline thereafter. The thickness of cartilage also decreases with age and especially with OA. [63]

Cartilage fissures are frequently documented in cadaver and animal research studies examining blunt impact. The number of fissures and their depth are related to the applied impact load and the contact pressure on the surface. They have also been shown to increase over time post impact in a rabbit model. [97] There are two theories for how OA initiation and progression occur. The first is that fissures and damage of the AC occur due to a mechanical insult that changes the ability to adequately absorb and transmit load. This initiates bone remodeling with increased stiffness that further damages the overlying cartilage and the cycle continues. The other theory involves a similar cycle, except that the mechanical insult causes trauma initially to the bone in the form of occult microcracks or "bone bruises". These cracks initiate remodeling of the subchondral bone, which in turn damages the AC by increasing the stresses seen in the overlying tissue and the chronic degradation cycle begins. [222]

The joints of the lower extremity are composed of a hard shell of cortical bone that forms the subchondral plate with trabecular bone filling in the diaphyseal ends. The thickness of the subchondral plate varies across the articular surfaces, particular ly between the medial and lateral tibial plateaus. The underlying trabecular bone also varies in material properties, especially centrally beneath the cruciate insertion points. The medial tibial plateau has a central region of increased strength, and while the lateral tibial plateau is generally weaker, the posterior region does have slightly elevated trabecular bone properties. [112] Loss of bone mineral density is the main factor in the decreased Young's modulus and ultimate stress of trabecular bone seen with aging. [63]

Occult injuries such as subchondral bone microcracks are documented in a number of impact studies with and without gross fracture of bone.[66,170,98] High rate impacts cause more microcracks than low rate impacts. [66] This microcracking is hypothesized to cause chronic subchondral bone thickening and remodeling post impact.

Biomechanical Function of the Knee Joint

The knee joint functions primarily in flexion and extension with a normal range of motion of approximately 130°. During passive flexion, the femoral condyles rotate and the contact point moves posteriorly on the tibial plateau. [179] Initially during flexion, there is also a small amount of internal tibial rotation. Articulation between the medial and lateral compartments of the knee, as well as the cruciate ligaments, guides this motion.

Biomechanics research has used two sectioning techniques to determine the primary and secondary contributions of the knee ligaments to preventing relative joint motion. One method is to apply known displacements prior to and after removal of a specific ligament and measure the amount of force required to produce the movement. This is known as the stiffness method. The other method is to apply known forces to the knee and to measure the resulting displacements before and after ligament sectioning. This is known as the flexibility method. When a primary restraint to a specific joint motion is sectioned, the force will decrease in the stiffness method or the displacement will increase in the flexibility method. If sectioning a specific ligament does not have one of these effects until after the primary restraint is removed, then it is a secondary restraint to that particular motion.

Ligament sectioning has been used to evaluate the ACL's role in preventing various types of joint displacement. [84,93,108,146,161] The ACL is a primary restraint to anterior tibial translation. [36,81,201,238] For an extended knee, the ACL is also considered a primary restraint to internal tibial rotation along with the MCL. [77,94,148,196] The ACL is also a secondary restraint to varus and valgus rotations of the femur [92,145,171], as well as external tibia rotation [172,203] and hyperextemsion [27,78,125,192]. Other primary restraints in the knee are as follows: the PCL resists posterior tibial subluxation, the MCL resists valgus rotation of the femur, the LCL resists varus rotation of the femur, and the posterior capsule resists knee hyperextension.

Other methods for determining a the role of a ligament in resisting specific joint motions include direct measurement of strain [26] or force [149] by implanting strain gauges, buckle transducers, or load cells. In subjects undergoing arthroscopic surgery with normal gait and an intact ACL, a strain transducer was implanted on the ACL and a variety of external loads were applied. [77] The results of this study show that an internal tibial torque of 10 Nm increased ACL strain, while a 10 Nm external torque did not. At 20° of knee flexion, weightbearing also significantly increased ACL strain. Combined loading of a 10 Nm internal torque and 40% of body weight, however, did not produce ACL strains higher than the isolated loading cases. This study also supports experimental investigations on cadaver knee specimens that document ligament forces of the knee under isolated and combined loading conditions. For knee flexion angles less than 30°, combined loading of a 10 Nm internal tibial torque and 100 N anterior tibial shear force produced ACL forces that exceeded the externally applied shear force. [148] In another study, two knees were flexed 30° with the tibia internally rotated 20°, resulting in the ACL providing 30-40% of the ligamentous restraining force. [194] In knees at 0° of flexion, an isolated 10 Nm internal torque produced an average ACL tensile force of 230 N. [94]

Normal in vivo weight bearing on the knee induces tensile strain in the ACL from anterior subluxation of the tibia. [77,141,146] The primary function (providing 85% of support) of the ACL is, in fact, to limit anterior tibial subluxation. [35,81,218] This motion occurs from compression of the TF joint for all knee flexion angles greater than 15° due to an inherent 10-15° posterior tilt of the tibial plateau (Figure 1). [60,86,87,141,218]

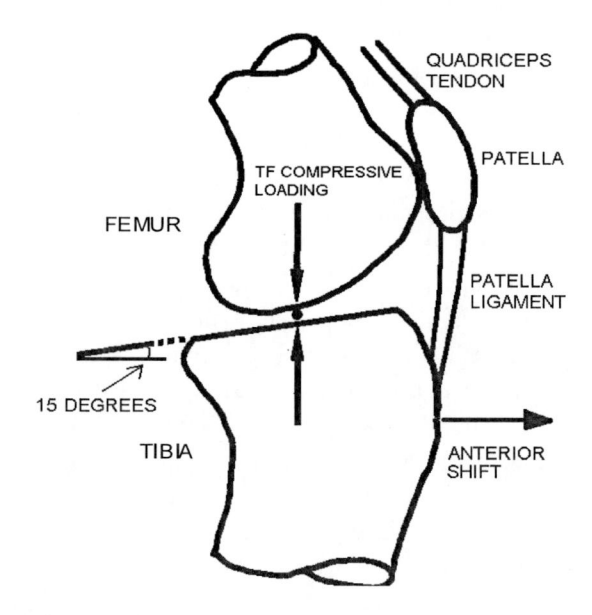

Figure 1. Posterior slope of the tibial plateau and TF compression to produce anterior displacement of the tibia (adapted from Meyer, 2005).

At 20° of knee flexion the average anterior/posterior (AP) laxity for a 200 N force applied to intact knees is 10 mm. [147] Using a commercially available clinical laxity measurement instrument, the KT-1000 (Medmetric Corp., San Diego, CA), the maximum anterior laxity of in vivo knees at 30° of knee flexion was 8.5 mm [55] or 5 mm for a 100 N anterior force. [213] After ACL sectioning, this anterior subluxation increased to 15 mm. [213] There is a high amount of scatter in comparing right-left AP laxity differences in both normal and ACL-deficient populations, but generally a difference in laxity >3 mm is indicative of an ACL disruption. [55] The AP laxity has been shown to be the greatest at 30° of knee flexion and increases when axial rotation of the tibia is allowed. [81] The sensitivity to diagnose a complete ACL disruption using this method is 96%. [55]

Acute Knee Injuries

Ligamentous Injury
An estimated annual cost (direct and indirect) for scholastic sports injuries is $1.3 billion. [102] The knee is one of the most frequently injured joints in the human body, accounting for 19-23% of all injuries. [7,59,107] Athletes in particular, suffer knee injuries at an even higher rate (nearly 40%) compared to other parts of the body. [144] The most common diagnosis for knee injuries in athletes is internal knee trauma at approximately 45%, followed by 34% for minor knee distortions, 11% for cartilage lesions, 5.5% for contusions, 3.3% for dislocations, and 1% for fractures. [144] Internal knee trauma is a classification that includes damage or tearing to the cruciate or collateral ligaments and menisci. The ACL, medial collateral ligament (MCL), and medial meniscus are the most frequently injured structures in the knee. [144] Epidemiological studies have shown there are 80,000-250,000 ACL tears in the USA each year, [91] with a total cost of two billion dollars. [105]

In professional football, knee sprains account for approximately 10% of injuries and while ACL rupture occurs in only 11% of cases, it represents a severe injury with a time loss of six months or more. [180] MCL injuries are more frequent (55-73% of knee injuries), and 45% of athletes with this injury miss more than three games. Other sports with high rates of ACL injuries include: squash, handball, volleyball, basketball, soccer, and skiing. [144]

The average age for ACL injured patients is 26 years of age, with males representing a majority of the cases due to higher levels of participation in sports and recreational activities. [54,87] One of the most important aspects of these injuries is the impact the injury has on a patient's ability to be active. The games and practices that are missed due to injury affect the player's skill development and personal satisfaction. [102] Injuries to high school athletes usually result in three to six days off, but approximately 45% of injuries require a week or more. [74] There is a significant difference in the percentage of season-ending injuries suffered by females (12.5%) versus males (8%). This is most likely due to internal knee trauma injuries, as females undergo surgery for this injury twice as frequently as males.

Following an ACL tear, most patients who undergo surgical reconstruction (65-88%) can return to their sport within the first year with even patients treated non-operatively return (19-82%) if they can regain knee stability in rehabilitation. [166] However, the rate of athletes competing at an elite level declines quicker than uninjured athletes, with only 30% of soccer players still competing three years after an ACL injury, versus 80% in the uninjured control population. [189] There is also a much higher rate of reinjury (2-13%) or injury to related structures such as the menisci, cartilage, or other ligaments (9-22%) if the athlete continues to compete after an ACL tear. [166]

The long-term cost of an acute injury may in fact be higher still, due to a significantly increased risk of developing chronic joint degeneration also known as post-traumatic osteoarthritis (OA). Following ACL rupture, approximately 50% of patients display signs of OA within ten years and nearly all patients have OA after 15-20 years. [166] Additionally, ACL reconstruction has been shown to have no effect on the high rate of post-traumatic OA. [76,165,224] Sports participation, in general, has also been shown to increase the rate of OA and certain sports such as weightlifting and team sports are associated with a higher risk of hip and knee OA, respectively. In contrast, moderate levels of exercise and activity appear safe and do not lead to OA. [230]

Analysis of Knee Injury Mechanisms

Most of the proposed ACL injury mechanisms are based on patient questionnaires and video analysis of the injury events. Approximately 91% of ACL injuries occur during sporting activities [178] and non-contact ACL injuries occur more frequently than injuries involving contact. [1,29,87,104,186,237] ACL injury results in immediate functional instability of the knee joint. A classic sign of an ACL tear is hearing a "pop" that occurs while cutting or pivoting that is followed by pain. [37,72] Following the injury, ACL-deficient patients may experience instability episodes and are more likely to develop additional injury to the knee joint, including meniscal tears [4,22,46] and osteoarthritis of the knee. [118]

Four mechanisms of noncontact isolated ACL rupture have been proposed in the clinical literature: The loading mechanisms are internal rotation of the tibia, [10,153] anterior shear of the tibia, [65] knee valgus bending, [29,133,176] and hyperextension of the knee. [101,160,205] Direct anterior shear of the tibia without contact from another player is quite uncommon, except in skiing when the entire bodyweight is on the tail of the ski, which can induce the "phantom-foot ACL injury mechanism". Hyperextension also may be more common in player-to-player contact scenarios, but has been documented to occur in noncontact situations with a large axial tibial load, such as jumping on a trampoline.[137]

Others propose that most ACL injuries occur in extended knees due to a combination of tibial rotation and valgus bending in the setting of an axial tibial load.[70,151,202,208] Many studies have emphasized the high frequency of ACL tears that occur during landing from a jump on one or both legs. [20,29,68,105,134]

In a recent ACL injury mechanism survey, the most common activities were basketball, football, and soccer (skiing injuries were excluded) and 38 out of 71 noncontact ACL injuries occurred while decelerating or just before a change in direction. [29] An additional 26 ACL injuries occurred during landing from a jump. In a study of only soccer related ACL injuries, 56 out of 105 players were changing direction towards the side of their injured knee, while 10 were turning towards the uninjured side. [70] An additional 26 players sustained their injuries when landing after jumping to head the ball, and the authors concluded that tackling and kicking did not contribute significantly to ACL ruptures in soccer. Skiing also has one of the highest rates of ACL injury, accounting for 25-30% of knee injuries. [183,208] These injuries are mainly associated with internal twisting or combined loading during a hard landing. [65,202]

Li et al. suggest that excessive compressive loads caused by impact load along the tibial shaft (e.g., landing from a jump) may contribute to injury of the ACL, especially when the knee is flexed. [141] While injury of the ACL has been documented in landings with the knee relatively straight, [207] the knee may also be flexed as much as 60-80° during a landing. [103]

Experimentally Produced Knee Injuries

Kennedy et al. tested five cadaver knees in internal rotation (at 20° of flexion) and premature fractures occurred at the bone clamps before ACL injuries. [127] Additional studies have been conducted in external tibial rotation to characterize MCL injury mechanisms. [126,200] Some of those specimens also had ACL injuries occur as the joints were externally rotated beyond the MCL failure point and impingement occurred against the medial edge of the lateral femoral condyle. [51,126] Kennedy also tested knees in hyperextension by applying an anteriorly directed force to the proximal femur with the tibia rigidly constrained. [125] They described tearing in the posterior capsule at approximately 30° of hyperextension, followed by complete anterior dislocation of the knee joint. [125] Other hyperextension studies either did not produce ACL injury [27] or used three-point bending with fixed pivot points that caused distraction between the tibia and femur.[78,192] The knee joint has also been tested with a valgus bending moment and those tests resulted in MCL rupture with one knee also suffering an ACL injury. [129] Isolated muscle force has also been shown to produce ACL injury at quadriceps forces of 4 kN. [61]

In cadaver experiments, excessive axial compression loads in the tibia will produce injury to the ACL when the knee joint is free to translate in the anterior-posterior direction. [114] In 4/5 joints at 60° and 4/5 joints at 90° of flexion, the ACL was ruptured at axial tibial loads of 4.4±1.1 kN and 4.6±1.2 kN respectively. Constrained experiments do not allow anterior-posterior (AP) or medial-lateral (ML) motion of the tibia with respect to the femur and result in fracture to the medial and lateral tibial plateau, medial femoral condyle and femoral notch at 8.0 ±1.8 kN. [21] Additionally, in constrained joints, the load to prevent anterior-posterior motion of the femur relative to the tibia is 1.2 ±0.5 kN. [114] This may be the tensile load in the ACL prior to rupture in unconstrained experiments. Recently, a porcine study confirmed that ACL injuries occur in unconstrained knees at 70° of flexion with TF compressive loads of approximately 3 kN. [235]

Knee Kinetics

The ground reaction force is approximately 2.5 times body weight when running. During controlled jump landings ground reaction forces (GRF) can be 4 or 6 times body weight for untrained females and males, respectively. [103] The internal loads in the knee joint are much higher than that due to the combined force of the contracting muscles in order to control knee flexion [68]. The TF contact force is estimated to be 15 times body weight when running. [89] Thus, for the average untrained male performing an uncontrolled jump landing on a relatively straight leg, joint compressive forces could well exceed 5 kN. This level of GRF may injure the ACL based on the above data from the cadaver experiments where the ACL injury-mitigating influences of neuromuscular joint control via the gastrocnemius and hamstrings muscles are not considered. [103] On the other hand, muscle forces also substantially increase the compressive force in the TF joint due to equilibrium and may contribute to ACL injuries by this mechanism.

Recent studies on the incidence of ACL rupture in female athletes have concentrated on potential differences in neuromuscular controls between the sexes and the training of hamstrings and quadriceps muscles in helping to aid in the limitation of anteriorly directed motion of the tibia, which appears to occur during a jump loading. [68,103] Quadriceps muscle force produces strain in the ACL. [229] Stop-jump landings include a posteriorly directed ground reaction force, but the necessary extension moment in the quadriceps needed to balance the knee produces an anterior shear force in the proximal tibia instead. [195] Lower extremity muscle fatigue may increase an athlete's risk for noncontact ACL injury. Increased injury rates occur during the latter portion of games in a variety of sports, which indicates that fatigue is a risk factor for injury. [83] The anterior shear force on the proximal tibia is significantly increased for both male and female subjects in the fatigued state during a stop-jump landing. [40] Previous studies have suggested that proximal tibial anterior shear force may be an indication of increased strain in the ACL. [110]

The goal of treatment for the ACL-injured patient is to prevent recurrent knee injury while allowing the patient to return to their desired level of work and sports participation. If left untreated, a torn ACL can cause an increased incidence of meniscal tears n addition to the anterior and rotary instability. [173,175] In patients who participate in frequent jumping or cutting sports, ACL reconstruction is usually recommended.

Post-Traumatic Osteoarthritis

Risk Factors and Epidemiology

Nearly 50% of Americans over the age of 65 have some form of arthritis with total costs of the disease approximating $80 billion per year. [39] Osteoarthritis (OA) is the most common musculoskeletal disease and the most common form of arthritis, affecting 20.7 million people in the USA alone. OA affects the cartilage and subchondral bone of diarthrodial joints. [139] It is characterized by irregular loss of cartilage in areas of high load, sclerosis of subchondral bone, subchondral cysts, and osteophytes.

Clinical diagnosis of osteoarthritis comes only when a significant reduction of the joint space is seen radiographically, [95] although MRI is proving to be a useful tool in diagnosing early OA. [106] From the patient's perspective, this disease is characterized by diarthrodial joint pain and tenderness, loss of range of motion, and localized inflammation around the affected joint. Since the main function of diarthrodial joints is to allow body movement and locomotion, this disease has grave consequences for a patient's quality of life.

Finding an association between end-stage OA and various causes has been difficult due to the long delay before chronic changes occur and radiographic evidence appears, which typically is at least 10 to 20 years. [232] In many patients, the disease is due to a lifetime of high stresses in a particular joint from a particular occupation or recreational activity. A significantly higher percentage of patients with ligament tears or sprains go on to develop OA, which may be a result of the change in the way forces are transferred through the joint after an injury. There is also the possibility of a single mechanical insult initiating the disease process, especially if there is fracture or soft tissue damage near the articulating surfaces. [40,58,167]

Sports participation in general has also been shown to increase the rate of OA, [49,139] and certain sports such as weightlifting and team sports[136] are associated with a higher risk of hip and knee OA, respectively.[40,57,58,85,214] In contrast, moderate levels of exercise and activity appear safe and do not lead to OA. [230] But, while moderate contact forces in the knee are safe and can even be beneficial for healthy joints,[220] excessive contact forces during an acute injury or applied repetitively during high impact sports induce long term joint degradation by damaging the articular cartilage and/or subchondral bone. History of a joint injury, particularly to the knee or hip, has been shown to increase the risk of OA in cross-sectional and case-control studies. [58,214] Furthermore, people who injure a knee before the age of 22 have a greater than threefold increased risk of diagnosed OA in that joint by their mid 50s. [85] Two specific types of injury are strongly associated with subsequent knee OA: cruciate ligament damage and meniscal tears. [73] In fact, 50-70% of patients with complete ACL rupture and associated injuries have radiographic changes consistent with chronic arthritis after 15 to 20 years. [88] Surgical reconstruction of the torn ACL is not effective in mitigating the incidence of joint OA, [166,224] as a significant proportion of these patients develop clinical symptoms of OA five to ten years post-injury. [11,79]

Bone Bruises

Subtle damage to cartilage and subchondral bone can occur without radiographic evidence of bone fracture. [182] Recent studies have focused on identifying occult bone trauma and relating it to clinical findings. These radiographically occult injuries to the bone, otherwise referred to as occult fractures or "bone bruises", may account for patient pain.[120] In over 80% of clinical ACL injury cases, a characteristic osteochondral lesion occurs in the tibial plateau and/or the femoral condyles. [162,207] These occult injuries have been shown to be accompanied by chondrocyte necrosis and surface lesions [69,116] and result in an overt loss of cartilage overlying geographic bone bruises in 48% of patients within six months of injury. [67,222] Bone bruises are associated with microcracks of the subchondral and/or trabecular bone [184,207] and may be caused by compressive trauma during the associated ligamentous injury. Radiographic images have also been used to relate bone marrow edema patterns with injury mechanisms via their characteristic "footprint". [121,122,191,223]

Osteochondral Microdamage

Lower extremity trauma causes acute pain followed by a chronic disease process that can lead to end-stage disease such as OA. [211] Biomechanically, the cartilage material properties including tensile, compressive, and shear moduli change. The hydraulic permeability of the cartilage also changes due to degradation of the collagen, causing increased water content and excessive swelling. Additionally, the subchondral bone thickness and stiffness both change as it undergoes remodeling due to changing stress levels. The progression of this disease involves chronic fragmentation of the cartilage surfaces and remodeling of subchondral bone. Histological methods are a common way of documenting subfracture injuries such as cartilage fissuring and occult microcracking at the calcified cartilage/subchondral bone interface. These studies use semi-quantitative scoring to analyze the condition of tissue as a result of impact and chronic degradation. Impact loading has been shown to initiate damage in articular cartilage between 11-36 MPa of contact pressure depending on the thickness, rate of loading, species, and location. [17,97,187,219] Haut documents that at the point of fracture, up to 60% of the human patellofemoral contact area exceeds 25 MPa. [97] This level of pressure was also shown to cause cartilage fissures in an in vitro cartilage explant model. [187]

Even when the ACL is not injured, presumably due to appropriate muscular contraction in the trained athlete, high TF contact forces would occur and may be sufficient to generate osteochondral microdamage. Histological microcracks of the subchondral plate occur in cadaver knees under high compressive loads, producing 18-21 MPa of contact pressure in the TF joint [21] and in a rabbit model at similar pressures. [113] Articular cartilage fibrillation and cell death have also been documented in explant studies when pressures exceed a critical threshold stress (25 MPa). [33,53,187,209,219]

Contact pressure distributions in the knee joint have been measured during physiological levels of TF compression,[2,32,80,188,216] varus-valgus bending, [152] and internal-external tibial rotation. [236] The TF contact pressures have also been computed by finite element analysis for a number of loading mechanisms, but not for failure level forces/moments. [23,24,115] Additional knee models have predicted the stress distributions that occur in the articular cartilage during TF contact, but they used rigid models for bone and are thus incapable of predicting damaged areas in the subchondral bone. [99,142] Experimental studies have documented osteochondral damage in the tibial plateau from TF compression in porcine [235] and rabbit knees. [113]

2. METHODS

Knee Specimens

All experiments were conducted on isolated tibiofemoral joints from fresh-frozen male cadavers (48±11 yrs) with no history of knee injury. The femur and tibia/fibula were sectioned approximately 15 cm proximal and distal to the center of the knee. The skin and muscle tissues were removed leaving the knee joint capsule and collateral ligaments intact. The femur and tibia/fibula shafts were cleaned with 70% alcohol and potted in cylindrical aluminum sleeves with room temperature curing epoxy. Knee joint specimen information is shown in Table 1 according to how the paired limbs were divided among loading conditions.

Data Recording and Statistics

The peak load, time to peak load, and actuator displacement corresponding to the peak load were recorded from the materials testing machine in each experiment. The relative joint displacements and rotations were documented with linear and rotary encoders. Certain measurements, such as hyperextension angle and valgus bending angle were also recorded using a motion capture system. Reflective markers were rigidly attached to the femur and tibia in four marker arrays. Pre-failure data from the test immediately prior to gross joint failure was compared to the results from the failure test. One way, repeated measure ANOVAs were used to compare the peak loads and the relative motions between the pre-failure and failure tests. SNK-post hoc tests were used where appropriate for multiple comparisons and significance was indicated for $p < 0.05$.

Table 1. Cadaver specimen information and experimental loading condition. Tibiofemoral compression (TFC), internal tibial torsion (ITT), hyperextension (HE) and valgus bending (VB)

Specimen	Age (yrs)	Height (m)	Weight (kg)	Experiment	
				TFCR	**ITT**
32057	50	1.67	64	Lt	Rt
32087	54	1.93	114	Rt	Lt
32153	59	1.78	100	Rt	Lt
32181	54	1.78	84	Lt	Rt
				TFCB	**HE**
32416	34	1.83	68	Lt	Rt
32284	53	1.83	111	Rt	Lt
32273	54	1.75	78	Lt	Rt
32302	59	1.78	86	Lt	Rt
32516	47	1.47	113	Rt	Lt
32388	NA	NA	NA	Lt	Rt
				VBO	**VBC**
32462	52	1.75	105	Rt	Lt
32498	47	1.78	64	Lt	Rt
32489	40	1.78	114	Rt	Lt
32532	19	1.88	86	Lt	Rt
Avg (SD)	**48 (11)**	**1.77 (0.11)**	**91 (19)**		

3. INJURIES DUE TO TIBIOFEMORAL COMPRESSION (TFC)

Biomechanical studies confirm that the ACL is a primary stabilizer of the knee for TFC. The tibial plateau surface has an inherent posterior slope of 10-15° relative to the long axis of the tibia [141] that varies across the medial and lateral compartments. This inclination creates a coupled anterior tibial translation and axial rotation which increases the distance between the tibial and femoral insertions of the ACL. [28] A similar effect, called "anterior neutral shift" of the tibia, has been described for externally applied TFC loads. [218] Few studies have documented force or relative joint displacements at failure levels under controlled loading of the knee joint. The goal of this experiment was to induce ACL rupture in the 30° flexed knee joint by TFC. The relative motions of the knee joint before and after failure of the ACL are important for injury mechanism identification from video analysis of clinical ACL tears.[131] The hypothesis of the study was that the magnitudes and types of motion observed after ACL rupture would significantly change from the relative joint displacements present just before ACL injury. Specifically, while the ACL is not a primary restraint to external tibia rotation, [148] this motion is frequently identified as a mechanism of injury in video analysis of ACL injuries. Valgus collapse of the knee is also commonly identified in videos of ACL rupture, but it is unknown if this is the cause of injury or simply a result of the ACL rupture itself.

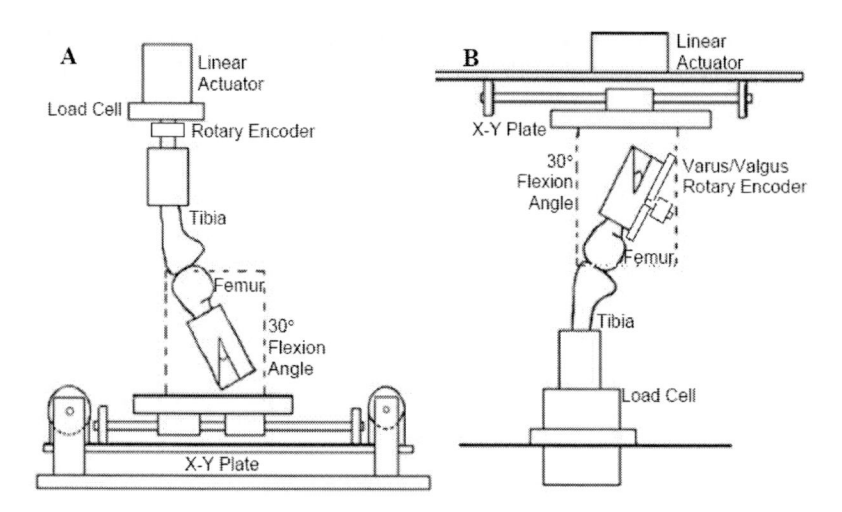

Figure 2. Knee specimens attached to the TFC testing fixtures. A) TFCR: Axial rotation of the tibia was allowed. B) TFCB: Varus/Valgus bending was allowed (adapted from Meyer and Haut, 2008).

Loading Methods

In one series of tibiofemoral compression experiments (TFCR, Table 1), a thrust bearing allowed axial, internal/external (IE) tibia rotation (Figure 2A). The potted femur was secured to a fixture with the knee joint flexion angle set at 30° and the varus/valgus angle adjusted and fixed in a position where the femoral condyles were perpendicular to the tibia. This fixture was attached to an X-Y translational plate to allow posterior/anterior (PA) and medial/lateral (ML) motions of the femur relative to the tibia during loading. [156] In the second series of experiments (TFCB, Table 1) the flexion angle was also set at 30° and femur varus/valgus (VV) rotation was unconstrained, but tibia axial rotation was prevented (Figure 2B). PA and ML displacement of the femur were also unconstrained relative to the tibia similar to the Series 1 experiments. Dynamic compressive loads were applied along the tibial axis by a linear hydraulic actuator with a single haversine waveform. All joints were repeatedly loaded with increasing TFC tests until gross failure of the knee joint.

Results

The peak posterior displacement of the femur in pre-failure tests was approximately 12 mm in both series of experiments (Table 2). In most TFCR specimens there was medial displacement of the femur. In TFCB experiments there was no clear medial or lateral displacement pattern. All TFCR experiments had internal rotation of the tibia develop during joint compression. TFCB experiments had a slight trend towards valgus femur rotation.

Failure tests showed an average higher peak compressive force than in the pre-failure tests (Table 3) and a slightly lower time to peak load (Figure 3). The peak posterior displacement of the femur was significantly increased in failure versus pre-failure tests with a combined mean value of 26±13 mm between both series of experiments. This maximum value occurred after most of the compressive load had been released due to the injury (Figure

4). In TFCR experiments, the peak ML displacement was not significantly changed after failure of the ACL, but followed the general pattern of displacement established in the pre-failure tests. In TFCB experiments there was a significant increase in the lateral displacement of the femur in the failure tests. The IE rotation of the tibia in TFCR was significantly different between failure and pre-failure tests. During early loading in failure tests the tibia rotated internally like in the pre-failure tests, but after the peak load and ACL failure, the direction of rotation changed rapidly (Figure 4) and the peak rotation was in the external direction for all specimens. In TFCB experiments there was a significant increase in the valgus femur rotation after failure (Figure 5).

Table 2. Data from TFC pre-failure experiments. ML indicates medial (+) and lateral (-), PA indicates posterior (+) and anterior (-), IE indicates internal (+) and external (-), VV indicates valgus (+) and varus (-)

	Specimen	Time to Peak Load (sec)	Peak TFC Load (kN)	Displacement at Peak Load (mm)	Peak ML Femur Motion (mm)	Peak PA Femur Motion (mm)	Peak IE Tibia Rotation (deg)	Peak VV Femur Rotation (deg)
TFCR	32057L	0.05	8.1	6.1	3.4	12	8.1	
TFCR	32087R	0.06	6.3	7.6	2.1	13	1.4	
TFCR	32153R	0.05	5.1	4.6	-5.6	13	3.7	
TFCR	32181L	0.21	4.9	6.4	3.9	23	8.4	
TFCB	32416L	0.21	7.7	8	0.1	18		1.3
TFCB	32284R	0.2	5.6	9	2.5	11		-0.4
TFCB	32273L	0.2	5.6	7	-2.4	16		1.0
TFCB	32302L	0.21	3.7	5	-1.3	9		1.3
TFCB	32516R	0.2	4.7	7	-1.6	7		7.0
TFCB	32388L	0.21	7.7	7	-2.3	14		2.6
			5.9 (1.5)	6.8 (1.3)	0.1 (3.1)	14 (4.6)	5.4 (3.4)	2.1 (2.6)

Table 3. Data from TFC failure experiments. ML indicates medial (+) and lateral (-), PA indicates posterior (+) and anterior (-), IE indicates internal (+) and external (-), VV indicates valgus (+) and varus (-). #Significant difference between pre-failure and failure tests

	Specimen	Time to Peak Load (sec)	Peak TFC Load (kN)	Displacement at Peak Load (mm)	Peak ML Femur Motion (mm)	Peak PA Femur Motion (mm)	Peak IE Tibia Rotation (deg)	Peak VV Femur Rotation (deg)
TFCR	32057L	0.05	8.6	6.8	5.9	34	-10.7	
TFCR	32087R	0.05	7.2	7.8	3.7	14	-1.7	
TFCR	32153R	0.05	4.5	7.2	-7.2	17	-5.5	
TFCR	32181L	0.2	5.8	7.4	3.7	52	-8.3	
TFCB	32416L	0.18	8.8	10	-8.7	33		4.9
TFCB	32284R	0.16	5.8	11	-5.5	28		11.2
TFCB	32273L	0.18	6.8	9	-10.4	31		8.0
TFCB	32302L	0.17	5.2	7	-5.9	26		6.5
TFCB	32516R	0.15	5.1	9	-1.4	8		13.3
TFCB	32388L	0.2	8.5	8	-3.5	16		6.5
			6.6 (1.6)#	8.3 (1.4)#	-2.9 (5.7)#	26 (13)#	-6.6 (3.9)#	8.4 (3.2)#

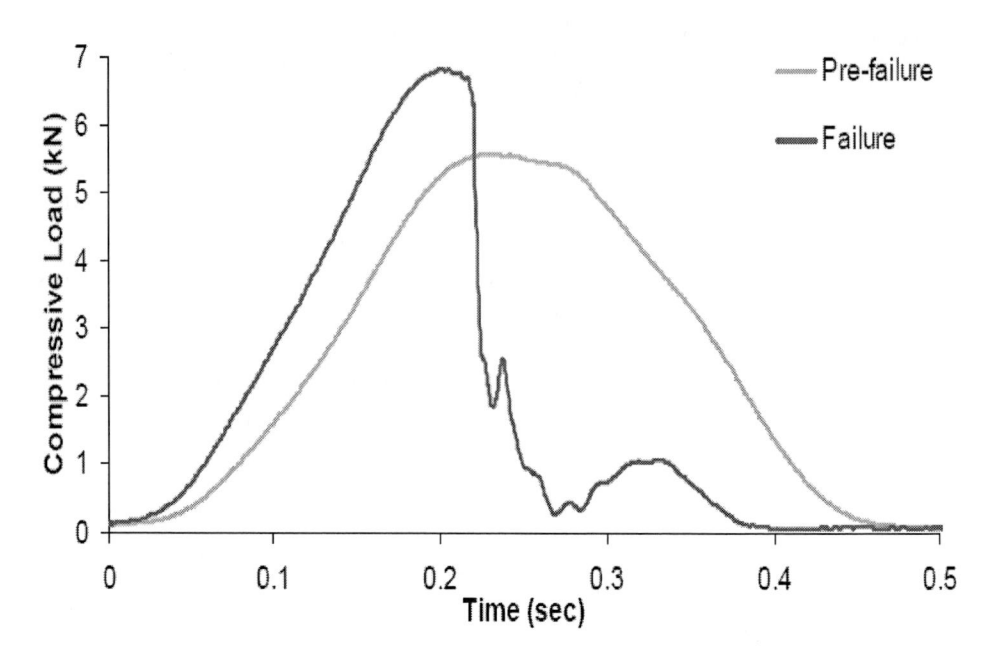

Figure 3. Representative load versus time plots for TFC pre-failure and failure tests.

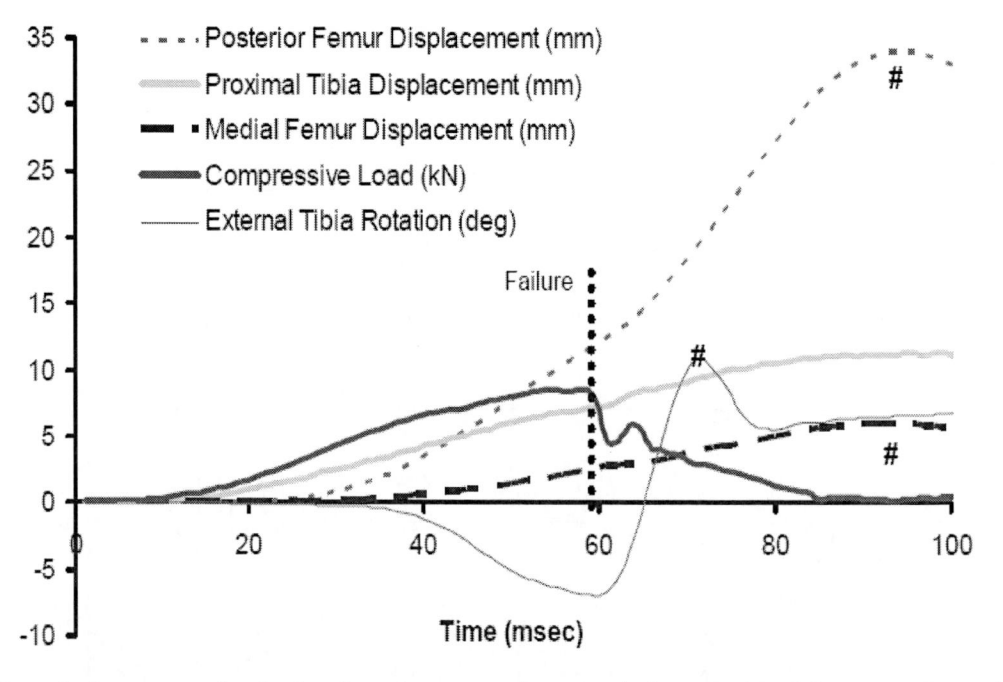

Figure 4. A representative load and motion versus time plot during a TFCR failure test. The peak compressive loads and the corresponding proximal tibia displacements occurred at the failure time point as marked. All other motions were measured at their peak values, indicated by #.

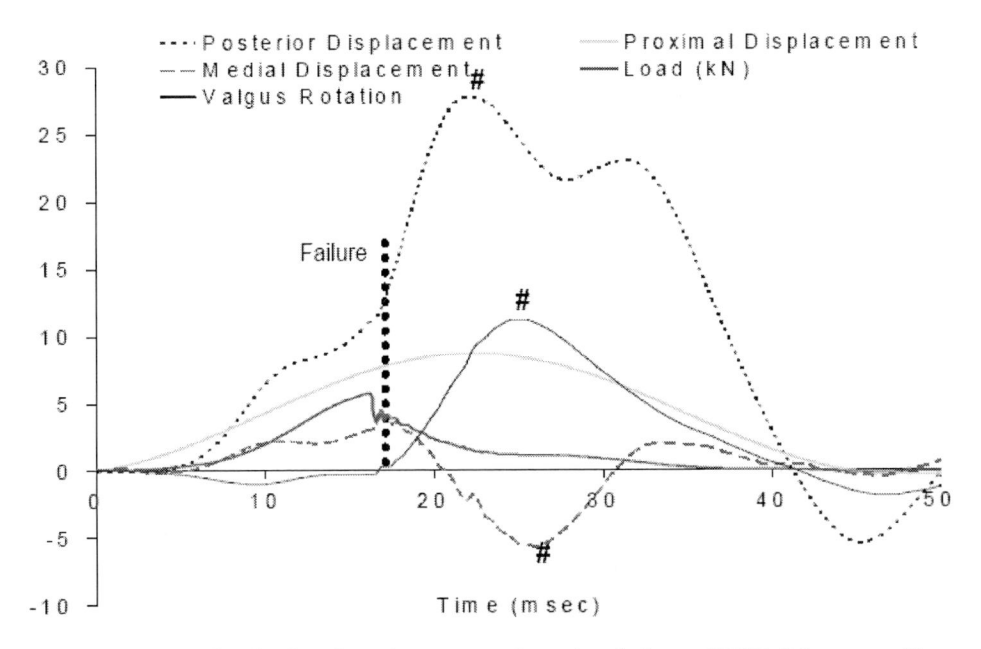

Figure 5. A representative load and motion versus time plot during a TFCB failure test. The peak compressive loads and the corresponding proximal tibia displacements occurred at the failure time point as marked. All other motions were measured at their peak values, indicated by #.

All failures involved the ACL, including 9/10 specimens with a complete or partial midsubstance ACL rupture, usually near the femoral insertion (Figure 6). In the cases of partial rupture, damaged fibers were largely observed in the posterolateral bundle of the ACL. One joint suffered an avulsion fractures at the insertion of the ACL into the tibia (Table 4).

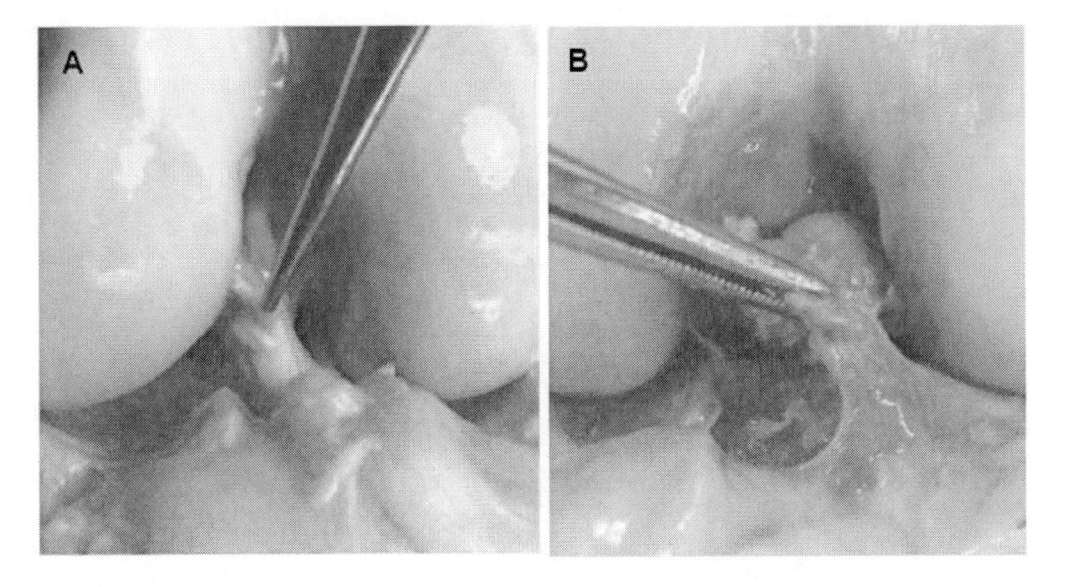

Figure 6. Anterior cruciate ligament rupture and avulsion specimens.

Table 4. Dissection documentation of injured structures following TFC failure tests. Complete tear (X), partial tear (/), avulsion (∧), tibia (T), femur (F)

	Specimen	ACL	PCL	MCL	LCL	Fracture
TFCR	32057L	/				
	32087R	/				
	32153R	/				
	32181L	X	∧ (T)		∧ (F)	
TFCB	32416L	/				
	32284R	X				
	32273L	X				
	32302L	/				
	32516R	∧ (T)				Lat Plateau
	32388L	/				Med Plateau

DISCUSSION

ACL injury occurred under excessive TFC as the femur displaced posterior relative to the tibia until ACL failure and continued afterwards. It was especially interesting that the direction of tibial rotation was changed from internal rotation in pre-failure tests to external rotation after failure of the ACL.

Most biomechanical evaluations of knee joint response under compressive external loading have been at low force levels, or comparisons of relative joint motion for intact and ACL sectioned knees. Isolated ACL rupture occurred in a previous study that applied high TF compressive loads to knees flexed 60, 90 and 120°. [154] The maximum force in those ACL failure experiments was 5.1 ± 2.1 kN compared with 6.6 ± 1.6 kN in the current study. In the previous experiments, allowing posterior displacement of the femur induced ACL rupture, while allowing other displacements while constraining posterior femur displacement produced femoral condyle and tibial plateau fractures. [114] Before ACL failure there was more relative displacement in the lateral compartment, producing internal tibial rotation in pre-failure tests. [150] After ACL rupture, anterior tibia subluxation continues to increase but with a higher magnitude in the medial compartment that produces external tibial rotation relative to the femur (Figure 7).

The isolated loading scenario applied to the knee joints in the current study was simplified in comparison to real world injury events. However, our goal was to reduce this complex problem to a couple of simple experimental conditions. Recent video analyses of ACL injuries conclude that plant-and-cut and landing maneuvers are the primary activities during injury, [134,176] and that they occur during the initial foot strike with only a small degree of knee flexion. [29] Olsen et al. estimate that the body weight distribution on the injured leg is more than 65% in most cases, and can reach 100%. [176] Axial compressive loading of the knee during landing from a jump is approximately six times body weight for males. [103] Therefore, in both the plant-and-cut and landing maneuvers, there are likely high levels of TFC that could be of similar magnitude to loads in the current study. Although this force was applied along the tibial axis in the current study, during a "stop-jump" landing there may also be a posteriorly directed ground reaction force at the foot. [41] Controversy exists as to whether this force component increases or decreases the amount of anterior subluxation of the proximal tibia because of confounding variables such as muscle force and knee flexion. [42,43] It is apparent, however, that the muscle forces needed to balance flexion moments at the knee will increase the TF compressive force beyond the vertical ground reaction force that is measured at the foot.

The current study shows that knee joint motions can vary in magnitude and direction following failure of the ACL. Biomechanical studies do not support external tibial rotation or valgus knee bending as mechanisms of isolated ACL rupture. The external rotation and valgus bending documented in video based studies of ACL injury cases could be occurring after ACL rupture when a large TFC load is present.

4. INJURIES DUE TO INTERNAL TIBIAL TORSION (ITT)

Clinical studies have proposed the mechanisms of ACL injury based on patient questionnaires and video analysis of the events. The most commonly referenced loading mechanism is internal tibial rotation. [10,29,153,176] In one study, athletes described internal tibial rotation as the injury mechanism in approximately 82% of cases. [10] Skiing has one of the highest rates of ACL injuries, accounting for 25-30% of knee injuries. [208] These injuries are mainly associated with internal twisting or combined torque and compression during a hard landing. [65,202] Biomechanical studies have also shown that internal tibial torque induces tensile forces in the ACL, [94,141,148, 194] especially when the knee is between full extension and 30° of flexion. The goal of this experiment was to induce ACL rupture in a 30° flexed knee joint by isolated internal tibial torsion.

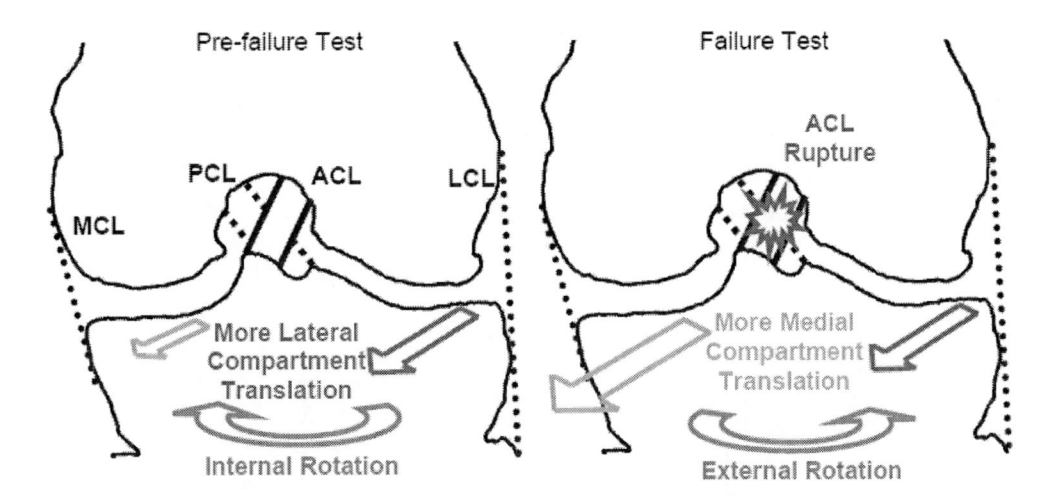

Figure 7. Coupled anterior tibial subluxation and internal rotation of the tibia.

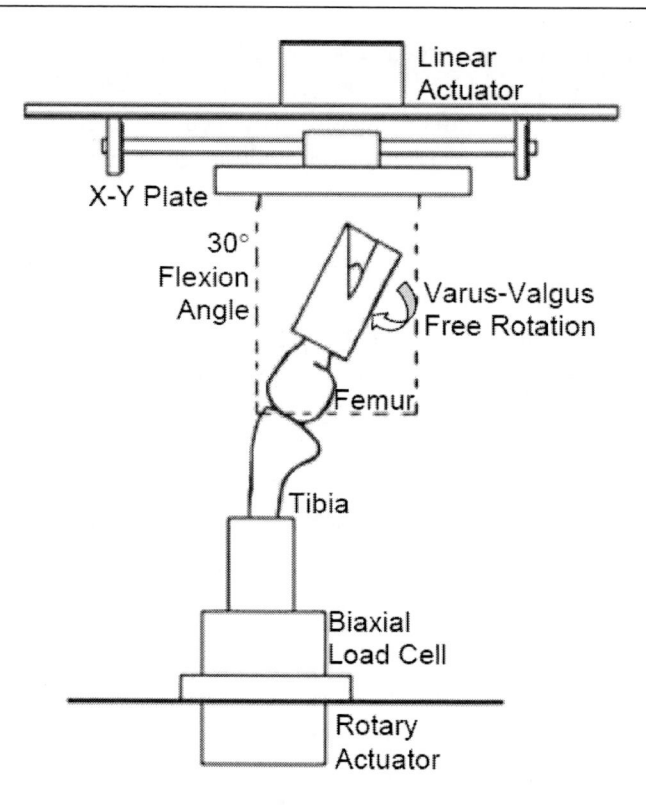

Figure 8. Diagram of the torsion testing fixture (adapted from Meyer et al., 2008.

Loading Methods

For internal tibial torsion experiments, the potted tibia was attached to a rotary hydraulic actuator through a biaxial (torsion-axial) load cell. [156] The potted femur was attached to a similar fixture and X-Y translational table as in the TFC experiments, with the main difference being that the whole device was attached to the rotation-locked, linear actuator (Figure 8). The joint flexion angle was also set to 30°, and for all but the first torsion specimen (32057R), the varus/valgus angle was left unconstrained. Compressive preloads were applied through the femur prior to the application of the internal torque on the tibia. Repeated, increasing levels of ITT were applied to each specimen until catastrophic injury of the joint.

Results

In the pre-failure tests the peak valgus rotation had a mean value of 10±3.7°, and in most specimens it was closely related to the level of applied internal rotation (Table 5). The peak posterior femur displacement had a mean value of 10±2 mm and this generally occurred early during the rotation. In some specimens, there was a decrease later in the test as valgus rotation peaked.

Table 5. Data from ITT pre-failure experiments. ML indicates medial (+) and lateral (-), PA indicates posterior (+) and anterior (-), VV indicates valgus (+) and varus (-)

Specimen	Time to Peak Torque (sec)	Peak Internal Torque (Nm)	Tibia Rotation at Peak Torque (deg)	Peak ML Femur Motion (mm)	Peak PA Femur Motion (mm)	Peak VV Femur Rotation (deg)
32057R	0.13	59.2	50	5.4	10.7	0 (locked)
32087L	0.19	46.8	62	6.7	9.2	7.6
32153L	0.24	23	37	1.7	8	14
32181R	1	31.1	32	-0.3	12.7	7.7
Avg (SD)		40 (16)	45 (14)	3.4 (3.2)	10 (2)	10 (3.7)

Failure tests showed a 16° increase in internal rotation to a maximum value of 61±19° (Table 6). The peak torque in the failure test was higher than in the pre-failure test (Figure 9). At the point of failure, there was a sharp drop in the torque (Figure 10). There was a significant increase between the failure and pre-failure tests for the peak valgus rotation and the peak lateral femur motion, but not the peak posterior femur motion. All torsional specimen failures involved the ACL, but 2/4 specimens also suffered MCL rupture (Table 7).

Table 6. Data from ITT failure experiments. ML indicates medial (+) and lateral (-), PA indicates posterior (+) and anterior (-), VV indicates valgus (+) and varus (-). #Significant difference between pre-failure and failure tests

Specimen	Time to Peak Torque (sec)	Peak Internal Torque (Nm)	Tibia Rotation at Peak Torque (deg)	Peak ML Femur Motion (mm)	Peak PA Femur Motion (mm)	Peak VV Femur Rotation (deg)
32057R	0.17	64.6	60	6.7	14.3	0 (locked)
32087L	0.18	49.2	85	13.2	12.2	18.1
32153L	1.1	29.7	60	6.5	6	22
32181R	0.87	39.2	39	13	13	23.5
Avg (SD)		46 (15)#	61 (19)#	10 (3.8)#	11 (3.7)	21 (2.8)#

Table 7. Injured structures following ITT failure tests. Complete tear (X), partial tear (/), avulsion (∧), tibia (T), fibula (fib)

Specimen	ACL	PCL	MCL	LCL	Fracture
32057R	/		X		
32087L	∧ (T)		/	∧ (fib)	
32153L	/				
32181R	/				

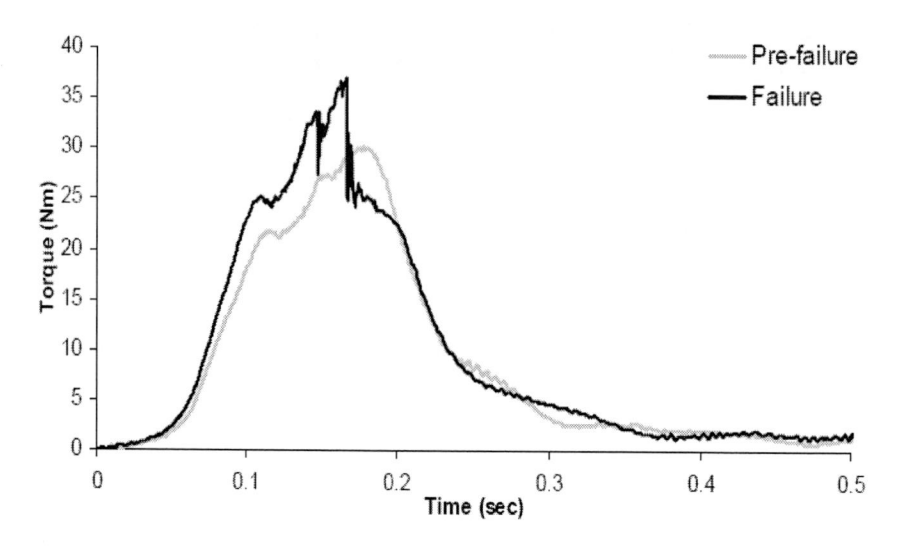

Figure 9. Representative torque versus time plots for ITT pre-failure and failure tests.

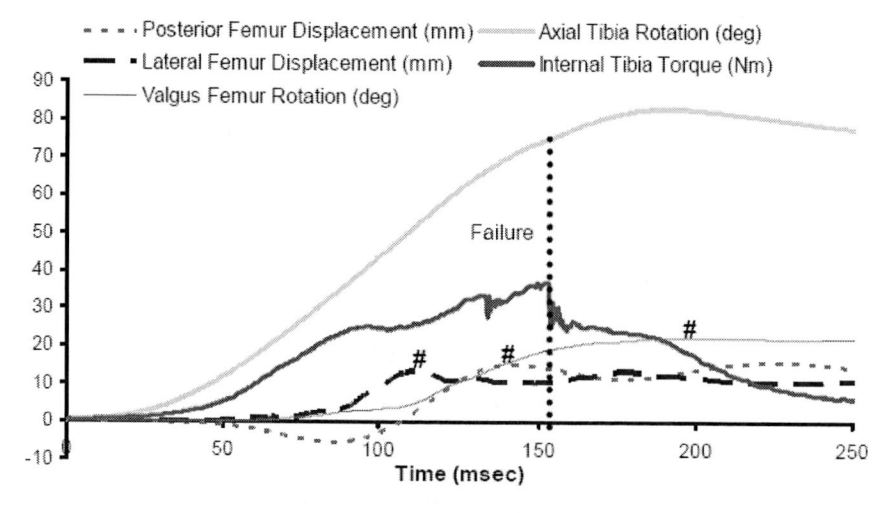

Figure 10. Representative torque and motion versus time during a ITT failure test. The peak internal torques and the corresponding axial tibia rotation occurred at the failure time point as marked. All other motions were measured at their peak values, indicated by #.

Discussion

Although internal tibial rotation is commonly suggested as the injury mechanism in clinical ACL ruptures, the current study is the first to consistently produce ACL injuries via excessive internal tibia rotation using cadaver knee joints. Kennedy et al. tested five cadaver knees in internal rotation (at 15-20° of flexion) and described the ACL becoming very taut, but they generated premature bone fracture at the clamps. [127] The ACL resists internal rotation by its orientation in the axial plane where it attaches slightly medial on the anterior tibial plateau and slightly lateral in the femoral notch. [5,9] An important factor in predicting

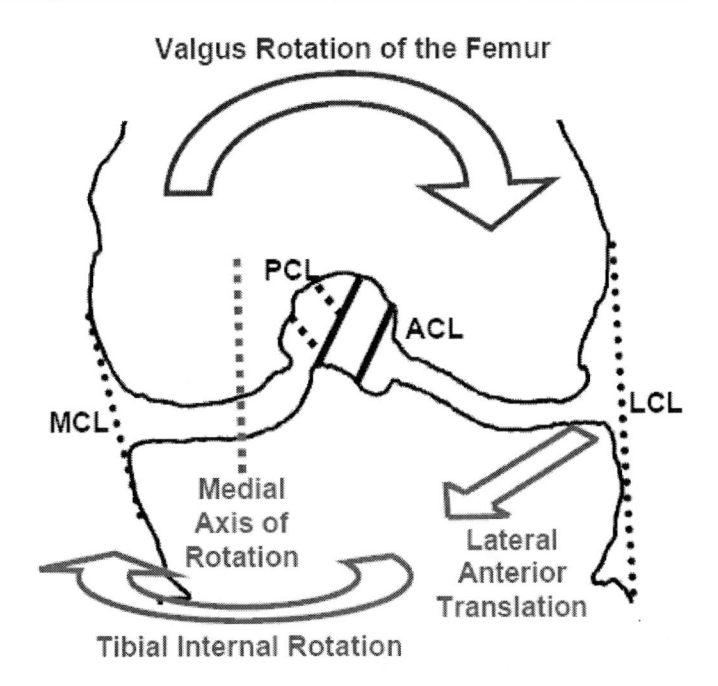

Figure 11. Coupled internal rotation of the tibia and valgus rotation of the femur.

tension in the ACL is the location of the axis of tibial rotation in the frontal plane. In the current study, the relative axis of rotation between the tibia and femur was not constrained by the experimental fixture. Since posterior displacement of the femur and posterior displacement of the medial tibial plateau occurred simultaneously, we concluded that the effective center of rotation was located medial to the ACL (Figure 11). In addition, these motions occurred on a posteriorly sloped tibia and produced a coupled motion between internal rotation of the tibia and valgus rotation of the femur. [151] Coupled internal tibial and valgus femur rotations have been previously documented for a 12.5 Nm valgus moment. [150] During those experiments, the axis of rotation was located near the MCL due to tension in that ligament as the primary restraint for VB moments. In the current study, valgus rotation of the femur may have also played a role in creating ACL tension and was significantly increased in magnitude after ACL failure. On the other hand, even with approximately 21° of valgus rotation of the femur, only two specimens had MCL damage.

5. INJURIES DUE TO HYPEREXTENSION (HE)

Isolated ACL injury occurs due to hyperextension approximately 6-25% of the time in sports. [7,29,143,176] Anterior dislocation of the knee (bicruciate injury) is also caused by hyperextension but occurs much less frequently than isolated ACL rupture. [31,101,160,198] A few case studies have described the scenario involved in both isolated ACL and bicruciate injuries from hyperextension, including non-contact jumping on a trampoline [137] and player to player contact during football. [225] Biomechanical studies have measured the tension in the ligaments of the knee for low hyperextension moments and show significantly more tension in the ACL than the PCL at 10 Nm. [226] The goal of this experiment was to induce ligament failure in isolated knees due to a pure hyperextension bending moment.

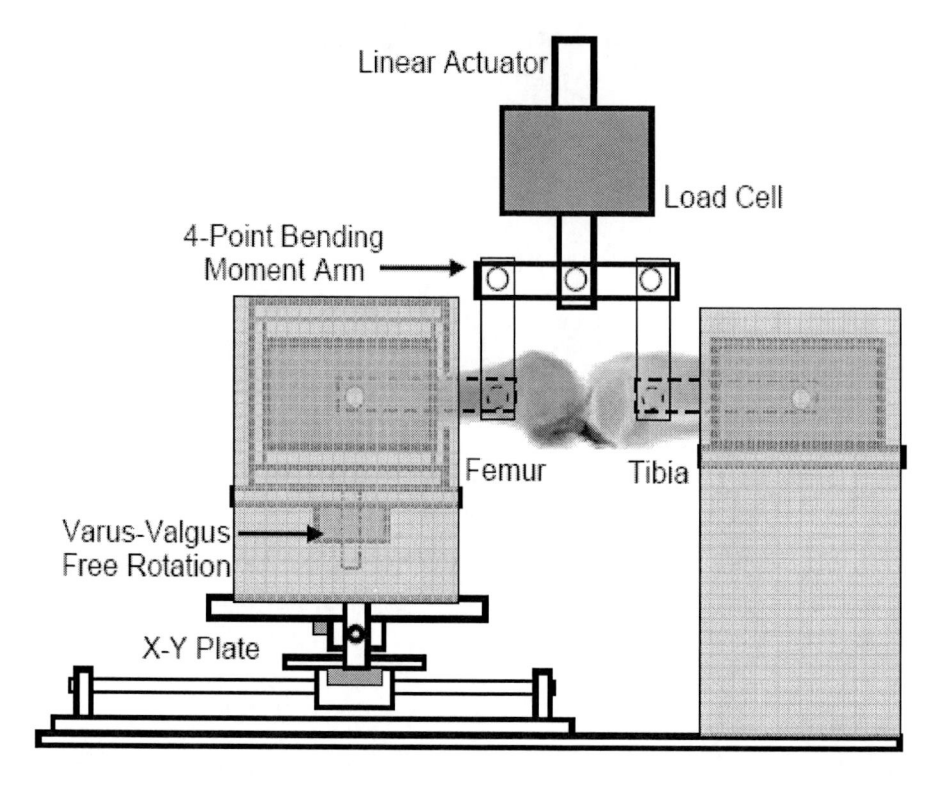

Figure 12. Diagram of the hyperextension testing fixture (adapted from Meyer et al., 2011).

Loading Methods

Hyperextension moments were applied via four-point bending with the moment applied to the potting cups (Figure 12). The femoral cup was mounted on an XY translational table to allow medial/lateral (ML) and proximal/distal (PD) motions. [159] In addition, varus/valgus (VV) angular rotation of the femur was unconstrained while axial tibia rotation was fixed in its neutral position. A linear hydraulic actuator was used to apply the bending moment. HE was applied to the joint with repeated increasing magnitudes until gross injury of the joint.

Results

The failure tests had significantly higher moments than the pre-failure tests, and exhibited a sudden drop in the force versus time plot (Figure 13) and a "popping" sound at the time of injury. All failures involved the ACL, PCL and posterior capsule (Table 8). The HE moment was 108±46 Nm at failure with a total extension angle of 34±11°. There was an unequal sharing of the rotation between the femur and tibia which produced an anterior subluxation of the tibia in all specimens (Figure 14). There was minimal lateral or valgus motion of the femur in any test (Figure 15).

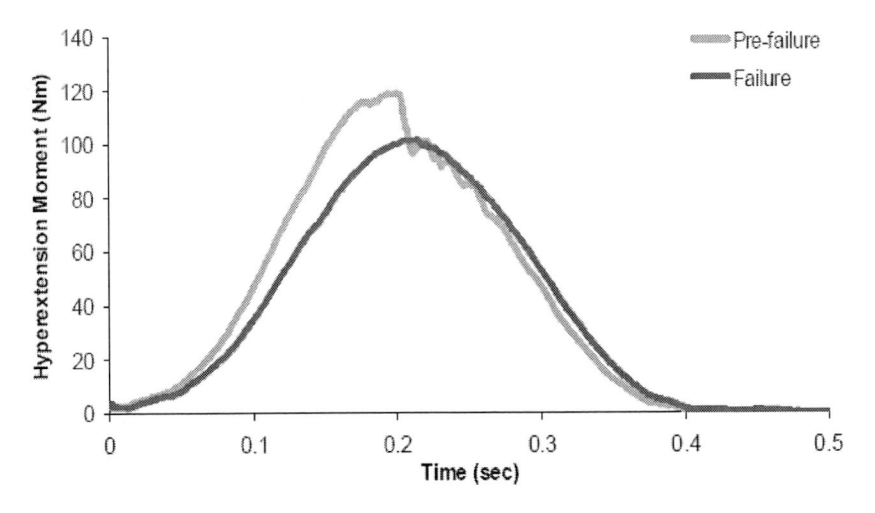

Figure 13. Representative bending moment versus time plot for HE pre-failure and failure tests.

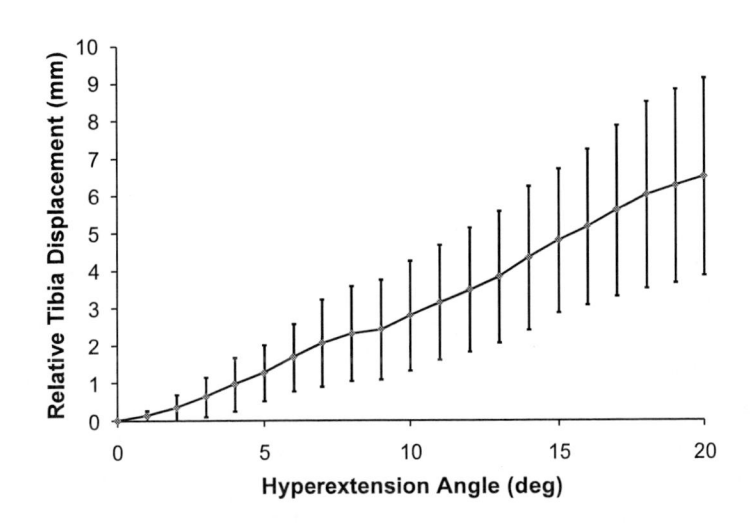

Figure 14. Relative anterior motion of the tibia with respect to the femur versus extension angle for HE failure tests.

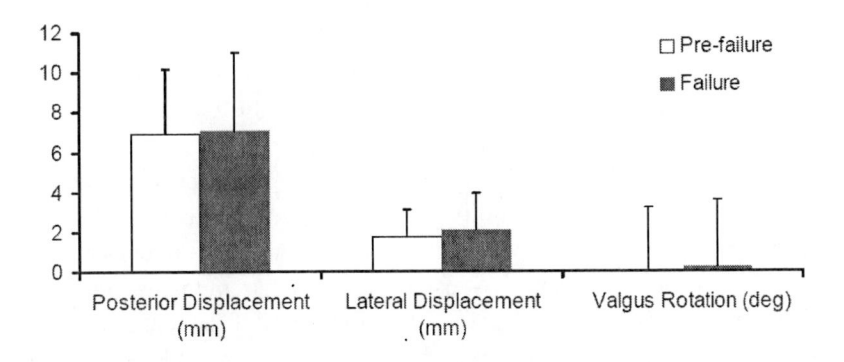

Figure 15. Joint displacements for pre-failure and failure tests.

Table 8. Peak force during HE pre-failure and failure tests and knee joint injury documented during dissection. Posterolateral bundle (PLB), Anteromedial bundle (AMB), Posteromedial bundle (PMB), Anterolateral bundle (ALB), Complete tear (X), Partial tear (/), Avulsion (∧). #Significant difference between pre-failure and failure tests

Specimen	Peak Moment (Nm)		ACL		PCL	
	Pre-failure	Failure	PLB	AMB	PMB	ALB
32416R	172	195	X	/		/
32284L	84	101	/			/
32273R	101	119		∧ (T)		/
32302R	73	80	/			/
32516L	63	70	∧ (F)			/
32388R	80	83	/			/
Avg (SD)	96 (40)	108 (46)#				

Discussion

The HE moments to cause gross failure in the human knee under four point bending have not been previously documented. Of the four experimental HE studies conducted to date by others, the most similar results to the current study were produced by Kennedy. [125] In that study the authors applied an anterior directed force to the proximal femur with the tibia rigidly constrained. They described tearing in the posterior capsule at approximately 30° of hyperextension followed by complete anterior dislocation of the knee joint. [125] After cruciate injury, the femur displaced posteriorly relative to the tibia similar to the current study. Additionally, the PCL was torn in 8/10 specimens, which correlates well with the PCL injury documented in the current study. In contrast, other previous studies did not produce ACL injury [27] or used three-point bending with fixed pivot points on the ends of the tibia and femur that limited the TF contact as the knee was hyperextended. [78,192] Bizot et al. likely produced posterior capsule and PCL injuries without any ACL ruptures because their method of applying 4-point bending consisted of displacing the tibia and femur equally in the posterior direction. [27] Instead, the current study applied equal bending moments to the tibia and femur, and did not constrain the extension angles for the two bones. This led to higher rotation of the femur than the tibia in all specimens which produced anterior subluxation of the tibia. Since the ACL is the primary restraint for anterior subluxation of the tibia, this motion was an important component of the ACL injuries.

The bending strength of the knee has been measured previously under lateral-medial bending moments that simulate automotive impacts on pedestrian lower limbs. [117,129] Although the injuries produced in those studies are different than the current study, Yamada predicted that lateral-medial and anterior-posterior bending strengths would be similar. [234] In fact, the current value of 108±46 Nm for joint failure in A-P bending compared well with three lateral-medial bending failures that occurred between 130 and 142 Nm in a previous study. [129] Slight differences in the failure moments may have been due to the high rates of loading used in the previous L-M experiments. The current experiments were conducted at a much lower loading rate (250 ms to peak), which might better simulate the loading rate that occurs in sports.

HE experiments produced bicruciate ligament injuries in all specimens. Additionally, the posterior capsule was damaged in all specimens. In a previous biomechanical study by another laboratory, ACL tension was significantly increased at 5° of hyperextension with the addition of either an internal torque or a varus moment, but was not increased with an external torque on the tibia or a valgus moment on the femur. [148] In sports injury scenarios, HE moments are likely combined with ITT[143] and/or TFC [224] that may produce isolated ACL injury. In noncontact injury scenarios, it would be difficult to produce a large HE moment without a significant TFC load occurring simultaneously (either from weight-bearing or muscle contraction force).

6. Injuries due to Valgus Bending (VB)

Valgus bending of the knee is one of the most commonly referenced loading mechanisms for ACL rupture in athletes. This type of motion is described in over 60% of non-skiing ACL injuries. [29] In basketball, approximately 37% of non-contact ACL injuries were termed "valgus collapse". [134] The importance of the ACL in restraining VB was demonstrated by a large force in the ACL at 30° of knee flexion. [82] Other biomechanical studies, however, have shown significantly more restraint from the MCL than the ACL during VB due to its anatomical location and orientation in the knee joint. [194,197] The goal of this experiment was to document the ligamentous failure due to VB moments applied to the knee. Additionally, in paired specimens, VB was combined with a compressive preload to better simulate an off-balance jump landing.

Loading Methods

Valgus moments were applied via four-point bending, with the moment applied to the potting cups (Figure 16). The femoral cup was mounted on an XY translational table to allow anterior/posterior (AP) and proximal/distal (PD) motions. [157] The flexion angle was fixed at 30°, while internal/external (IE) rotation of the femur was unconstrained. A linear hydraulic actuator was used to apply VB with magnitudes until gross injury of the joint. For one limb from each pair (Table 1), no tibiofemoral compressive preload was used (VBO) while the other limb was subjected to combined valgus bending (VBC) with a tibiofemoral compression pre-load applied immediately before each VB experiment. The tibiofemoral compression preload was applied by hand using a lever arm that was connected to the femoral fixture through extension springs, to produce 2-4 times body weight (xBW).

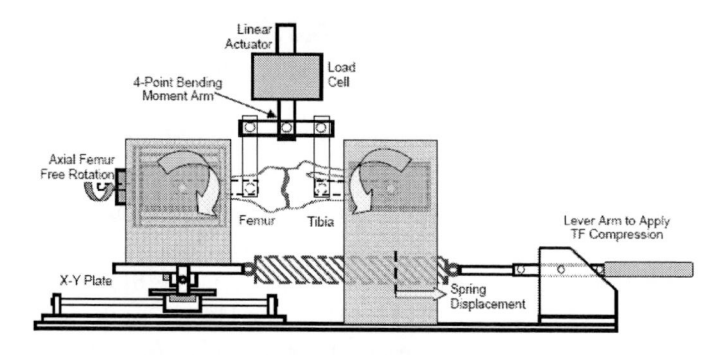

Figure 16. Knee specimen, potted and attached to the valgus bending test fixture (adapted from Meyer et al., 2009).

Results

The application of a VB moment resulted in internal femoral rotation and valgus rotation of the knee joint (Table 9). No significant differences in the amount of valgus rotation or internal femoral rotation were documented between the VBO group and VBC group. The average valgus rotation at failure was 29±7.2 degrees, and the average internal femur rotation was 38±14 degrees. The data presented in Table 9 was recorded only during the application of the VB moment. The initial application of the compression pre-load in the VBC experiments resulted in approximately 2.5° of varus knee joint rotation, 5° of external femoral rotation, and 4 mm of posterior femoral subluxation. No posterior displacement was noted during the application of the VB moment. All failures, except for one specimen, involved the MCL. There were also three cases of partial rupture or avulsion of the ACL (Table 9). The average failure VB moment was similar between the VBO and the VBC experiments, yielding an average of 107±52 Nm.

Table 9. Maximum VB moment, knee motion at peak moment and knee joint injuries documented during dissection. Complete tear (X), partial tear (/), avulsion (/\\), tibia (T), fibula (F)

		Peak Moment (Nm)	Valgus (+) Rotation (deg)	Internal (+) Femur Rotation (deg)	Injuries			
					MCL	ACL	PCL	LCL
VBO	32462R	39	36	48	/			
	32498L	225	20	22	X			
	32489R	91	35	32	X			
	32532L	68	35	35	X	/		
Avg (SD)		106 (82)	32 (7.7)	34 (11)				
VBC	32462L	184	27	53	/			/\ (F)
	32498R	96	36	59		/		
	32489L	63	20	23	X			
	32532R	93	24	31	X	/\ (T)		
Avg (SD)		109 (52)	27 (6.8)	42 (17)				

Discussion

Seven out of eight of the VB experiments resulted in MCL rupture, and three out of eight experiments generated ACL injury. There was no difference in the gross injury patterns produced by the two experimental loading conditions. Epidemiological studies have also document similar rates for combination MCL and ACL injuries for both non-contact and contact injury mechanisms. [71] Knee VB moments causing gross failure in four point bending have been previously documented. [30,129] In one study, three knees were tested at full extension with only distal motion of the femur allowed that resulted in MCL rupture at approximately 137 Nm and 12° of VB. [129] One specimen in that study also had an injury documented to the ACL. Another study tested knee joints in either four point bending or combined bending and shear. [30] The average four point bending failure moment was 121±26 Nm at a valgus angle of 14±2°. The injuries were not grouped by the type of experiment, but most of the joints suffered MCL injury and 12.5% also had an ACL injury. The bending moments from those studies compare relatively well with the current study at 107 Nm, but the failure angles were lower than the 29° of VB in the current study. This difference may be attributable to the large amount of axial femoral rotation that was coupled with the VB in the current study. In most descriptions of valgus collapse in sports there are similar references to coupled valgus bending, axial rotation, and even knee flexion during the injury. [47,134] The lack of isolated ACL injuries without a significant TF compressive load may suggest that TFC is in fact a primary component of sports ACL injury mechanisms.

7. CONTACT PRESSURES

Rupture of the ACL is associated with degeneration of the joint that can eventually lead to posttraumatic osteoarthritis. [73] In over 80% of ACL injury cases, a characteristic osteochondral lesion occurs in the tibial plateau and/or the femoral condyle. [162,207,209] Vellet et al. documents an overt loss of cartilage overlying geographic bone bruises in 48% of patients within six months of injury. [222] These "bone bruises" are associated with occult microcracks of the subchondral and/or trabecular bone and may be caused by compressive loading during the associated ligamentous injury [184,207] Additionally, chondrocyte necrosis and surface lesions of articular cartilage occur in regions overlying bone bruises in clinical cases of ACL rupture. [116] Our laboratory has previously shown histological microfractures of the subchondral plate in isolated, flexed human knees under high compressive loads producing 18-21 MPa of average peak contact pressure in the TF joint. [21] Articular cartilage fibrillation and cell death have also been documented in explant studies when pressures exceed a critical threshold stress (25 MPa). [53,187,214] However, the compressive loads (pressure) that are developed in the human knee during ligamentous injury have not been measured. The goal was to document the levels of contact pressure developed in the human knee joint during gross ligamentous injuries induced by sports loading scenarios.

Methods

During each test in the previous four types of loading experiments, pressure sensitive film packets were inserted into the medial and lateral compartments of the TF joint to record the contact area and pressures. [155,157,159] To insert the pressure film packets, the patella was removed and two small incisions were made in the posterior capsule in the center of each compartment. Low (0-10 MPa) and medium (10-50 MPa) range pressure films were stacked together and sealed between two sheets of polyethylene (0.04 mm thick) to prevent exposure to synovial fluid. [17] Using the previously documented procedure, the film was scanned and converted to pressures using a dynamically calibrated density-to-pressure scale. For comparison purposes, only the medium film contact areas and average pressures were reported except when the medium film area was zero; then the average pressure from the low pressure film was used. Additionally, the area over 25 MPa was computed to show the region of joint contact that was at the most risk of articular cartilage and underlying subchondral bone damage. Pressure film data from the experiment immediately prior to failure and during the failure experiment were documented to compare the locations of potentially microdamaged cartilage and subchondral bone in the medial and lateral compartments.

Results

For pre-failure TFC experiments, there were no significant differences in the average contact area or pressure between the lateral and medial compartments (Table 10). In the medial compartment there were significant increases in all the measured variables between the pre-failure and failure tests (Table 11). For the lateral compartment, the maximum pressure was increased between pre-failure and failure tests. The pressure distribution of the region over 25 MPa occurred posterior on the tibial plateau. The pressure distributions were

Table 10. Contact pressure data from TFC pre-failure experiments

		Medial Compartment				Lateral Compartment			
		Area	Area > 25 MPa	Avg Pressure	Max Pressure	Area	Area > 25 MPa	Avg Pressure	Max Pressure
		(mm²)		(MPa)		(mm²)		(MPa)	
TFCR	32057L	137	36	21	33	285	35	19	39
	32087R	161	19	18	36	281	0	12	21
	32153R	149	0	13	22	39	0	11	19
	32181L	36	0	11	19	164	26	18	46
	Avg (SD)	121 (57)	14 (17)	16 (5)	28 (8)	192 (117)	15 (18)	15 (4)	31 (13)
TFCB	32416R	217	4	16	31	228	0	16	25
	32284R	65	0	12	19	8	0	11	16
	32273L	0	0	7	10	8	0	11	17
	32302L	0	0	7	10	0	0	6	10
	32516R	0	0	7	10	189	2	17	29
	32388L	228	51	20	39	1	0	11	14
	Avg (SD)	85 (109)	9 (20)	12 (6)	20 (13)	72 (106)	0 (1)	12 (4)	19 (7)

also similar between the pre-failure and failure tests. TFCB failure experiments generated slightly higher contact area in the medial compartment than in the lateral compartment (Figure 17).

Table 11. Contact pressure data from TFC failure experiments

		Medial Compartment				Lateral Compartment			
		Area (mm²)	Area > 25 MPa	Avg Pressure	Max Pressure (MPa)	Area (mm²)	Area > 25 MPa	Avg Pressure	Max Pressure (MPa)
TFCR	32057L	306	88	21	37	230	72	20	39
	32087R	278	61	19	50	260	0	12	23
	32153R	159	3	15	33	23	0	11	23
	32181L	281	11	16	36	246	50	20	50
	Avg (SD)	256 (66)	41 (41)	18 (3)	39 (7)	190 (112)	30 (36)	16 (5)	34 (13)
TFCB	32416R	240	51	20	44	250	6	18	30
	32284R	173	0	14	28	66	0	14	22
	32273L	85	0	14	24	150	0	12	24
	32302L	148	1	16	30	3	0	11	18
	32516R	14	0	12	18	195	7	17	30
	32388L	246	61	21	39	12	0	12	23
	Avg (SD)	151 (90)	19 (29)	16 (4)	31 (10)	113 (101)	2 (3)	14 (3)	25 (5)

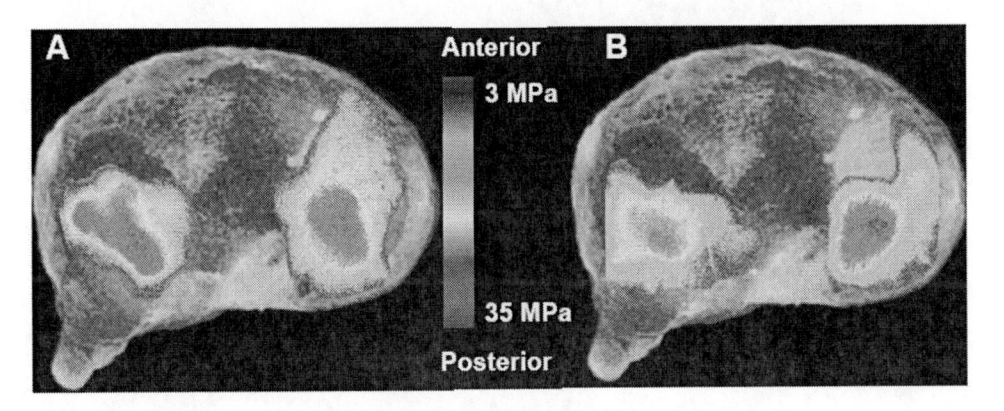

Figure 17. Representative shape and magnitude of pressure distributions in failure tests for TFCR or TFCB experiments.

Table 12. Contact pressure data from ITT pre-failure experiments

	Medial Compartment				Lateral Compartment			
	Area (mm²)	Area > 25 MPa	Avg Pressure	Max Pressure (MPa)	Area (mm²)	Area > 25 MPa	Avg Pressure	Max Pressure (MPa)
32057R	183	73	26	50	0	0	0	0
32087L	49	2	14	25	69	0	12	20
32153L	0	0	6	10	86	0	12	20
32181R	133	1	14	37	113	0	13	14
Avg (SD)	61 (67)	1 (1)	11 (5)	24 (14)	89 (22)	0 (0)	12 (1)	18 (3)

Table 13. Contact pressure data from ITT failure experiments

	Medial Compartment				Lateral Compartment			
	Area	Area > 25 MPa	Avg Pressure	Max Pressure	Area	Area > 25 MPa	Avg Pressure	Max Pressure
	(mm²)		(MPa)		(mm²)		(MPa)	
32057R	245	78	25	50	0	0	0	0
32087L	80	5	17	34	0	0	6	10
32153L	33	4	16	32	61	0	15	24
32181R	107	3	13	31	95	0	13	23
Avg (SD)	73 (37)	4 (1)	15 (2)	32 (2)	52 (48)	0 (0)	11 (5)	19 (8)

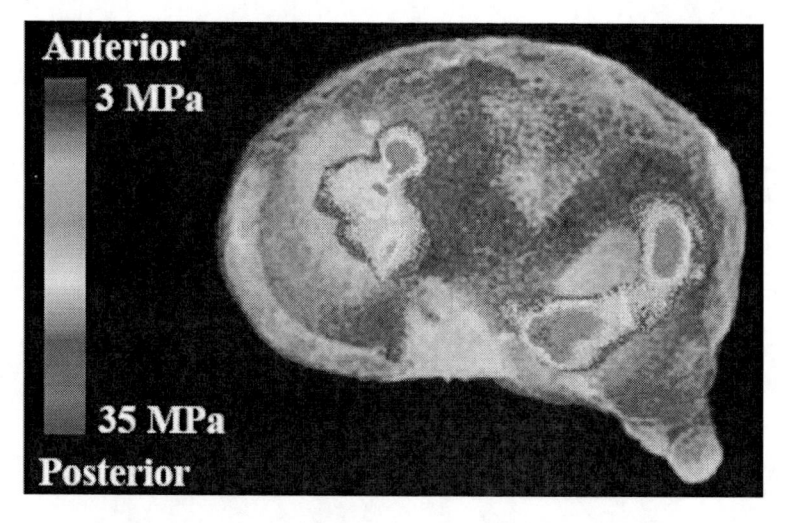

Figure 18. Representative shape and magnitude of the pressure distribution in ITT failure experiments.

Table 14. Contact pressure data from HE pre-failure experiments

	Medial Compartment				Lateral Compartment			
	Area	Area > 25 MPa	Avg Pressure	Max Pressure	Area	Area > 25 MPa	Avg Pressure	Max Pressure
	(mm²)		(MPa)		(mm²)		(MPa)	
32416R	65	9	19	37	45	0	12	19
32284R	47	0	13	23	88	0	15	22
32273L	101	0	17	29	26	0	12	19
32302L	71	2	17	29	66	9	19	35
32516R	35	6	19	41	65	9	14	21
32388L	119	0	13	23	1	9	12	15
Avg (SD)	73 (32)	3 (4)	16 (3)	30 (7)	48 (31)	1 (3)	14 (3)	22 (7)

For ITT pre-failure (Table 12) and failure tests (Table 13), there were no differences in the average contact area or pressure between the lateral and medial compartments. In the medial compartment, the pressure distribution was located more anterior for ITT experiments

(Figure 18). In the lateral compartment, the location of highest pressures occurred more posteriorly.

The HE experiments generated high contact pressure and maximum pressure in the anterior medial and lateral compartments (Tables 14 and 15). The contact area in the medial compartment was slightly higher than in the lateral compartment (Figure 19).

Table 15. Contact pressure data from HE failure experiments

	Medial Compartment				Lateral Compartment			
	Area	Area > 25	Avg	Max	Area	Area > 25	Avg	Max
	(mm²)		(MPa)		(mm²)		(MPa)	
32416R	80	28	22	44	106	0	15	24
32284R	54	0	17	25	127	0	16	25
32273L	155	49	21	38	48	0	12	18
32302L	79	9	19	34	68	3	17	37
32516R	44	7	18	40	68	0	14	23
32388L	130	0	13	23	7	0	12	17
Avg (SD)	90 (44)	15 (19)	18 (3)	34 (8)	71 (42)	1 (1)	14 (2)	24 (7)

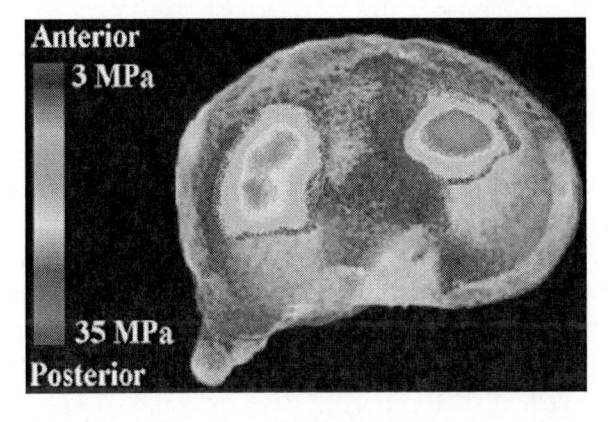

Figure 19. Representative shape and magnitude of the contact pressure distribution in HE failure experiments.

Table 16. Contact pressure data from VB failure experiments

		Medial Compartment				Lateral Compartment			
		Area	Area Over 25 MPa	Avg Pressure	Max Pressure	Area	Area Over 25 MPa	Avg Pressure	Max Pressure
		(mm²)		(MPa)		(mm²)		(MPa)	
VBO	32462R	0	0	0	0	56	0	11	15
	32498L	0	0	0	0	245	11	16	33
	32489R	0	0	5	7	166	16	16	32
	32532L	0	0	5	9	104	0	13	22
	Avg (SD)	0 (0)	0 (0)	3 (3)	4 (5)	143 (82)	7 (8)	14 (2)	26 (8)
VBC	32462L	19	0	11	15	257	63	20	39
	32498R	96	0	12	20	167	1	15	26
	32489L	130	0	15	22	345	17	16	34
	32532R	12	0	11	20	536	15	16	32
	Avg (SD)	64 (58)	0 (0)	12 (2)	19 (3)	326 (158)	24 (27)	17 (2)	33 (6)

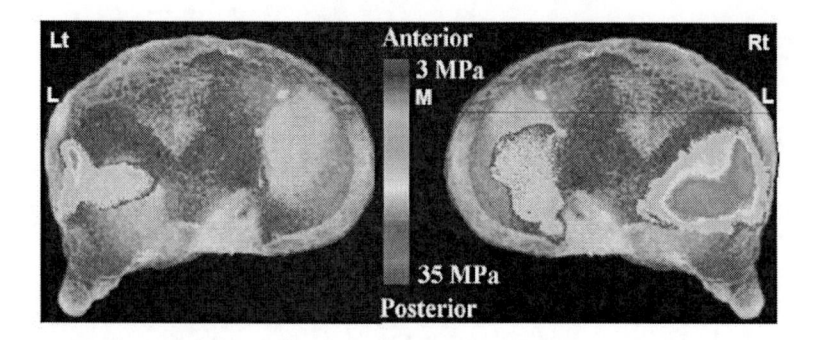

Figure 20. Representative shape and magnitude contact pressure distributions for VBO (Lt) and VBC (Rt) experiments. Lateral (L), medial (M).

In the VBO experiments, there were no pressures recorded by the medium pressure film in the medial compartment for any specimen. The low pressure film was then considered, but two specimens still exhibited no medial pressure (Table 16). There were high contact pressures in the lateral compartment regardless of the level of compressive preload (Figure 20).

Discussion

TFC experiments resulted in regions of high contact pressure in the posterior medial and lateral tibial plateaus. A common injury scenario for ACL rupture during a jump landing includes abduction of the femur that results in high stresses in the lateral compartment.[121] However, the current contact pressures were distributed over both the medial and lateral tibial plateaus. In subfailure experiments there were higher forces in the lateral compartment, but in failure experiments the higher contact pressures and areas occurred in the medial compartment.

ITT experiments produced relatively smaller and less severe contact regions posteriorly on the lateral plateau and anteriorly on the medial plateau than were seen for TFC. The contact pressures in this case were indirectly caused by a balance of forces due to high tensile forces generated in the ACL and other ligamentous structures of the knee. In one specimen where varus-valgus rotation was prevented, there were high contact pressures developed on the medial plateau and the lateral aspect of the knee joint separated with negligible contact pressure. In the subsequent unconstrained specimens, valgus rotation occurred and the contact pressures were distributed evenly between the medial and lateral compartments.

The hyperextension mechanism of ACL rupture has been associated clinically with bone bruises in the anterior aspect of the tibial plateau and anterior aspect of the femoral condyle.[191,223] This clinical "footprint" compares well to the current contact pressure results in the central and anterior tibial plateau. An important finding of this experiment was that the HE moments required to produce ligamentous injury generated similar magnitudes of contact pressure to those produced during ACL rupture under TFC. The increase in average contact area, average contact pressure, and maximum pressure in pre-failure to failure experiments was relatively low, suggesting that the contact pressures needed to create osteochondral microdamage may be present at pre-failure levels as well. This is in contrast to the pattern of contact pressures documented in TFC where there was a much larger increase in pressure levels for pre-failure tests than tests that produced ACL failure.

VB experiments produced an average maximum contact pressure of approximately 30 MPa, similar to the magnitude in TFC experiments. However, VBO experiments resulted in contact pressures located only in the lateral compartment. One clinical injury mechanism that likely produces contact only in the lateral compartment is a forced valgus moment from contact with another player that impacts the lateral side of the knee.[191,223] This sports scenario may be similar to the VBO experiments. In the VBC experiments, the contact was distributed slightly more to the medial side but remained significantly higher in the lateral compartment than the medial compartment. There was a statistically significant difference in the maximum pressure in the medial compartment between the two experimental groups, but not for the lateral compartment.

8. COMPUTATIONAL MODELING OF JOINT INJURY

Contact pressure distributions in the TF joint have been measured [2,216] and computed by finite element analysis [24,25,99,115,142] for a number of loading mechanisms. One limitation with these previous studies is that the contact pressures are from physiological levels of loading and therefore not relevant for injury level forces/moments. In addition, these computational models of the knee generally consist of rigid bones that cannot predict when and where microdamage will occur to the articular cartilage and subchondral bone. For high levels of contact pressure, a rigid subchondral bone would also cause concentrated stress in the cartilage.

The previous section documented the distinct contact pressure distributions in the TF joint produced by each loading mechanism. There were similarities between the maximum pressures developed in TFC, HE and VB. The maximum pressures in those experiments were greater than 30 MPa for at least one region. TFC had the most distributed pattern of severe contact pressure over the central and posterior regions of the lateral and medial compartments. For the HE experiments, the severe pressures were located in the central and anterior regions of the lateral and medial compartments. In VB experiments, the maximum contact pressure was in the central and posterior regions of the lateral compartment. The ITT experiments, on the other hand, had maximum pressures of only 25 MPa in the anterior region of the medial compartment and they were even lower on the posterior region of the lateral compartment. The goal of these simulation studies was to use an anatomically-correct 3D finite element model to determine stresses in the articular cartilage and underlying bone for various loading mechanisms presented in the previous sections. The computational model would then be used to predict the osteochondral damage caused by the TF contact pressures in each of the experimental loading conditions.

The high TF contact forces developed during ACL rupture have been linked with acute trauma to the articular cartilage and underlying subchondral bone in cadaver and clinical studies. Load induced articular cartilage damage occurs either with or without simultaneous disruption of the underlying bone. [16] Cartilage damage that occurs without subchondral bone damage includes fissures that begin at the cartilage surface and extend downwards at approximately 45°. Damage that includes the subchondral bone occurs as microcracks at the interface between cartilage and bone, also called the tidemark. [15] Both types of damage have been explained using a Tresca, or maximal shear stress criterion. [8,13,14,64,228] How the contact pressure distributions affect the tissues depends on the structural and material properties of the tissues themselves. The lateral tibial plateau has a thicker layer of cartilage [164] but lower subchondral bone material properties than the medial plateau. [109] Even when there is an equal distribution of pressure between the medial and lateral plateaus, the stress in the cartilage may be reduced and the stress in the subchondral bone may be increased on the lateral versus the medial side due to these differences in tissue properties. This effect may help explain the frequent occurrence of bone bruises in the lateral tibial plateau. Yet because higher physiological loads pass through the medial compartment, the clinical literature reports a higher rate of post-traumatic OA in the medial tibial plateau following ACL rupture.

Methods

The model geometry used in the current study was based on a subject-specific CT scan of a tibial plateau that most closely represented a healthy middle-aged individual. The left tibial plateau of a 54 year old male (32273) with a height of 69 inches and weight of 171 lbs was chosen for the study. The subject had no history of lower extremity injury or arthritis. An axial CT scan of the knee was acquired prior to testing with an in-plane resolution of .33 mm and slice thickness of .625 mm. The tibia had been potted in epoxy and the potting material was included in the CT scan. To create a computational model of this geometry, the DICOM images were imported into Mimics (v12.11 Materalise, Leuven, Belgium) and a standard CT bone density threshold value (>226 Hu) was used to create 3D surface objects of the tibial and femoral bones. Remeshing tools were employed to create a simplified and smooth final surface mesh before it was converted into a volume mesh of tetrahedral elements. The resultant bone models were exported into ABAQUS CAE (v 6.8 Hibbit, Karlsson & Sorensen Inc., Pawtuchet, RI) for finite element analysis. The cartilage layers were created in ABAQUS by selecting the articular surface and creating additional elements to get the desired thickness (Figure 21). Since cartilage is not clearly distinguishable in CT scans, these thicknesses were based on documented values from the literature and vary between 1.3 and 4.5 mm across the medial and lateral plateaus (Figure 22).[164]

The material properties of subchondral bone have been shown to vary widely across the medial and lateral plateau,[109] as well as from the anterior to posterior compartment.[90] Therefore, subchondral bone regions were divided by medial and lateral plateau and areas covered or uncovered by the meniscus. Trabecular bone regions were separated and the Young's modulus (E) was based on bone mineral density.[45] The overlying cartilage layer varies in thickness. Although cartilage is typically modeled as a biphasic material,[199] the viscous relaxation time is relatively large (1500 sec) so that it can be reduced to an elastic material for the short loading times in the current model (50-250 msec).[64] The material properties of cartilage and bone are given in Figure 22. [12,52,132,135,199] The damage criterion thresholds were based on the relationship between shear strength (Tresca stress) and bone mineral density from the literature and are also given in Figure 22. [45,212] The threshold for Tresca stress that initiates cartilage fissures is approximately 5.5 MPa. [16]

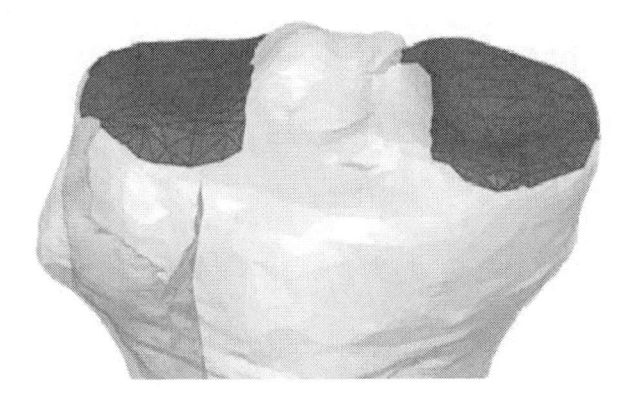

Figure 21. Layer of articular cartilage created on the medial and lateral surfaces of the tibial plateau.

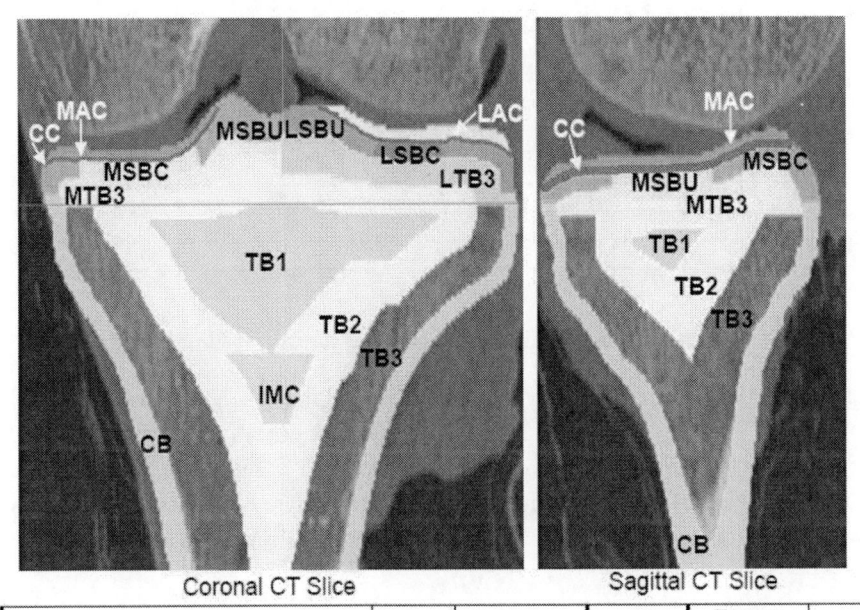

Tissue Zone	Abb.	Thickness (mm)	E (MPa)	Tresca Criterion (MPa)	v
Medial Articular Cartilage	MAC	1.5	35	5.5	.49
Lateral Articular Cartilage	LAC	2	35	5.5	.49
Calcified Cartilage	CC	.2	350	4	.3
Medial Subchondral Bone Covered	MSBC	3.5	3500	35	.3
Medial Subchondral Bone Uncovered	MSBU	3	3250	34	.3
Lateral Subchondral Bone Covered	LSBC	2.5	2750	31	.3
Lateral Subchondral Bone Uncovered	LSBU	2	2500	30	.3
Medial High Density Trabecular Bone	MTB3	3	1250	15	.3
Lateral High Density Trabecular Bone	LTB3	4	1250	15	.3
Cortical Bone	CB	NA	14000	68	.3
High Density Trabecular Bone	TB3	NA	1250	15	.3
Medium Density Trabecular Bone	TB2	NA	750	9	.3
Low Density Trabecular Bone	TB1	NA	350	4	.3
Intramedulary Canal	IMC	NA	0	NA	NA

Figure 22. Tissue zones and material properties for bone and cartilage. Subchondral bone was divided into regions covered or uncovered by the meniscus.

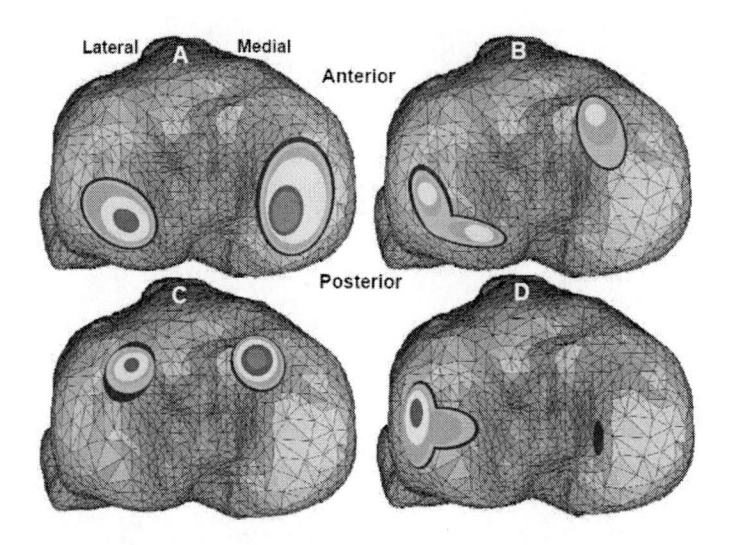

Experiment		Lateral Compartment		Medial Compartment	
		Contact Area (mm^2)	Max Pressure (MPa)	Contact Area (mm^2)	Max Pressure (MPa)
TFC	A	125	25	150	30
ITT	B	50	20	50	20
HE	C	50	25	75	30
VB	D	125	25	0	5

Figure 23. Generalized contact pressure distribution patterns for each loading condition.

Four generalized pressure distributions were applied directly to the tibial plateau representing the loading experiments (Figure 23). The location, contact area, maximum pressure, and pressure distribution were matched on each compartment for each simulation. The tibia was rigidly constrained at the potting interface. The maximum Tresca stress in each region was converted into pass/fail data depending on the failure criteria.

Results

The generalized pressure distribution analyses produced a maximum Tresca stress in the articular cartilage of approximately 6 MPa for TFC, HE and VB and 4.5 MPa for ITT. The patterns of Tresca stresses on the articular surfaces are shown in Figure 24, where a threshold of 5.5 MPa was considered the failure criterion for cartilage (presented as dark red). In the TFC analysis there were similar maximum shear stresses produced in each compartment, but the area exceeding the damage criterion threshold was slightly larger in the medial cartilage than in the lateral cartilage. In both compartments there was also a distinguishable horseshoe shaped pattern of high Tresca stress that matched the uncovered regions of increased modulus in the underlying subchondral bone. For HE and VB there were clear differences between the maximum Tresca stresses in the medial and lateral compartments. Damage was predicted in the anterior region of the medial compartment during HE experiments and the central region of the lateral compartment for VB experiments. In each region, the articular cartilage was classified as damaged if the Tresca stress failure criteria was exceeded (Table 17).

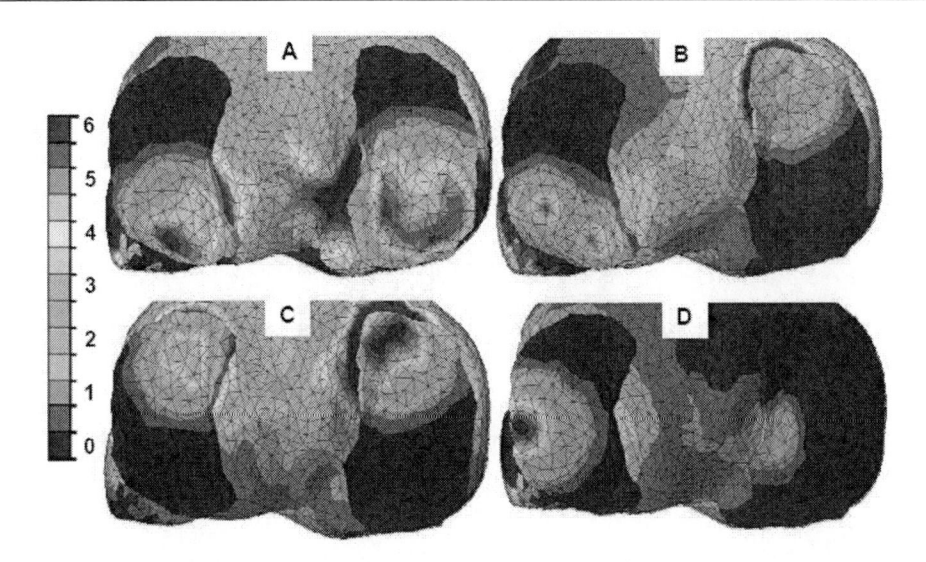

Figure 24. Cartilage surface Tresca stress (MPa) distributions for TFC (A), ITT (B), HE (C), and VB (D) simulations.

Table 17. Maximum Tresca stresses (MPa) in the articular cartilage. Highlights indicate that tissue region that exceeded the Tresca damage criterion threshold of 5.5 MPa

Region	TFC Lateral	TFC Medial	ITT Lateral	ITT Medial	HE Lateral	HE Medial	VB Lateral	VB Medial
Anterior	-	0.5	-	4.5	5	6	1.5	-
Central	4	5.5	4	2.5	4.5	4	6	2.5
Posterior	6	6	5	-	-	-	3.5	1.5

The Tresca stresses in the cartilage were highest along the articular surfaces and decreased towards the subchondral bone (Figure 25). The subchondral bone stress, on the other hand, was distributed evenly with depth. In the medial covered region, the maximum Tresca stress damage threshold was exceeded only under TFC, while the lateral covered region was exceeded only for the applied VB contact pressures (Table 18). The damage criterion threshold was exceeded for TFC for both the medial and lateral compartments not covered by the menisci (uncovered), as well as for HE in the medial uncovered region. The trabecular bone had the highest Tresca stresses at the interface with the subchondral bone and decreased with depth away from the surface. The damage threshold was exceeded in both compartments during TFC, the medial compartment for HE, and the lateral compartment for VB. When comparing the Tresca stress pattern in the medial and lateral compartments during TFC, there was slightly higher stress in the medial compartment but the lateral compartment had a deeper extending pattern of stress that exceeded the damage criterion threshold.

Table 18. Maximum Tresca stresses (MPa) in the subchondral bone. Highlights indicate that tissue region that exceeded the Tresca damage criterion threshold

Region	Tresca Criterion (Mpa)		TFC		ITT		HE		VB	
	Lateral	Medial	Lateral	Medial	Lateral	Medial	Lateral	Medial	Lateral	Medial
Covered Subchondral Bone	31	35	25	40	15	20	10	30	32	5
Uncovered Subchondral Bone	30	34	30	50	20	30	20	35	15	10
Trabecular Bone	15	15	16	18	12	12	14	16	18	4

Discussion

These simulations demonstrate a model of the knee for computing the stress in the cartilage and bone to predict regions of damage caused by different contact pressure distributions that occur during knee injuries. The maximum articular cartilage shear stresses produced in the current study were between 4.5-6 MPa. The damage threshold (5.5 MPa) was shown in a previous study of direct impact onto cartilage correlated to a 2-D FEM. [16] Most other studies have computed much lower values of maximum shear stress in computational models of TFC at much lower magnitudes of input force. [99,142,228]

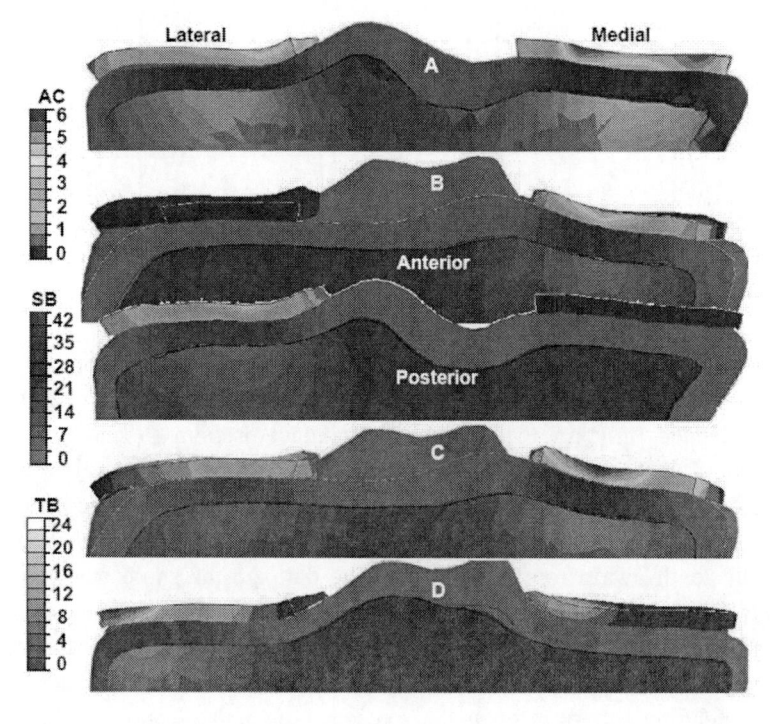

Figure 25. Coronal slices through the tibial plateau at the point of maximum Tresca stress (MPa) for TFC (A), ITT (B), HE (C), and VB (D).

In failure TFC experiments there were slightly higher contact pressures in the medial compartment than the lateral compartment. These values were used for the generalized pressure distribution analysis and produced higher Tresca stress in the medial compartment cartilage. Similar stresses were produced in the subchondral and trabecular bone between the two compartments, however. This lends support to the idea of medial bone bruises occurring from a "countercoup" effect suggested by Kaplan et al. [122] In this scenario, the lateral compartment contusion occurs first just prior to the ACL failure. Then for ACL injuries that occur with large TF compressive forces, a medial compartment contusion occurs during the compensatory varus bending that takes place as the knee forces are lessening. A limitation of the current study was the lack of temporal contact pressure distributions to use in the knee model to investigate this effect further. On the other hand, it is clear that a bone bruise in the posterior medial compartment must occur with a large TF compressive force due to the lack of stress in this region from the other loading conditions used in the current study.

The HE and VB experiments also produced regions with high Tresca stress in trabecular bone. These areas of damage compare well with the characteristic bone bruise patterns described in clinical studies for these ACL injury mechanisms. [100] Isolated ITT, on the other hand, likely does not produce significant cartilage or subchondral bone damage, based on the current analysis. In clinical cases when a patient cites internal twisting and bone bruises are documented, it might be suggested that there must also have been a large axial force in the tibia generated by the ground reaction forces. Most of the video analyses of these events show that these injuries typically occur with a large percentage of the ground reaction force being carried by the injured limb, and these values are usually several times body weight during running, cutting, or landing from a jump. [134,176]

The current study used linear elastic materials, which do not represent most biological materials. Although the instantaneous response has been shown to be equivalent to an incompressible elastic material, this approach does not allow for the decomposition of stress into its fluid and solid phases. [8,14] Cartilage fissuring would be more closely related with the amount of stress carried by the solid phase. Additionally, for bone there are other failure criteria than Tresca stress that might be more appropriate such as a maximum principal stress or strain criteria. The Tresca or the maximum shear stress criterion applied to all types of tissue simplified the interpretation of the results. This was deemed appropriate because the focus was placed on scaling the elastic modulus and damage threshold based on bone mineral density. Many studies have shown approximately linear relationships between bone mineral density and material properties of both cortical and trabecular bone. [45,52,111,206] However, little data exists for the subchondral plate, other than the differences between the covered and uncovered areas of the meniscus. [34] An assumption was made that the material properties for subchondral bone would follow a linear relationship between trabecular and cortical bone, based on the bone mineral density.

9. CONTACT INDUCED OSTEOCHONDRAL MICROTRAUMA

In over 80% of ACL injury cases, a characteristic osteochondral lesion occurs in the tibial plateau and/or the femoral condyle. [162,207,209] Vellet et al. documented an overt loss of cartilage overlying geographic bone bruises in 48% of patients within six months of injury.

[222] These "bone bruises" are associated with occult microcracks of the subchondral and/or trabecular bone and may be caused by compressive loading during the associated ligamentous injury. [184,207] Additionally, chondrocyte necrosis and surface lesions of articular cartilage occur in regions overlying bone bruises in clinical cases of ACL rupture. [116] The goal was to relate microdamage in the articular cartilage and underlying subchondral bone with the loading mechanism producing ligamentous injury to the knee. Regions of high contact pressure and Tresca stress exceeding the failure criterion for cartilage or subchondral and trabecular bone are at increased risk of suffering osteochondral microdamage.

Methods

Surface fissures on the articular surfaces were highlighted for photographic documentation by wiping India ink across the surfaces. Histology was used to quantify cartilage and subchondral bone damage after a careful gross dissection of the joint. [18] TFC, ITT and HE specimens were cut into 8 micron thick slices on a rotary microtome from anterior to posterior at locations near the center of the medial and lateral compartments. [155,159] Two sections from each compartment were chosen for staining with Safranin O-Fast Green. The samples were examined independently with light microscopy by two blinded investigators. Each slice was divided by thirds across the anterior, central, and posterior regions of each compartment. Specific microdamage that was recognized were horizontal and vertical microcracks along the cartilage-subchondral bone interface, superficial and deep zone cartilage damage, and cartilage compression lines (Figure 26).

The VB specimens were scanned using a GE Explore Locus microCT system (General Electric, Fairfield, CT, USA) at a voxel resolution of 90 μm obtained from 400 views. [157] The beam angle of increment was 0.5, and the beam strength was set at 80 kvp and 450 μA. The volumetric image data was visualized with the GE Healthcare MicroView software application to document subchondral bone microdamage in the medial and lateral compartments. Potential damage was identified in the anterior, central and posterior regions of each compartment.

Results

Analysis of the histological samples revealed occult injuries for all TFC specimens following gross failure. Cartilage (Figure 27) and subchondral bone (Figure 28) microdamage was located in central to posterior regions in both compartments. There were similar amounts of damage in the two series of TFC experiments and between medial and lateral compartments. Specific types of damage that were noted were vertical microcracks located in the deep cartilage zone extending into the subchondral bone, and horizontal microcracks located along the tidemark running parallel with the articular surface. There were also fissures of the articular cartilage in both compartments and in similar locations as the subchondral bone damage.

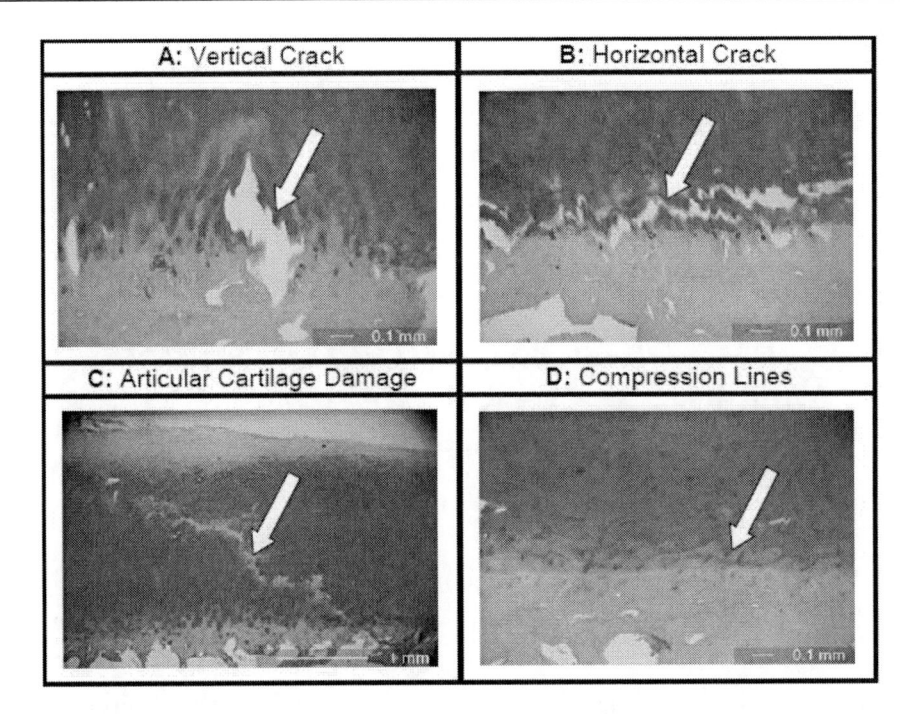

Figure 26. Photographs of representative cartilage and subchondral bone microtrauma (adapted from Meyer et al., 2008).

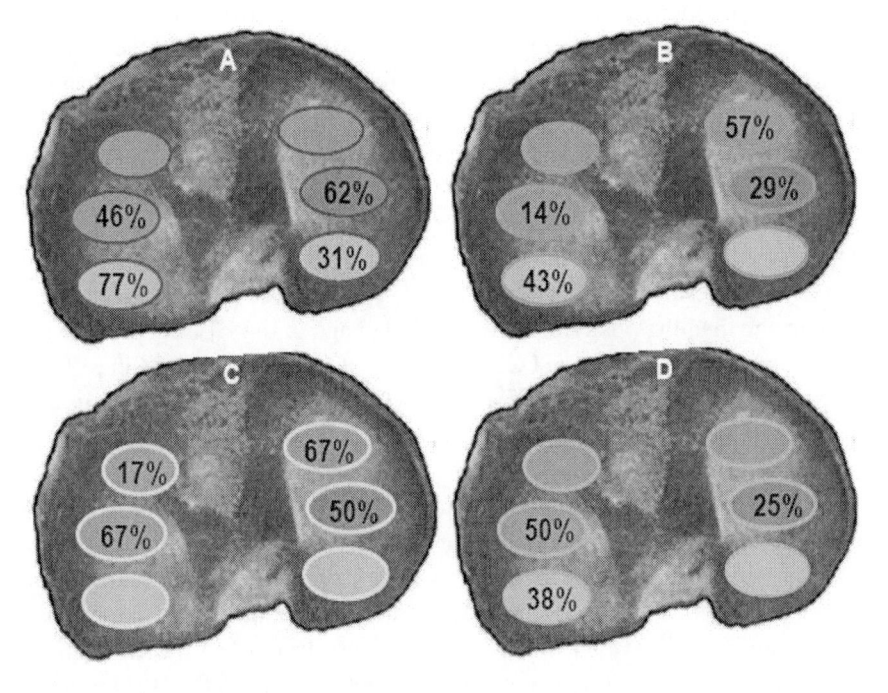

Figure 27. Percentage of specimens with cartilage microdamage in each region for TFC (A), ITT (B), HE (C), and VB (D) experiments.

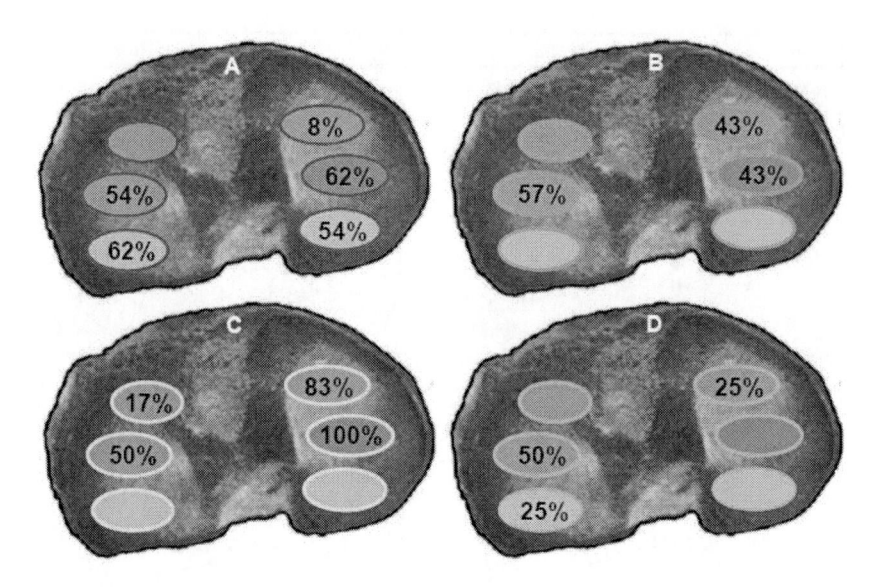

Figure 28. Percentage of specimens with subchondral bone microdamage in each region for TFC (A), ITT (B), HE (C), and VB (D) experiments.

Following ITT failure experiments, occult injuries were documented for all specimens. There was damage in the anterior region of the medial compartment and posterior in the lateral compartment. In addition to horizontal microcracks in the lateral compartment, the ITT specimens also had cartilage damage in the central lateral and central and anterior medial regions. The damage in the torsion specimens was not as extensive as in the paired specimens from TFCR experiments. In fact, there was significantly more damage in the posterior regions of both compartments for TFC experiments, but more damage in the anterior medial region for torsion experiments.

The HE experiments produced subchondral bone and cartilage microdamage in the central to anterior regions across each compartment. In the lateral compartment there were no differences between the microdamage documented in the anterior, central, and posterior regions. In the medial compartment, there was more microdamage recorded in the central region than in the anterior and posterior regions. The anterior region also had significantly more microdamage than the posterior region. The damage in the HE specimens was as severe as in the paired specimens from the TFCB experiments. In fact, there was more damage in the anterior regions of both compartments for HE experiments, but less damage in the posterior regions than TFCB experiments.

Following VB experiments there were articular cartilage fissures in all specimens, except for one specimen from the VBO group. A majority of the articular cartilage damage was noted in the lateral compartment, with only two specimens also displaying medial fissures and both of those were from the VBC experiments. The subchondral bone damage was documented using microCT (Figure 29). Microcracks under the lateral compartment of the tibial plateau were identified in all four of the specimens from the VBC experiments. Lateral microcracks were also identified in two of the four specimens from the VBO experiments.

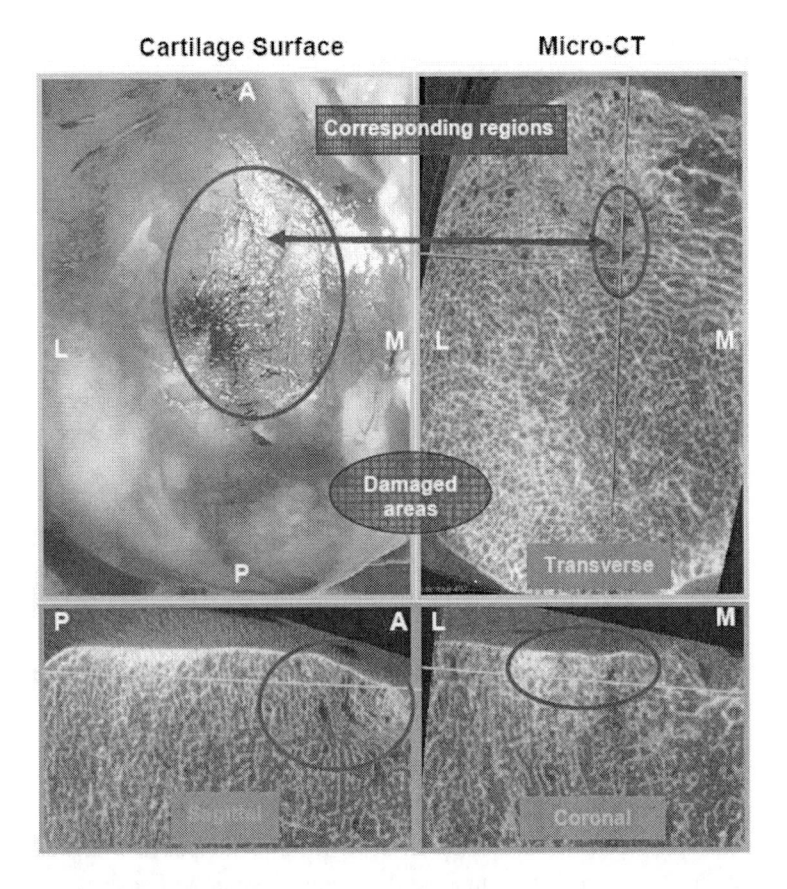

Figure 29. Gross cartilage damage and corresponding subchondral bone damage on the lateral tibial plateau. Reference lines in microCT images indicated the relative slice location between planes. Lateral (L), medial (M), anterior (A), posterior (P).

Discussion

TFC experiments resulted in regions of high contact pressure on the posterior medial and lateral tibial plateaus. While bone bruises in the medial tibial plateau are less common than in the lateral compartment, [121] medial compartment knee OA is a more frequent and conspicuous condition. In pre-failure experiments there were higher forces in the lateral compartment, but in failure experiments, the higher contact pressures and areas occurred in the medial compartment. A "countercoup" effect after ACL failure was suggested by Kaplan et al. to explain the mechanism that produces medial compartment bone contusions during ACL injuries. [122] In this scenario the medial compartment contusion occurs after a lateral compartment contusion during the compensatory varus bending that may occur as the knee forces are reducing. The authors' conclusion that only injuries with large forces could result in medial bone contusions is also supported by the current data where differences in contact force distribution between pre-failure and failure tests were documented in compression specimens. The histological analysis revealed vertical microcracks at the interface between cartilage and subchondral bone on both the medial and lateral plateaus, without signs of gross tibial plateau fracture. These regions of microdamage generally coincided with areas that developed the highest contact pressures. To our knowledge, this is the only study to document controlled experimentally-induced occult microcracks at the cartilage-bone interface in ACL injured human cadaver knees. In a previous study, occult microcracks were also documented in the tibial plateau of knee specimens subjected to TF impacts at similar compressive loads. [21] Those experiments simulated automotive accidents. The knee joint was therefore flexed 90° and relative motion between the tibia and femur was constrained to prevent injury to the ACL. [114] The current study also documented additional damage and matrix compression lines in regions of the cartilage overlying microcracks at the cartilage-bone interface in compression specimens. This demonstrated how localized chondral or osteochondral fracture may occur in patients with a torn knee ligament.

Osteochondral microdamage was also documented due to ITT. These microdamages were usually in the form of horizontal microcracks on the lateral tibial plateau and could be due to excessive shear stress. Since TFC did not result in as many horizontal microcracks, this suggests that alternate loading conditions may have influenced the type of microdamage generated in the subchondral bone. An additional factor for the location of subchondral and cartilage damage may be the intrinsic structural and material properties of the tissues. Contact in the posterior lateral compartment during ITT occurred as the lateral femoral condyle was displaced towards the posterior-center of the tibial plateau. The central area of the tibial plateau has material properties that can be orders of magnitude lower than the lateral plateau, [90] and this infrequent location for joint contact may have produced microdamage at a relatively low level of force in the current study.

HE has been associated clinically with bone bruises in the anterior aspect of the tibial plateau and anterior aspect of the femoral condyle. [191,223] The contact pressures in pre-failure tests were similar to the contact pressures in failure experiments, suggesting that the contact pressures needed to create osteochondral damage may be present at pre-failure levels as well. In fact, bone bruises can occur in clinical patients during severe knee hyperextension resulting in either bicruciate dislocations, [50] isolated ACL rupture, [185] isolated PCL rupture, [221] or without any associated ligamentous damage. [233]

The valgus bending mechanism of ACL rupture is associated with bone bruises in the lateral aspect of the tibial plateau and lateral femoral condyle. [100,191] This clinical "footprint" compares well with the current results showing cartilage damage and subchondral bone microcracks in cadavers. All of the VBC specimens had cartilage damage and subchondral bone microcracks, and three of the VBO specimens had cartilage damage with two of those also having subchondral bone microcracks. These osteochondral microcracks were located in the lateral tibial plateau. Bone bruises occur in the lateral compartment three to five times more frequently than in the medial compartment. [190,207,209] Based on these results, while the risk of osteochondral damage in the lateral compartment may be slightly reduced for VB without a substantial axial load, the likelihood of medial compartment damage may be significantly increased in cases with a combined axial tibial compression component.

Although histology has been commonly used to document subchondral bone microcracks, this method is somewhat limited by providing only a 2D slice of the tissue in selected regions. MicroCT, on the other hand, has also been previously used to document subchondral bone microcracks after a severe impact on the surface of cartilage. [217] In the VB specimens, a microCT scan was used to identify microcracks in the lateral facet of six out of eight specimens. Articular cartilage fissures were documented over the medial and lateral facets by wiping India ink over the tibial surface. There was good agreement between the location of stained cartilage fissures and microCT subchondral bone microcracks. This data compares favorably to clinical studies showing damage to articular cartilage overlying bone bruises. [116,222]

10. DISCUSSION AND CONCLUSION

Isolated ACL Injury

The first goal of these experiments was to identify the relative knee joint motions that cause ligamentous injury to occur. Therefore, this study measured the pre-failure and failure characteristics of different loading mechanisms in order to determine the cause-and-effect relationship in the relative motion between the tibia and femur and the types of ligamentous injuries sustained. TFC induced a large amount of anterior tibia subluxation in pre-failure tests (Table 19). Since the ACL is the primary restraint for anterior tibial subluxation, this motion was expected to produce tension in the ACL and eventually lead to failure. There was 50% less anterior tibial subluxation produced in the ITT and HE than TFC experiments. In the VB experiments, there was a small amount of anterior tibial subluxation that occurred during the compressive preload of VBC experiments, but very little during the bending moment application. ITT and VB experiments both had strongly coupled internal and valgus rotations. In the TFC and HE experiments there was very little internal tibial rotation or valgus bending of the knee.

After gross failure of the knee joint, the primary motions were significantly increased for each type of experiment. In the TFC experiments the magnitude of anterior tibial subluxation was more than doubled after ACL failure. In the ITT and VB experiments, internal and valgus rotations were significantly increased after combined ACL and MCL failure, but little additional motion was observed in the other directions. There was a significant increase in the hyperextension bending angle after ACL and PCL failure as would be expected for those experiments. Therefore, these are likely the most important motions for correlating knee joint injury with the loading mechanisms from sports scenarios.

Table 19. Joint motions prior to failure for each loading mechanism.
#Significant difference between pre-failure and failure tests

	TFC	ITT	HE	VB
Post/Ant Motion (mm)	14 (4.6)#	10 (2.0)	6.9 (3.3)	NA
Med/Lat Motion (mm)	0.1 (3.1)	3.4 (3.2)#	1.7 (1.4)	NA
Int/Ext Angle (deg)	5.4 (3.4)#	40 (16)#	0	38 (14)#
Valg/Var Angle (deg)	2.1 (2.6)#	10 (3.7)#	-0.1 (3.3)	29 (7.2)#
Flex/Ext Angle (deg)	30	30	-34 (11)#	30

An interesting result was documented for internal/external tibial rotation and valgus/varus bending during TFC failure tests. These motions were observed in two separate series of experiments, due to the problems associated with applying large TF compressive forces when they were simultaneously unconstrained. In the pre-failure tests there were small internal and valgus rotations, but in the failure tests there was either external tibial rotation or valgus rotation was significantly increased depending on the motion constrained. These results showed that the motions observed after ACL failure were not representative of the relative displacements that produce tension in the ACL. Prior to failure there was more relative displacement in the lateral compartment, producing small amounts of internal tibial rotation. After ACL rupture, relative displacement in the medial compartment was released which produced a net external rotation of the tibia. In the case of VB, the motion was limited in the pre-failure tests for all loading mechanisms except direct VB. After failure in both the TFC and ITT experiments, there was more than double the amount of valgus rotation as in the pre-failure test.

Video analyses have identified the timing, body positioning, and activities most frequent during sports ACL injuries. The injury timing is usually during the initial foot strike and the position is an extended, slightly valgus, and externally rotated knee. The most frequent activities are plant-and-cut and landing maneuvers with most of the body weight distribution on the injured leg. Therefore, in both the plant-and-cut and landing maneuvers there are likely high levels of TFC that could be of similar magnitude to loads in the current study. Similar injury mechanism characteristics have been noted in patient surveys following their ACL injury, but one area of conflict noted in these studies is the direction of tibial rotation. In many cases, the patient recalls internal tibial rotation rather than external tibia rotation. This disagreement is explained based on the motion observed in the TFC experiments. The exact time when the ACL injury occurs cannot be recorded from a video analysis and the body position can change rapidly after failure.

A common problem encountered in biomechanical testing to failure occurs when the applied force is substantially higher than the failure tolerance of the tissues. In that case, the loading causes a total joint dislocation or complex fracture without a clear indication of when a particular tissue was damaged. The force and displacement data obtained for such an experiment is called right censored data, because failure occurred but it is not apparent what the exact values were at the time of failure. In the opposite scenario, a single experiment with an applied force that is too low could result in no tissue damage (left-censored data). In this case it is unclear how much more force or displacement could have been applied before the tissue failed. The alternative is to use repeated tests at increasing load levels, as was done in the current series of experiments. Frequently in these studies, failure is a force-limiting event and therefore both the peak force and tissue failure occur at the same moment (uncensored data). However, the joint displacements may continue to increase after failure due to the increased laxity available from the damaged structures. [128] In the current study, the pre-failure tests were left-censored data points, but the forces were not very far off from the failure forces, so the peak displacement data in those tests may represent the maximum joint displacements that can be withstood without an injury. The failure test peak displacements were right-censored, but only for the injuries reported (i.e. the rest of the joint remained intact but did not prevent the large documented motions). In contrast, the forces dropped sharply in failure tests so the peak values likely correspond to the actual knee ligament injury tolerance (uncensored data).

Table 20. Failure forces and injuries sustained by the ligaments of the knee for each loading mechanism. #Significant difference between pre-failure and failure tests

	TFC	ITT	HE	VB
Failure Load or Moment (kN or Nm)	6.6 (1.6)#	46 (15)#	108 (46)#	106 (63)
Anterior Cruciate Ligament	100%	100%	100%	38%
Posterior Cruciate Ligament	10%	0%	100%	0%
Medial Collateral Ligament	0%	50%	0%	88%
Lateral Collateral Ligament	10%	25%	0%	13%
Frequently Injured Knee Ligaments ▬ACL ▬LCL PCL MCL				

Tibiofemoral Compression

The second goal was to identify the loading mechanisms that produce anterior tibial subluxation and isolated ACL injuries. The results provide evidence that compressive load in the TF joint is a primary component of the loading mechanism for non-contact, isolated ACL injuries in the extended knee. ACL injuries were produced under all four of the loading conditions, although these injuries were frequently combined with injuries to other ligamentous structures as well (Table 20). In the TFC experiments, ACL injuries were produced in all of the specimens and combined ligamentous injuries occurred in only one specimen. ITT also produced injuries to the ACL, but these were frequently combined with an injury to one or both of the collateral ligaments. ITT produced ligamentous injury in the knee at lower torques than are required to produce injury in the ankle.[158] HE caused a complete anterior dislocation of the knee (injury to both the ACL and PCL). Finally, VB produced ACL failure in three specimens and MCL failure in seven specimens. Therefore, in the current study it is apparent that the only loading mechanism that produced isolated failure of the ACL was TFC.

Complex injuries of the knee are frequent in all levels of sports and they usually occur as a result of multiple forces applied to the knee simultaneously. The isolated loading mechanisms applied to the knee joints in the current study was a way of simplifying this complex problem to more straightforward experimental conditions. The primary loading mechanisms important in cases of isolated ACL injury were identified as internal rotation of the tibia, valgus knee bending, hyperextension of the knee, and axial loading through the tibia. Varus bending, external tibial rotation, hyperflexion and anterior shear of the tibia were not tested in the current series of experiments. It is possible to have all of these loading mechanisms occur during noncontact sports injury scenarios with the exception of anterior tibial shear, which only occurs during contact with another player or object. However, the only loading mechanisms that were tested were the ones expected to produce ACL failure based on previous biomechanical studies.

Most biomechanical evaluations of knee joint response for external loading mechanisms have been at low force levels or comparisons of relative joint motions for intact and ACL sectioned knees. One other study that produced isolated ACL injuries did so with a 4500 N quadriceps muscle force.[61] At 20° of knee flexion, the patellar tendon has a slight anterior directed force component which produced anterior subluxation of the tibia during quadriceps muscle contraction. An additional loading mechanism that was not tested was distraction of the tibia and femur. Although this is a common experimental technique for measuring the stiffness and failure strength of the ACL in biomechanical studies, it was not considered relevant to the current study due to the complete lack of TF joint contact. In the real world it might be expected that more complicated combined loading mechanisms would also produce isolated ACL injury. Several possible loading combinations might be internal tibial torsion with combined valgus bending and/or combined hyperextension moments, or any of the previously mentioned loading mechanisms combined with a significant axial tibial load component.

Compressive loads in the knee joint during running and landing from a jump can be up to fifteen times body weight. These TF joint contact forces are combinations of both the ground reaction and muscle contraction forces. Therefore, it is possible that the quadriceps muscle contraction in the DeMorat et al. experiments produced high TF compressive loads and anterior tibial subluxation occurred due to the posterior slope of the tibial plateau.[61] The combined experimental results of the current study and effect of quadriceps force provide substantial evidence for the importance of sagittal plane motion in non-contact ACL injury mechanisms, which has been previously overlooked in the clinical literature.

Post-Traumatic Osteoarthritis

The final goal was to correlate clinical patterns of knee injuries and bone bruises to the loading mechanism and distributions of contact pressure. There is evidence that post-traumatic osteoarthritis is due, in part, to osteochondral microdamage that occurs at the time of the acute ligamentous injury. Each loading mechanism produced a distinct contact pressure distribution in the TF joint. There were similarities between the magnitudes of contact pressure developed in three of the loading mechanisms. The maximum pressures were greater than 30 MPa for at least one location on the tibial plateau for the TFC, HE, and VB experiments (Figure 30). For ITT experiments, the maximum pressure was approximately 25 MPa in the anteromedial compartment and even lower in the posterolateral compartment. In the computational models, all but the ITT model produced maximum shear stresses in the articular cartilage, subchondral bone, and trabecular bone which exceeded the thresholds for predicted tissue damage. The locations of this predicted tissue damage were variable depending on the applied pressure distribution, but cartilage damage was predicted in all loading mechanisms and subchondral and trabecular bone damage was predicted for all mechanisms except ITT.

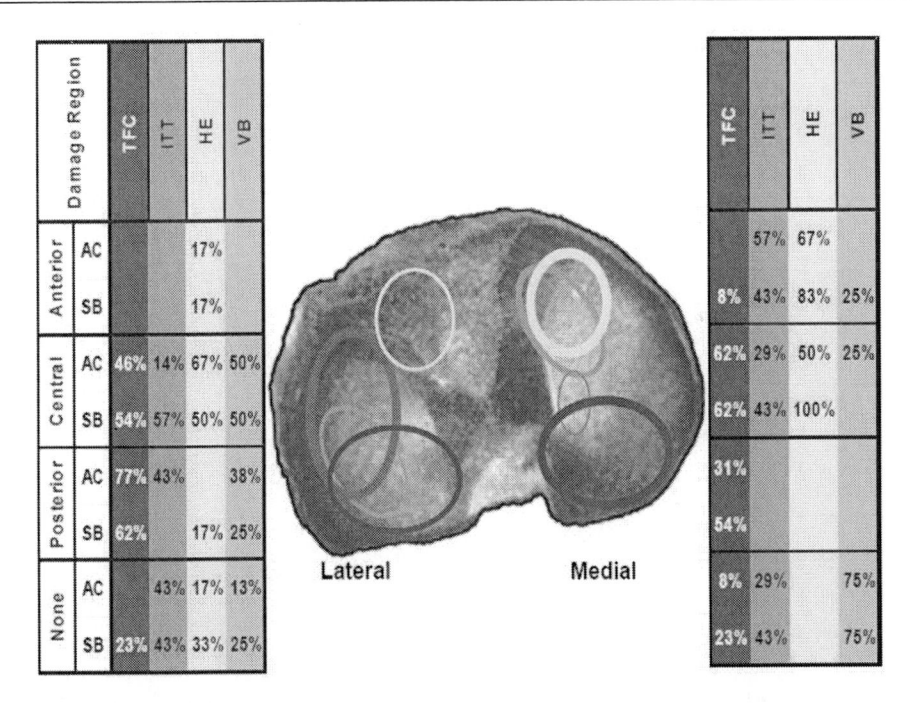

Figure 30. Percentage of specimens with articular cartilage (AC) and subchondral bone (SB) microdamage in each region for each loading mechanism. Circles represent regions of contact pressure and their line thickness represents the pressure magnitude.

The pressure distributions and computational model predictions correlated well with the location of osteochondral damage, both in the form of cartilage fissures and subchondral bone microcracks. In the central and posterior regions of the lateral and medial compartments of TFC specimens, there was osteochondral damage in at least one of these regions and sometimes multiple regions were damaged. For the HE specimens, the damage was limited to the central and anterior regions of the lateral and medial compartments. In VB, nearly all of the damage was in the central and posterior regions of the lateral compartment, with very few specimens suffering damage in the central medial compartment. Finally, ITT produced damage primarily in the posterolateral and anteromedial compartments, but the percentage of specimens without any damage was elevated.

Bone bruise patterns in certain knee injuries, such as ACL rupture, have been linked to a characteristic "footprint" of the injury loading mechanism. These osseous injuries may be caused by a direct blow to the bone or by tensile forces that occur during an avulsion injury. During ACL injuries, however, bone bruises are frequently "kissing" contusions which are produced in the tibia and femur at the site where the opposing articular surfaces are in contact at the moment of injury. The bone bruise pattern is a static representation of the impact forces that occurred at the time of injury and provides clues to the associated soft-tissue injuries as well as the mechanism of rupture. Radiologists have used this information to construct a mechanism-based classification system to relate the patterns of bone bruising and ligament damages for complex, clinical cases of knee injury (Table 21).

The ligamentous injury patterns described for each loading mechanism in Table 21 are similar to the injury results for the failure experiments in the current study (Table 20). Based on previous biomechanical studies at physiological force levels and a limited number of

Table 21. Classification of loading mechanism, bone bruise patterns and gross ligament injuries (adapted from Hayes et al., 2000)

Loading Mechanism	Bone Bruise Location	Ligament Injuries
Pure hyperextension	Anterior central tibia, anterior femoral condyles	ACL, PCL, posterior capsule
Pure valgus	Lateral tibia, lateral femoral condyle	ACL, MCL
Valgus, external rotation, axial tibia compression	Posterior lateral tibia, lateral femoral condyle, medial tibia, medial femoral condyle	ACL, MCL
Internal tibial rotation, valgus	Posterior lateral tibia, lateral femoral condyle	ACL, MCL
Internal tibia rotation, axial tibia compression	Posterior lateral tibia, lateral femoral condyle, medial tibia, medial femoral condyle	ACL, MCL, LCL
Axial tibia compression	Posterior lateral tibia, lateral femoral condyle, posterior medial tibia, medial femoral condyle	ACL

cadaver experiments at failure load level, a correlation between these loading mechanisms and ligamentous injuries was expected. However, the main purpose of the current series of experiments was not just to cause gross failures of the knee joint, but to use the injury mechanisms as models for understanding patterns of osteochondral damage and evaluating the risk of developing post traumatic osteoarthritis. Contact pressure distributions in the TF joint have been measured and computed by finite element analysis for a number of loading mechanisms, but not at failure level forces. Additionally, osteochondral damage has also been documented in the tibial plateau from a direct impact or from TFC, but this chapter represents the first series of experiments to relate osteochondral damage with contact pressures to a variety of injury mechanisms.

In HE the pre-failure contact pressure magnitudes were comparable to the failure pressures. For the other loading mechanisms, the magnitude of pressure was slightly lower but still exceeded 30 MPa. In these scenarios, there may be the potential for osteochondral microdamage to occur without gross ligamentous knee injury. This occurs frequently in the clinical literature, as bone bruises are often identified on MRI without a corresponding ACL or other soft tissue injury. [19]

CONCLUSION

Isolated ACL injuries occur from TFC, but ITT and VB caused combined MCL injuries and HE caused combined PCL injuries. TFC produced anterior tibial subluxation leading up to isolated ACL injury. After failure, there were significant increases in external tibial rotation and valgus knee bending. Based on the current studies, the magnitude of vertical ground reaction forces and muscle contraction forces producing compression of the TF joint should be considered as an important mechanism in sports ACL injury scenarios. In addition, each loading mechanism produced a distinct contact pressure distribution that correlated well with the location of osteochondral microdamage. Importantly, TFC, HE and VB mechanisms of joint injury produced regions of contact pressure exceeding 30 MPa. In the computational model, this level of contact pressure produced maximum shear stresses in the articular cartilage, subchondral bone, and trabecular bone that exceeded the threshold for predicted tissue damage. There is a long-term risk of developing post-traumatic osteoarthritis from these failure levels of joint loading. In addition, however, the fact that maximum contact pressure was also severe in certain pre-failure tests suggests that there may still be an enhanced risk of chronic joint degeneration even if ligamentous injury is absent.

REFERENCES

[1]   Agel J, Arendt E, Bershadsky B. Anterior cruciate ligament injury in National Collegiate Athletic Association basketball and soccer. *Am. J. Sports Med.* 2005;33(4):524-531.

[2]   Ahmed A, Burke D. In-vitro measurement of static pressure distribution in synovial joints- Part 1: Tibial surface of the knee. *J. Biomech. Eng.* 1983;105:216-225.

[3]   Akizuki S, Mow V, Muller R, et al. Tensile properties of human knee joint cartilage: I. Influence of ionic conditions, weight bearing, and fibrillation on the tensile modulus. *J. Orthop. Res.* 4:379-392, 1986.

[4]   Allen C, Wong E, Livesay G, Sakane M, Fu F, Woo S. Importance of the medial meniscus in the anterior cruciate ligament-deficient knee. *J. Orthop. Res.* 2000;18:109-115.

[5]   Amis A, Dawkins G. Functional anatomy of the anterior cruciate ligament: fibre bundle actions related to ligament replacements and injuries. *J. Bone Jt. Surg.* 1991;73:260-267.

[6]   Andreasson G, Lindenberger U, Renstrom P, et al. Torque developed at simulated sliding between sport shoes and an artificial turf. *Am. J. Sports Med.* 1986;14(3):225-230.

[7]   Arendt E, Dick R. Knee injury patterns among men and women in collegiate basketball and soccer: NCAA data and review of literature. *Am. J. Sports Med.* 1995;23(6):694-701.

[8]   Armstrong C, Lai W, Mow V. An analysis of the unconfined compression of articular cartilage. *J. Biomech. Eng.* 1984;106:165-173.

[9]   Arnoczky S. Anatomy of the anterior cruciate ligament. *Clin. Orthop. Rel. Res.* 1983;172:19-25.

[10]   Arnold J, Coker T, Heaton L, Park J, Harris W. Natural History of Anterior Cruciate Tears. *Am. J. Sports Med.* 1979;7:305-313.

[11]   Asano H, Muneta T, Ikeda H, Yagishita K, Kurihara Y, Sekiya I. Arthroscopic evaluation of the articular cartilage after anterior cruciate ligament reconstruction: a short-term prospective study of 105 patients. *Arthroscopy.* 2004;20:474-481.

[12]   Ashman RB, Cowin SC, Van Bruskirk WC, Rice JC. A continous wave technique for the measurement of the elastic properties of bone. *J. Biomech.* 1984;17:349-361.

[13]   Askew M, Mow V. The biomechanical function of the collagen fibril ultrastructure of articular cartilage. *J. Biomech.* 1978;100:105-115

[14] Ateshian G, Lai W, Zhu W, Mow V. An asymptotic solution for the contact of two biphasic cartilage layers. *J. Biomech.* 1994;37:1347-1360.

[15] Atkinson PJ, Haut RC. Subfracture insult to the human cadaver patellofemoral joint produces occult injury. *J. Orthop. Res.* 1995;13:936-944.

[16] Atkinson T, Haut R, Alterio N. Impact-induced fissuring of articular cartilage: an investigation of failure criteria. *J. Biomech. Eng.* 1998a;120:181-187.

[17] Atkinson P, Newberry W, Atkinson T, Haut R. A method to increase the sensitive range of pressure sensitive film. *J. Biomech.* 1998b;31:855-859.

[18] Atkinson P, Walsh J, Haut R. The human patella: A comparison of three preparation methods. *J. Histotech.* 1998c;21:151-153.

[19] Atkinson P, Cooper T, Anseth S, Walter N, Kargus R, Haut R. Association of knee bone bruise frequency with time postinjury and type of soft tissue injury. *Orthop.* 2008;31:440.

[20] Bahr R, Krosshaug T. Understanding injury mechanisms: a key component of preventing injuries in sport. *Br. J. Sports Med.* 39;2005:324-329.

[21] Banglmaier R, Dvoracek-Driksna D, Oniang'o T, Haut R. Axial compressive load response of the 90° flexed human tibiofemoral joint. *43rd Stapp. Car. Crash Conf. Proc.* 1999;43:127-139.

[22] Bellabarba C, Bush-Joseph C, Bach B. Patterns of meniscal injury in the anterior cruciate-deficient knee: a review of the literature. *Am. J. Orthop.* 1997;26:18-23.

[23] Bendjaballah M, Shirazi-Adl A, Zukor D. Biomechanics of the human knee joint in compression: reconstruction, mesh generation and finite element analysis. *Knee.* 1995;2:69-79.

[24] Bendjaballah M, Shirazi-Adl A, Zukor D. Finite element analysis of human knee joint in varus-valgus. *Clin. Biomech.* 1997;12:139-148.

[25] Bendjaballah M, Shirazi-Adl A, Zukor D. Biomechanical response of the passive human knee joint under anterior-posterior forces. *Clin. Biomech.* 1998;13:625-633.

[26] Beynnon B, Howe J, Pope M, Johnson R, Fleming B. The measurement of anterior cruciate strain in vivo. *Int. Orthop.* 1992;16:1-12.

[27] Bizot P, Meunier A, Christel P, Witvoet J. Experimental passive hyperextension injuries of the knee: biomechanical aspects and their consequences (French). *Revue de Chirurgie Orthop.* 1995;81:211-220.

[28] Blankevoort L, Huskies R. A mechanism for rotational restraints in the knee joint. *J. Orthop. Res.* 1996;14:676-679.

[29] Boden B, Dean G, Feagin J, Garrett W. Mechanisms of anterior cruciate ligament injury. *Orthop.* 2000;23:573-578.

[30] Bose D, Bhalla K, Untaroiu C, Ivarsson B, Crandall J, Hurwitz S. Injury tolerance and moment response of the knee joint to combined valgus bending and shear loading. *J. Biomech. Eng.* 2008;130:031008 1-8

[31] Brautigan B, Johnson D. The epidemiology of knee dislocations. *Clin. Sports Med.* 2000;19:387-397.

[32] Brown T, Shaw D. In vitro contact stress distribution on the femoral condyles. *J. Orthop. Res.* 1984;2:190–199.

[33] Buckland-Wright J, Lynch J, Dave B. Early radiographic features in patients with anterior cruciate ligament rupture. *Ann. Rheum. Dis.* 2000;59:641-646.

[34] Burr D, Schaffler M. The involvement of subchondral mineralixed tissues in osteoarthrosis: Quantitative microscopic evidence. *Micro Res. Tech.* 1998;37:343-357.

[35] Butler D, Noyes F, Grood E. Ligamentous restraints to anterior-posterior drawer in the human knee. A biomechanical study. *J. Bone Jt. Surg.* 1980;62A:259-270.

[36] Butler D. Anterior Cruciate Ligament; Its Normal Response and Replacement. *J. Orthop. Res.* 1989;7:910-921.

[37] Cameron M, Mizuno Y, Cosgarea AJ. Diagnosing and managing anterior cruciate ligament injuries. *J. Musculoskeletal Med.* 2000;17:47-53.

[38] Cavanagh P, Lafortune M. Ground reaction forces in distance running. *J. Biomech.* 1980;13:397-406.

[39] Centers for Disease Control. Guidelines for schools and communities for promoting lifelong physical activity. 1997

[40] Chapchal G. Posttraumatic Osteoartritis After Injury of the Knee and Hip Joint. *Reconstr. Surg. Trauma.* 1978;16: 87-94.

[41] Chappell J, Yu B, Kirkendall D, Garrett W. A comparison of knee kinetics between male and female recreational athletes in stop-jump tasks. *Am. J. Sports Med.* 2002;30:261-267.

[42] Chappell J, Herman D, Knight B, Kirkendall D, Garrett W, Yu B. Effect of fatigue on knee kinetics and kinematics in stop-jump tasks. *Am. J. Sports Med.* 2005;33:1022-1029.

[43] Chaudhari A, Andriacchi T, van den Bogert A, McLean S, Yu B, Chappell J, Garrett W. Letters to the editor. *Am. J. Sports Med.* 2006;34:312-315.

[44] Chen E, Black J. Materials design analysis of the prosthetic anterior cruciate ligament. *J. Biomat. Res.* 1980;14:567-586.

[45] Ciarelli MJ, Goldstein SA, Kuhn JL, Cody DD, Brown MB. Evaluation of orthogonal mechanical properties and density of human trabecular bone from the major metaphyseal regions with materials testing and computed tomography. *J. Orthop. Res.* 1991;9:674-682.

[46] Cipolla M, Scala A, Gianni E, Puddu G. Different patterns of meniscal tears in acute anterior cruciate ligament ruptures and in chronic ACL-deficient knees: classification, staging and timing of treatment. *Knee Surg. Sports Traumatol. Arthrosc.* 1995;3:130-134.

[47] Cochrane J, Lloyd D, Buttfield A, Seward H, McGivern J. Characteristics of anterior cruciate ligament injuries in Australian football. *J. Sci. Med. Sports.* 2007;10:96-104.

[48] Conn J, Annest J, Gilchrist J. Sports and recreation related injury episodes in the US population, 1997-99. *Inj. Prev.* 2003;9:117-123.

[49] Cosgarea A, Schatzke M. Knee problems in the young athlete: A clinical overview. *J. Musculoskeletal. Med.* 1997;14(8):96-109.

[50] Crotty JM, Snow RD, Brogdon BG, DeMouy EH. Magnetic resonance imaging of trauma patterns in the knee. *Emergency Rad.* 1998;5:237-244.

[51] Csintalan R, Ehsan A, McGarry M, Fithian D, Lee T. Biomechanical and Anatomical Effects of an External Rotation Torque Applied to the Knee; A Cadaveric Study. *Am. J. Sports Med.* 2006;34:1623-1629.

[52] Cuppone M, Seedhom BB, Berry E, Ostell AE. The longitudinal Young's modulus of cortical bone in the midshaft of human femur and its correlation with CT scanning data. *Calcif. Tissue Int.* 2004;74:302-309.

[53] D'Lima DD, Hashimoto S, Chen PC, Colwell CW, Lotz MK. Human chondrocyte apoposis in response to mechanical injury. *Osteoarthritis Cart.* 2001;9:712-719.

[54] Daniel D, Fithian DC. Indications for ACL surgery. *Arthroscopy.* 1994;10:434-441.

[55] Daniel D, Stone M, Sachs R, Malcom L. Instrumented measurement of anterior knee laxity in patients with acute anterior cruciate ligament disruption. *Am. J. Sports Med.* 1985;13:401-407.

[56] Daniel D, Stone M, Dobson B, Fithian D, Rossman D, Kaufman K. Fate of the ACL injured patient: A prospective outcome study. *Am. J. Sports Med.* 1994;22:632-644.

[57] Davies-Tuck M, Wluka A, Wang Y, Teichtahl A, Jones G, Ding C, Cicuttini F. The natural history of cartilage defects in people with knee osteoarthritis. *Osteoarthritis Cart.* 2008;16:337-342.

[58] Davis M, Ettinger W, Neuhaus J, Cho S, Hauck W. The association of knee injury and obesity with unilateral and bilateral osteoarthritis of the knee. *Am. J. Epidem.* 1989;130(2):278-288.

[59] Deitch J, Starker C, Walters S, Moseley J. Injury risk in professional basketball players: A comparison of Women's National Basketball Association and National Basketball Association Athletes. *Am. J. Sports Med.* 2006;34(&):1077-1083.

[60] DeJour H, Bonnin M. Tibial translation after anterior cruciate ligament rupture. Two radiological tests compared. *J. Bone Jt. Surg.* 1994;76B:745-749.

[61] DeMorat G, Weinhold P, Blackburn T, Chudik S, Garrett W. Aggressive quadriceps loading can induce noncontact anterior cruciate ligament injury. *Am. J. Sports Med.* 2004;32:477-483.

[62] Ding M. Age variations in the properties of human tibial trabecular bone and cartilage. *Acta Orthop. Scand. Suppl.* 2000;292:1-45.

[63] Eberhardt A, Lewis J, Keer L. Normal contact of elastic spheres with two elastic layers as a model of joint articulation. *J. Biomech. Eng.* 1990;113:410-417.

[64] Ettlinger C, Johnson R, Shealy J. A method to help reduce the risk of serious knee sprains incurred in alpine skiing. *Am. J. Sports Med.* 1995;23:531-537.

[65] Ewers B, Jayaraman V, Banglmaier R, Haut R. The effect of loading rate on the degree of acute injury and chronic conditions in the knee after blunt impact. *Stapp. Conf. Proc.* 2000;44:299-314.

[66] Faber K, Dill J, Amendola A, Thain L, Spouge A, Fowler P. Occult osteochondral lesions after anterior cruciate ligament rupture six-year magnetic resonance follow-up study. *Am. J. Sports Med.* 1999;27(4):489-494.

[67] Fagenbaum R, Darling W. Jump landing strategies in male and female college athletes and the implications of such strategies for anterior cruciate ligament injury. *Am. J. Sports Med.* 2003;31:233-240.

[68] Fang C, Johnson D, Leslie MP, Carlson CS, Robbins M, Cesare PE. Tissue distribution and measurement of cartilage oligomeric matrix protein in patients with magnetic resonance imaging-detected bone bruises after acute anterior cruciate ligament tears. *J. Orthop. Res.* 2001;19:634-641.

[69] Fauno P, Wulff Jakobsen B. Mechanism of Anterior Cruciate Ligament Injuries in Soccer. *Int. J. Sports Med.* 2004;27:75-79.

[70] Fayad L, Parellada J, Parker L, Schweitzer M. MR imaging of anterior cruciate ligament tears: is there a gender gap? *Skeletal. Radiol.* 2003;32:639-646.

[71] Feagin J. The syndrome of the torn anterior cruciate ligament. *Orthop. Clin. North Am.* 1979;10:81-90.

[72] Felson D. An update on the pathogenesis and epidemiology of osteoarthritis. *Radiologic Clinics N. Am.* 2004;42:1-9.

[73] Fernandez W, Yard E, Comstock R. Epidemiology of lower extremity injuries amoung U.S. high school athletes. *Acad. Emergency Med.* 14;2007:641-645.

[74] Ferretti A, Papandrea P, Conteduca F, Mariani PP. Knee ligament injuries in volleyball players. *Am. J. Sports Med.* 1992;20:203-207.

[75] Fink C, Hoser C, Hackl W, Navarro R, Benedetto K. Long-term outcome of operative or nonoperative treatment of anterior cruciate ligament rupture – Is sports activity a determining variable? *Int. J. Sports Med.* 2001;22:304-309.

[76] Fleming B, Renstom P, Beynnon B, Engstrom B, Peura GD, Badger GJ, Johnson RJ. The effect of weight-bearing and external loading on anterior cruciate ligament strain. *J. Biomech.* 2001;34:163-170.

[77] Fornalski S, McGarry MH, Csintalan RP, Fithian DC, Lee TQ. Biomechanical and anatomical assessmendt after knee hyperextension injury. *Am. J. Sports Med.* 2008;36:80-84.

[78] Friederich N, O'Brien W. Gonarthrosis after injury of the anterior cruciate ligament. *Unfallchir Versicherungsmed.* 1993;86:81-89.

[79] Fukubayashi T, Kurosawa H. The contact area and pressure distribution pattern of the knee: A study of normal and osteoarthrotic knee joints. *Acta Orthop. Scand.* 1980;51:871-879.

[80] Fukubayashi T, Torzilli PA, Sherman MF, Warren RF. An in vitro biomechanical evaluation of AP motion of the knee. *J. Bone Jt. Surg.* 1982;64A:258-264.

[81] Fukuda Y, Woo S, Loh J, Tsuda E, Tang P, McMahon P, Debski R. A quantitative analysis of valgus torque on the ACL: A humen cadaveric study. *J. Orthop. Res.* 2003:21:1107-1112.

[82] Gabbett T, Dumrow N. Risk factors for injury in subelite rugby league players. *Am. J. Sports Med.* 2005;33:428-434.

[83] Gabriel M, Wong E, Woo S, Yagi M, Debski R. Distribution of in situ forces in the anterior cruciate ligament in response to rotatory loads. *J. Orthop. Res.* 2004;22:85-89.

[84] Gelber A, Hochberg M, Mead L, Wang N, Wigley F, Klag M. Joint injury in young adults and risk for subsequent knee and hip osteoarthritis. *Annals Internal. Med.* 2000;133:321-328.

[85] Genin P, Weill G, Julliard R. The tibial slope. Proposal for a measurement method. *J. Radiol.* 1993;74:27-33.

[86] Giffen J, Vogrin T, Zantop T, Woo S, Harner C. Effects of increasing tibial slope on the biomechanics of the knee. *Am. J. Sports Med.* 2004;32:376-382.

[87] Gillquist J, Messner K. Anterior cruciate ligament reconstruction and the long-term incidence of gonarthritis. *Sports Med.* 1999;27:143-156.

[88] Glitsch U, Baumann W. The three-dimensional determination of internal loads in the lower extremity. *J. Biomech.* 1997;30:1123-1131.

[89] Goldstein S, Wilson D, Sonstegard D, Matthews L. The mechanical properties of human tibial trabecular bone as a function of metaphyseal location. *J. Biomech.* 1983;16:965-969.

[90] Griffin L, Agel J, Albohm M: Non-contact anterior cruciate ligament injuries: risk factors and prevention strategies. *J. Am. Acad. Orthop. Surg.* 2000;8:141-150.

[91] Grood E, Noyes F, Butler D, Suntay W. Ligamentous and capsular restraints preventing straight medial and lateral laxity in intact human cadaver knees. *J. Bone Jt. Surg.* 1981;63A:1257-1269.

[92] Hallen L, Lindahl O. Rotation in the knee-joint in experimental injury to the ligaments. *Acta Orthop. Scand.* 1965;36:400-407.

[93] Hame S, Oakes D, Markolf K. Injury to the Anterior cruciate ligament during alpine skiing; A biomechanical analysis of tibial torque and knee flexion angle. *Am. J. Sports Med.* 2002;30:537-540.

[94] Hamerman D. The biology of osteoarthritis. *New Eng. J. Med.* 1989;320:1322-1330

[95] Hammer D. Artificial playing surfaces. *Athletic Training.* 1981;16:127-129.

[96] Haut RC. Contact Pressures in the Patello-Femoral Joint During Impact Loading on the Human Flexed Knee. *J. Orthop. Res.* 1989;7:272-280.

[97] Haut RC, Atkinson PJ. Insult to the Human Cadaver Patello-Femoral Joint: Effects of Age on Fracture Tolerance and Occult Injury. *Stapp. Car Crash J.* 1995;39:281-294.

[98] Haut-Donahue T, Hull M, Rashid M, Jacobs C. A finite element model of the human knee joint for the study of tibio-femoral contact. *J. Biomech. Eng.* 2002;124:273-280.

[99] Hayes C, Brigido M, Jamadar D, Propeck T. Mechanism-based pattern approach to classification of complex injuries of the knee depicted at MR imaging. *RadioGraphics.* 2000;20:S121-S134.

[100] Heinrichs A. A review of knee dislocations. *J. Ath. Train.* 2004;39:365-369.

[101] Hergenroeder A. Prevention of sports injuries. *Pediatrics.* 1998;101(6):1057-1063.

[102] Hewett T, Stroupe A, Nance T, Noyes F. Pylometric training in female athletes: Decreased impact forces and increased hamstrings torques. *Am. J. Sports Med.* 1996;24:765-773.

[103] Hewett T, Lindenfeld T, Riccobene J, Noyes F. The effect of neuromuscular training on the incidence of knee injury in female athletes: A prospective study. *Am. J. Sports Med.* 1999;27:699-706.

[104] Hewett T, Myer G, Ford K. Anterior cruciate ligament injuries in female athletes: Part 1, Mechanisms and risk factors. *Am. J. Sports Med.* 2006;34:299-311.

[105] Hodgson R, Carpenter T, Hall L. Magnetic Resonance Imaging of Osteoarthritis. *Articular Cart and Osteoarthritis Raven Press Ltd*, NY. 1992:629-667.

[106] Hootman J, Macera C, Ainsworth B, Addy C, Martin M, Blair S. Epidemiology of musculoskeletal injuries among sedentary and physically active adults. *Med. & Sci. Sports Exercise.* 2002;34:838-844.

[107] Hull M. Analysis of skiing accidents involving combined injuries to the medial collateral and anterior cruciate ligaments. *Am. J. Sports Med.* 1997;25:35-40.

[108] Hurwitz D, Sumner D, Andriacchi T, Sugar D. Dynamic knee loads during gait predict proximal tibial bone distribution. *J. Biomech.* 1998;31:423-430.

[109] Hutchinson M, Ireland M. Knee injuries in female athletes. *Sports Med.* 1995;19:288-302.

[110] Hvid I, Hansen S. Trabecular bone strength patterns at the proximal tibial epiphysis. *J. Orthop. Res.* 1985;3:464-472.

[111] Hvid I. Trabecular bone strength at the knee. *Clin. Orthop.* 1988;227:210-221.

[112] Isaac DI, Meyer EG, Haut RC. Contact pressures and associated chondrocyte damage in the rabbit tibiofemoral joint under impact. *J. Biomech. Eng.* 2008;130:041018 1-5.

[113] Jayaraman V, Sevensma E, Kitagawa M, Haut R. Effects of anterior-posterior constraint on injury patterns in the human knee during tibiofemoral joint loading from axial forces through the tibia. *45th Stapp Car Crash Conf. Proc.* 2001;45:449-468.

[114] Jilani A, Shirazi-Adl A, Bendjaballah M. Biomechanics of human tibio-femoral joint in axial rotation. *Knee.* 1997;4:203-213.

[115] Johnson D, Urban W, Caborn D, Canarthos W, Carlson C. Articular cartilage changes seen with magnetic resonance imaging-detected bone bruises associated with acute anterior cruciate ligament rupture. *Am. J. Sports Med.* 1998;26:409-414.

[116] Kajzer J, Matsui Y, Ishikawa H, Schroeder G. Shearing and Bending Effects At the Knee Joint At Low-Speed Lateral Loading. *SAE Paper.* 1999-01-0712.

[117] Kannus P, Javinen M. Conservatively treated tears of the anterior cruciate ligament: long-term results. *J. Bone Jt. Surg.* 1987;69A:1007-1012.

[118] Kapandji I. The physiology of the joints: Vol. 2, *Lower Limb.* 1987. Churchill-Livingstone, Edinburg, UK.

[119] Kapelov R, Teresi L, Bradley WG, Bucciarelli NR, Murakami DM, Mullin WJ, Jordan JE. Bone Contusions of the Knee; Increased Lesion Detection with Fast Spin-echo MR Imaging with Spectroscope Fat Saturation. *Radiology.* 1993;189:901-904.

[120] Kaplan P, Walker C, Kilcoyne R, Brown D, Tusek D, Dussault R. Occult fracture patterns of the knee associated with anterior cruciate ligament tears: Assessment with MR imaging. *Musculoskeletal Rad.* 1992;183:835-838.

[121] Kaplan P, Gehl R, Dussault R, Anderson M, Diduch D. Bone contusions of the posterior lip of the medial tibial plateau (Countercoup injury) and associated internal derangements of the knee at MR imaging. *Radiology.* 1999;211:747-753.

[122] Kempson G. Relationship between the tensile properties of human articular cartilage from the human knee and age. *Ann. Rheum. Dis.* 1982;41:508-511.

[123] Kempson G. Age-related changes in the tensile properties of human articular cartilage: a comparitive study between the femoral head of the hip joint and the talus of the ankle joint. *Biochem. Biophys. Acta.* 1991;1075:223-230.

[124] Kennedy JC. Complete dislocation of the knee joint. *J. Bone Jt. Surg.* 1963;45:889-904.

[125] Kennedy J, Fowler P. Medial and anterior instability of the knee: An anatomical and clinical study using stress machines. *J. Bone Jt. Surg.* 1971;53-A:1257-1270.

[126] Kennedy J, Weinberg H, Wilson A. The anatomy and function of the anterior cruciate ligament: As determined by clinical and morphological studies. *J. Bone Jt. Surg.* 1974;56-A:223-235.

[127] Kent R, Funk J. Data censoring and parametric distribution assignment in the development of injury risk functions from biomechanical data. SAE World Cong, Detroit, Michigan, SAE Technical Paper No. 2004 01 0317.

[128] Kerrigan J, Bhalla K, Madeley J, Funk J, Bose D, Crandall J. Experiments for establishing pedestrian-impact lower limb injury criteria. *SAE Paper.* 2003-01-0895.

[129] Klein T, Chaudhry M, Bae W, Sah R. Depth-dependent biomechanical and biochemical properties of fetal, newborn, and tissue-engineered articular cartilage. *J. Biomech.* 40:182-190, 2007

[130] Koga H, Nakamea A, Shima Y, Iwasa J, Myklebust G, Engebretsen L, Bahr R, Krosshaug T. Mechanisms for noncontact anterior cruciate ligament injuries: Knee joint

kinematics in 10 injury situations from female team handball and basketball. *Am. J. Sports Med.* 2010;38:2218-2225.

[131] Knets I, Malmeister A. Deformability and strength of human compact bone tissue. *Mechanics of Biological Solids, Bulgarian Academy of Sciences.* 1977:133.

[132] Krosshaug T, Andersen T, Olsen O, Myklebust G, Bahr R. Research approaches to describe the mechanisms of injuries in sport: limitations and possibilities. *Br. J. Sports Med.* 2005;39:330-339.

[133] Krosshaug T, Nakamae A, Boden B, Engebretsen L, Smith G, Slauterbeck J, Hewett T, Bahr R. Mechanisms of anterior cruciate ligament injury in basketball: Video analysis of 39 cases. *Am. J. Sports Med.* 2007;35:359-367.

[134] Kuhn JL, Goldstein SA, Ciarelli MJ, Matthews LS. The limitations of canine trabecular bone as a model for human: A biomechanical study. *J. Biomech.* 1989;22:95-107.

[135] Kujala U, Kettunen J, Paananen H. Knee osteoarthritis in former runners, soccer players, weight lifters and shooters. *Arthritis Rheum.* 1995;38(4):539-546.

[136] Kwolek CJ, Sundaram S, Schwarcz TH, Hyde GL, Endean ED. Popliteal artery thrombosis associated with trampoline injuries and anterior knee dislocations in children. *Am. Surg.* 1998;64:1183-1187.

[137] Lambson R, Barnhill B, Higgins R. Football Cleat Design and its Effect on Anterior Cruciate Ligament Injuries. A Three Year Prospective Study. *Am. J. Sports Med.* 1996;24(2):155-159.

[138] Lane N. Physical activity at leisure and risk of osteoarthritis. *Annals Rheumatic Diseases.* 1996;55:682-684.

[139] Lee I, Paffenbarger R. Associations of light, moderate and vigorous intensity physical activity with longevity: The Harvard alumni health study. *Am. J. Epidem.* 151;2000:293-299.

[140] Li G, Rudy T, Allen C. Effect of combined axial compressive and anterior tibial loads on in situ forces in the anterior cruciate ligament: a porcine study. *J. Orthop. Res.* 1998;16:122-127.

[141] Li G, Lopez O, Rubash H. Variability of a three-dimensional finite element model constructed using magnetic resonance images of a knee for joint contact stress analysis. *J. Biomech. Eng.* 2001;123:341-346.

[142] Lohmander L, Stenberg A, Englund M, Roos H. High prevalence of knee osteoarthritis, pain, and functional limitations in female soccer players twelve years after anterior cruciate ligament injury. *Arth. Rheum.* 2004;50: 3145-3152.

[143] Majewski M, Susanne H, Klaus S. Epidemiology of athletic knee injuries: A 10-year study. *Knee.* 2006;13:184-188.

[144] Markolf K, Mensch J, Amstutz H. Stiffness and laxity of the knee- the contributions of the supporting structures. A quantitative in vitro study. *J. Bone Jt. Surg.* 1976;63A:570-585.

[145] Markolf K, Bargar W, Shoemaker S, Amstutz H. The role of joint load in knee stability. *J. Bone Jt. Surg.* 1981;63:570-585.

[146] Markolf K, Kochan A, Amstutz H. Measurement of knee stiffness and laxity in patients with documented absence of the anterior cruciate ligament. *J. Bone Jt. Surg.* 1984;66-A:242-252.

[147] Markolf K, Burchfield D, Shapiro M, Shepard M, Finerman G, Slauterbeck J. Combined knee loading states that generate high anterior cruciate ligament forces. *J. Orthop. Res.* 1995;13:930-935.

[148] Markolf K, Gorek J, Kabo J, Shapiro M. Direct measurement of resultant forces in the anterior cruciate ligament: An in vitro study performed with a new experimental technique. *Am. J. Bone Jt. Surg.* 1999;72:557-567.

[149] Matsumoto H. Mechanism of the pivot shift. *J. Bone Jt. Surg.* 1990;72-B:816-821.

[150] Matsumoto H, Suda Y, Otani T, Niki Y, Seedhom B, Fujikawa K. Roles of the anterior cruciate ligament in preventing valgus instability. *J. Orthop. Sci.* 2001;6:28-32.

[151] McKellop H, Sigholm G, Redfern F, Doyle B, Sarmiento A, Luck Sr J. The effect of simulated fracture-angulations of the tibia on cartilage pressures in the knee joint. *J. Bone Joint Surg. Am.* 1991;73:1382–1391.

[152] McNair P, Marshall R, Matheson J. Important features associated with acute anterior cruciate ligament injury. *New Zealand Med. J.* 1990;103:537-539.

[153] Meyer E, Haut R. Excessive compression of the human tibio-femoral joint causes ACL rupture. *J. Biomech.* 2005;38:2311-2316.

[154] Meyer E, Baumer T, Slade J, Smith W, Haut R. Tibiofemoral contact pressures and osteochondral microtrauma during ACL rupture due to excessive compressive loading and internal torque of the human knee. *Am. J. Sports Med.* 2008a;36:1966-1977.

[155] Meyer E and Haut R. Anterior cruciate ligament injury induced by internal tibial torsion of tibiofemoral compression. *J. Biomech.* 2008b;41:3377-3383.

[156] Meyer E, Villwock M, Haut R. Tibiofemoral contact pressures that induce cartilage damage and subchondral bone microcracks during valgus bending of the human knee. *Clin. Biomech.* 2009;24:577-582.

[157] Meyer E, Villwock M, Powell J, Fouty A, Haut R. Rotational injuries of the lower extremity and the use of an in situ risk assessment tool for rotational traction. *STARSS Conf. Proc.* 2010.

[158] Meyer E, Baumer T, Haut R. Pure passive hyperextension of the human cadaver knee generates simultaneous bicruciate ligament rupture. *J. Biomech. Eng.* 2011;133:011012(1-5).

[159] Meyers M, Harvey P. Traumatic Dislocation of the knee joint. *J. Bone Jt. Surg.* 1971;53-A:16-29.

[160] Mills O, Hull M. Rotational flexibility of the human knee due to varus/valgus and axial moments in vivo. *J. Biomech.* 1991;24(8):673-690.

[161] Mink J, Deutsch A. Occult cartilage and bone injuries of the knee: Detection, classification, and assessment with MR imaging. *Radiology.* 1989;170:823-829.

[162] Morrison J. The mechanics of the knee joint in relation to normal walking. *J. Biomech.* 1970;3:51-61.

[163] Muhlbauer R, Lukasz S, Faber S, Stammberger T, Eckstein F. Comparison of knee joint cartilage in triathletes and physically inactive volunteers based on magnetic resonance imaging and three-dimensional analysis. *Am. J. Sports Med.* 2000;28:541-546.

[164] Myklebust G, Holm I, Maehlum S, Engelbretsen L, Bahr R. Clinical, functional and radiologic outcome in team handball players 6 to 11 years after anterior cruciate ligament injury. A follow-up study. *Am. J. Sports Med.* 2003;31:981-989.

[165] Myklebust G, Bahr R. Return to play guidelines after anterior cruciate ligament surgery. *Br. J. Sports Med.* 39;2005:127-131.

[166] Nagel D, States J. Dashboard and bumper knee – Will arthritis develop? *Am. Auto Accident Med.* 1977;21:272-278.

[167] National Collegiate Athletic Association. *NCAA injury surveillance system summary.* Indianapolis IN. 2001:80-89.

[168] National Federation of State High School Associations. 2007–2008 *Athletics Participation Summary.* Indianapolis, IN. 2008.

[169] Newberry W, Haut R. The Effects of Subfracture Impact Loading on the Patello-Femoral Joint in a Rabbit Model. *Stapp. Car Crash J.* 1996;40:149-159.

[170] Nielsen S, Ovesen J, Rasmussen O. The anterior cruciate ligament on the knee: An experimental study of its importance in rotatory knee instability. *Arch. Orthop. Trauma Surg.* 1984;103:170-174.

[171] Nielsen S, Helmig P. Instability of knees with ligament lesions: Cadaver studies of the anterior cruciate ligament. *Acta Orthop. Scand.* 1985;56:426-429.

[172] Noyes F, Delucas J, Torvik P. Biomechanics of anterior cruciate ligament failure: An analysis of strain-rate sensitivity and mechanisms of failure in primates. *J. Bone Jt. Surg.* 1974;56:236-253.

[173] Noyes F, Grood E. The strength of the anterior cruciate ligament in humans and Rhesus monkeys. *J. Bone Jt. Surg.* 1976;58:1074-1082.

[174] Noyes F, Matthews D, Mooar P, Grood E. The symptomatic anterior cruciate-deficient knee. Part II: the results of rehabilitation, activity modification, and counseling on functional disability. *J. Bone Jt. Surg.* 1983;65:163-174.

[175] Olsen O, Myklebust G, Engebretsen L, Bahr R. Injury mechanism for anterior cruciate ligament injuries in team handball: A systematic video analysis. *Am. J. Sports Med.* 2004;32:1002-1012.

[176] Pate R, Pratt M, Blair S, Haskell W, Macera C, Bouchard C, Buchner D, Ettinger W, Heath G, King A. Physical activity and public health. A recommendation from the Centers for Disease Control and Prevention and the American College of Sports Medicine. *J. Am. Med. Assoc.* 1995;275:402-407.

[177] Paul J, Spindler K, Andrish J, Parker R, Secic M, Bergfeld J. Jumping versus nonjumping anterior cruciate ligament injuries: A comparison of pathology. *Clin. J. Sport Med.* 2003;13:1-5.

[178] Pinskerova V, Johal P, Nakagoawa S, Sosna A, Williams A, Gedroyc W, Freeman M. Does the femur roll-back with flexion? *Br. J. Bone Jt. Surg.* 2004;86:925-931.

[179] Powell J, Schootman M. A Multivariate Risk Analysis of Selected Playing Surfaces in the National Football League: 1980-1989. An Epidemiological Study of Knee Injuries. *Am. J. Sports Med.* 1992;20(6):686-694.

[180] Powell J, Barber-Foss, K. Sex-related injury patterns among selected high school sports. *Am. J. Sports Med.* 2000;28:385-391.

[181] Pritsch M, Comba D, Frank G, Horoszowski H. Articular Cartilage Fractures of the Knee. *J. Sports Med.* 1984;24:299-302.

[182] Pujol N, Blanchi M, Chambat P. The incidence of anterior cruciate ligament injuries among competitive alpine skiiers. A 25-year investigation. *Am. J. Sports Med.* 2007;35:1070-1074.

[183] Rangger C, Kathrein A, Freund M, Klestil T, Kreczy A. Bone bruise of the knee: Histology and cryosections in 5 cases. *Acta Orthop. Scand.* 1998;69:291-294.

[184] Remer EM, Fitgerald SW, Friedman H. Anterior cruciate ligament injury: MR imaging diagnosis and patterns of injury. *RadioGraphics.* 1992;12:901-915.

[185] Renstrom P, Ljungqvist A, Arendt E, Beynnon B, et al. Non-contact ACL injuries in female athletes: an International Olympic Committee current concepts statement. *Br. J. Sports Med.* 2008;42:394-412.

[186] Repo R, Finlay J. Survival of Articular Cartilage after Controlled Impact. *Am. J. Bone Jt. Surg.* 1977;59:1068-1076.

[187] Riegger-Krugh C, Gerhart T, Powers W, Hayes W. Tibiofemoral contact pressures in degenerative joint disease. *Clin. Orthop.* 1998;348:233-245.

[188] Roos H, Adalberth T, Dahlberg L, Lohmander LS. Osteoarthritis of the knee after injury to the anterior cruciate ligament or meniscus: the influence of time and age. *Osteoarth. Cart.* 1995;3:261-267.

[189] Rosen M, Jackson D, Berger P. Occult osseous lesions documented by magnetic resonance imaging associated with anterior cruciate ligament ruptures. *Arthroscopy.* 1991;7:45-51.

[190] Sanders T, Medynski M, Feller J, Lawhorn K. Bone contusion patterns of the knee at MR imaging: Footprint of the mechanism of injury. *RadioGraphics.* 2000;20:S135-S151.

[191] Schenck RC, Kovach IS, Agarwal A, Brummelt R, Ward RA, Lanetot D, Athanasiou KA. Cruciate injury patters in knee hyperextension: A cadaveric model. *Arthroscopy.* 1999;15:489-495.

[192] Schinagl R, Gurskis D, Chen A, Sah R. Depth-dependent confined compression modulus of full-thickness bovine articular cartilage. *J. Orthop. Res.* 15:499-506, 1997.

[193] Seering W, Piziali R, Nagel D, Schurman D. The function of primary ligaments of the knee in varus-valgus and axial rotation. *J. Biomech.* 1980;13:785-794.

[194] Sell T, Ferris C, Abt J, Tsai Y, Myers J, Fu F, Lephart S. Predictors of proximal tibia anterior shear force during a vertical stop jump. *J. Orthop. Res.* 2007;25:1589-1597.

[195] Senter C, Hame S. Biomechanical analysis of tibial torque and knee flexion angle: Implications for understanding knee injury. *Sports Med.* 2006;36(8):635-641.

[196] Shapiro M, Markolf K, Finerman G, Mitchell P. The effect of section of the medial collateral ligament on the force generated in the anterior cruciate ligament. *Am. J. Bone Jt. Surg.* 1991;73:248-256.

[197] Shelbourne KD, Klootwyk TE. Low-velocity knee dislocation with sports injuries: Treatment principles. *Clin. Sports Med.* 2000;19:443-456.

[198] Shepard D, Seedhom B. The 'Instantaneous' compressive modulus of human articular cartilage in joints of the lower limb. *Rheumatology.* 1999;38:124-132.

[199] Shoemaker S, Markolf K. In Vivo Rotary Knee Stability; Ligamentous and Muscular Contributions. *J. Bone Jt. Surg.* 1982;64-A:208-216.

[200] Shoemaker S, Markolf K. Effects of joint load on the stiffness and laxity of ligament-deficient knees: An in vitro study of the anterior cruciate and medial collateral ligaments. *J. Bone Jt. Surg.* 1985;67-A:136-146.

[201] Shoemaker S, Markolf K, Dorey F, Zager S, Namba R. Tibial torque generation in a flexed weight-bearing stance. *Clin. Orthop. Relat. Res.* 1988;228:164-70.

[202] Shoemaker S, Daniel D. The limits of knee motion: in vitro studies. Eds. Daniel DM, Akeson WH, O'Connor JJ. *Knee ligaments: structure, function, injury and repair.* NY: Raven Press. 1990:153-161.

[203] Shorten M, Hudson B, Himmelsbach J: Shoe-surface traction of conventional and in-filled synthetic turf football surfaces. *Proc XIX International Congress of Biomechanics, University of Otago,* Dunedin, New Zealand: 2003.

[204] Snearly W, Kaplan P, Dussault R. Lateral-compartment bone contusions in adolescents with intact anterior cruciate ligaments. 1996;198:205-208.

[205] Snyder S, Schneider E. Estimation of mechanical properties of cortical bone by computed tomography. *J. Orthop. Res.* 1991;9:422-431.

[206] Speer K, Spritzer C, Basset F, Feagin J, Garrett W. Osseous injury associated with acute tears of the anterior cruciate ligament. *Am. J. Sports Med.* 1992;20:382-389.

[207] Speer K, Warren R, Wickiewicz T, Horowitz L, Henderson L. Observations on the injury mechanism of anterior cruciate ligament tears in skiers. *Am. J. Sports Med.* 1995;23:77-81.

[208] Spindler K, Schils J, Bergfeld J, Andrish J, Weiker G, Anderson T, Piraino D, Richmond B, Medendorp S. Prospective study of osseous, articular, and meniscal lesions in recent anterior cruciate ligament tears by magnetic resonance imaging and arthroscopy. *Am. J. Sports Med.* 1993;21:551-557.

[209] Stanitski C, McMaster J, Ferguson R: Synthetic turf and grass: A comparative study. *Am. J. Sports Med.* 1974;2(1):22-26.

[210] States JD. Adult occupant injuries of the lower limb. *Proc. Symp. Biomech.* 1986:97-107.

[211] Stone J, Beaupre G, Hayes W. Multiaxial strength characteristics of trabecular bone. *J. Biomech.* 1983;16:743-752.

[212] Sullivan D, Levy I, Sheskier S, Torzilli P, Warren RF. Medial restraints to anterior-posterior motion of the knee. *J. Bone Jt. Surg.* 1984;66A:930-936.

[213] Tepper S, Hochberg M. Factor associated with hip osteoarthritis: data from the First National Health and Nutrition Examination Survey. *Am. J. Epidemiol.* 1993;137:1081-1088.

[214] Thambyah A. A hypothesis matrix for studying biomechanical factors associated with the initiation and progression of posttraumatic osteoarthritis. *Med. Hypoth.* 2005;64:1157-1161.

[215] Thambyam A, Goh J, Das De S. Contact stress in the knee joint in deep flexion. *Med. Eng. Phys.* 2005;27:329-335.

[216] Thambyah A, Shim V, Chong L, Lee V. Impact-induced osteochondral fracture in the tibial plateau. *J. Biomech.* 2008;41:1236-1242.

[217] Torzilli P, Deng X, Warren R. The effect of joint-compressive load and quadriceps muscle force on knee motion in the intact and anterior cruciate ligament-sectioned knee. *Am. J. Sports Med.* 1994;22:105-112.

[218] Torzilli P, Grigiene R, Borrelli J, Helfet DL. Effect of impact load on articular cartilage: Cell metabolism and viability and matrix water content. *J. Biomech. Eng.* 1999;121:433-441.

[219] U.S. Department of Health and Human Services. Physical activity and health: A report of the Surgeon General. Sudbury, Ma: Jones & Bartlett Pub. 1998:173-208.

[220] Vanhoenacker FM, Snoeckx A. Bone marrow edema in sports: General concepts. *Euro J. Rad.* 2007;62:6-15.

[221] Vellet A, Marks P, Fowler P, Munro T. Occult posttraumatic osteochondral lesions of the knee: Prevalence, classification, and short-term sequelae evaluated with MR imaging. *Radiology.* 1991;178:271-276.

[222] Viskontas DG, Giuffre BM, Duggal N, Graham D, Parker D, Coolican M. Bone bruises associated with ACL rupture: Correlation with injury mechanism. *Am. J. Sports Med.* 2008;36: 927-933.

[223] Von Porat A, Roos E, Roos H. High prevalence of osteoarthritis 14 years after an anterior cruciate ligament tear in male soccer players: *A study of radiographic and patient relevant outcomes.* 2004;63:269-273.

[224] Wang J, Rubin R, Marshall J. A mechanism of isolated anterior cruciate ligament rupture. *Am. J. Bone Jt. Surg.* 1975;57:411-413.

[225] Washer DC, Markolf KL, Shapiro MS, Finerman GA. Direct in vitro measurement of forces in the cruciate ligaments. *J. Bone Jt. Surg.* 1993;75A:377-386.

[226] Williamson A, Chen A, Masuda K, et al. Tensile mechanical properties of bovine articular cartilage: variations with growth & relationships to collagen network components. *J. Orthop. Res.* 21:872-880, 2003.

[227] Wilson W, van Rietbergen B, van Donkelaar C, Huiskes R. Pathways of load-induced cartilage damage causing cartilage degeneration in the knee after meniscectomy. *J. Biomech.* 2003;36:845-851.

[228] Withrow T, Huston L, Wojtys E, Ashton-Miller J. The relationship between quadriceps muscle force, knee flexion, and anterior cruciate strain in an in vitro simulated jump landing. *Am. J. Sports Med.* 2006;34:269-274.

[229] Wolf B, Amendola A. Impact of Osteoarthritis on sports careers. *Clin. Sports Med.* 24;2005:187-198.

[230] Woo S, Hollis J, Adams D, Lyon R, Takai S. Tensile properties of the human femur-anterior cruciate ligament-tibia complex: The effect of specimen age and orientation. *Am. J. Sports Med.* 1991;19(3):217-225.

[231] Wright V. Post-traumatic osteoarthritis- A medico-legal minefield. *J. Rheum.* 1990;29:474-478.

[232] Wright RW, Phaneuf MA, Limbird TJ, Spindler KP. Clinical outcome of isolated subcortical trabecular fractures (bone bruise) detected on magnetic resonance imaging in knees. *Am. J. Sports Med.* 2000;28:663-667.

[233] Yamada H. Strength of biological materials. Baltimore, MD: The Williams and Wilkings Co. 1970.

[234] Yeow CH, Cheong CH, Ng KS, Lee PVS, Goh SCH. Anterior cruciate ligament failure and cartilage damage during knee joint compression: A preliminary study based on the porcine model. *Am. J. Sports Med.* 2008;36:934-942.

[235] Yildirim G, Walker P, Susman-Fort J, Aggarwal G, White B, Klein G. The contact locations in the knee during high flexion. *Knee.* 2007;14:379-384.

[236] Yu B, Garrett W. Mechanisms of non-contact ACL injuries. *Br. J. Sports Med.* 2007;47:i47-i51.

[237] Zantop T, Herbort M, Raschke M, Fu F, Peterson W. The role of the anteromedial and posterolateral bundles of the anterior cruciate ligament in anterior tibial translation and internal rotation. *Am. J. Sports Med.* 2007;35:223-227.

In: The Knee
Editor: Randy Mascarenhas

ISBN: 978-1-61942-268-1
© 2012 Nova Science Publishers, Inc.

Chapter II

3D COMPUTATIONAL MODELING OF THE HUMAN KNEE IN PHYSIOLOGICAL STATE

M. H. Doweidar, R. M. Sánchez, E. Peña, B. Calvo and M. Doblaré

Group of Structural Mechanics and Materials Modeling (GEMM).
Aragón Institute of Engineering Research (I3A), University of Zaragoza,
Betancourt Building, María de Luna, Zaragoza, Spain
Biomedical Research Networking center in Bioengineering,
Biomaterials and Nanomedicine (CIBER-BBN), Spain

ABSTRACT

Although the knee is probably the most studied joint in the human body, the work carried out to date is still far from predicting true mechanical behavior and has not yet solved many of the doubts about the origin of several injuries. This is due mainly to the high cost involved with experimentation, technical difficulties in the measurement of stress and strain, and the inability to faithfully reproduce certain diseases and degenerative states in vivo. Faced with these difficulties, numerical simulation is an alternative fast, accurate and economical method capable of providing information that is often very difficult to otherwise obtain. The main objective of this study was to develop a knee three-dimensional computational model to analyze the role of joint ligaments and menisci in load transmission and joint stability. We present a computational model of a healthy adult male in full extension to other three different scenarios: flexion of 60 degrees on the femur (simplified model), static compression load of 1150 N on the tibia (full model) and flexion of 10 degrees to the tibia (full model). In the developed model, bones were considered to be rigid. Articular cartilage and menisci were considered to be linearly elastic, isotropic and homogeneous. Ligaments were considered hyperelastic and transversely isotropic. Initial strains on the ligaments and patellar tendon were also considered and the model was validated using experimental and numerical results obtained by other authors. The results obtained reproduce the complex, nonuniform stress and strain fields that occur in the soft tissue of the knee as a result of the kinematics of the human knee joint under a physiologic external load.

Keywords: Numerical simulation, Finite element method, Large deformations, Hyperelasticity, Soft tissues, Human ligaments, Human knee joint

1. Introduction

The knee is the largest and one of the most mechanically complex joints in the human skeleton. Its design reconciles two seemingly contradictory aspects: high stability in maximum extension and high mobility that permitting a wide range of phsyiological activity. This mobility originates from a complex mechanism composed of bones, menisci, cartilage, tendons, ligaments and muscles. A good understanding of the biomechanical behavior of the knee is an invaluable tool for improving diagnosis, treatment and surgical planning. Due to the relative incongruence of the articular surfaces, ligaments play a key role in providing passive stability to the joint throughout a complete arc of motion. Each ligament provides stability and restrains knee motion in more than one degree of freedom, while the overall joint stability depends both on the contributions of the individual ligaments as well as their interactions. A full understanding of the restraint role of each individual ligament is essential to adequate diagnosis and assessment for surgical procedures [1]. The menisci are another important multifunctional component of the knee with a fundamental role in load transmission, shock absorption, proprioception, improvement of stability and lubrication [2]. Load distribution over an incongruent joint surface is effectively redistributed by the menisci to maintain maximum congruency [3]. Functionality of the menisci and their role in load transmission have been discussed by Fairbank et al. [9], as well as many others [3, 4, 5]. Articular cartilage forms a thin tissue layer that lines the articulating ends of all diarthrodial joints in the body , including the knee. The primary function of these cartilage layers is to minimize contact stresses generated during joint loading via lubrication of the joint [10].

A proper understanding of knee joint biomechanics is therefore essential to improve the prevention and treatment of its disorders and injuries. Despite the many investigations developed, the exact mechanical behavior and etiology of injury of the knee joint not completely known. This is partially due to inherent limitations in current experimental studies including high costs, difficulties with obtaining accurate measures of strain and stress and the difficulty with reproduction of pathological or degenerative conditions of the knee. Finite element (FE) models have been proven to provide deep insight into the physiologic and mechanical properties of biological tissues and organs while reducing both cost and time. An appropriately developed finite element model is a powerful tool in predicting the effects of the different parameters involved and to provide information otherwise difficult to obtain from experiments. It is important to note that the reliability of these models strongly depends on appropriate geometrical reconstruction and accurate mathematical descriptions of the behavior of the biological tissues involved, as well as their interactions with the surrounding environment. With this in mind, we still need to improve our understanding regarding the constitution of the more common biological tissues such as ligaments, tendons, cartilage and menisci.

The knee is probably the most studied joint in the human body [2, 3, 4, 5, 6, 7]. Peña et al. [6] published a computational analysis that included incorporation of stress on the menisci, articular cartilage, and all the main ligaments (patellar tendon (PT), anterior cruciate (ACL), posterior cruciate (PCL), medial collateral (MCL) and lateral collateral (LCL)). Prior to this, the vast majority of previous studies used one-dimensional representations of the knee ligaments [11, 1, 12, 13, 14]. This approach proved to be useful for predicting joint kinematics, but non-uniform 3D stress and strain could not be predicted. Other researchers developed 3D finite element models of individual human ligaments such as the ACL [15, 16] or the MCL [17]. Finally, other papers presented specific computational models of parts of the human knee to discuss different aspects of its biomechanical behavior [18]. In [19] a three-dimensional model has developed to analyze the human patella biomechanics during passive knee flexion. Beynnon et al. [23] presented an analytical sagittal plane model of the knee to study how cruciate ligament bundles control joint kinematics. In [20, 11] and [21] several nonlinear finite element models of the entire human joint were presented to investigate the biomechanics of the passive tibiofemoral joint in full extension under anterior-posterior drawer forces and internal-external torques.

Perie et al. [22] and Li et al. [13] considered joint contact stresses and contact areas on human knee menisci. In these latter models, ligaments were modeled as non-linear springs. We present a complete three-dimensional model of the healthy human knee joint (See Fig. 1). This included all relevant ligaments, menisci and articular cartilage. Different experimental and numerical results were used to validate it initially [14, 20, 24, 25, 27]. Once sufficiently validated, our main goal was to analyze the combined role of cartilage, menisci and ligaments in load transmission and stability. We present a model of a healthy adult male knee in full extension as well as three different scenarios: (i) Flexion of 60 degrees of the femur (simplified model); (ii) static compression load of 1150 N of the tibia (full model) and (iii) flexion of 10 degrees of the tibia (full model).

2. MATERIAL AND METHODS

2.1. Knee Joint Geometry

It is important to note that the reliability of these models strongly depends on appropriate geometric reconstruction and accurate mathematical description of the behavior of the biological tissues involved, and their interactions with the surrounding environment. In this

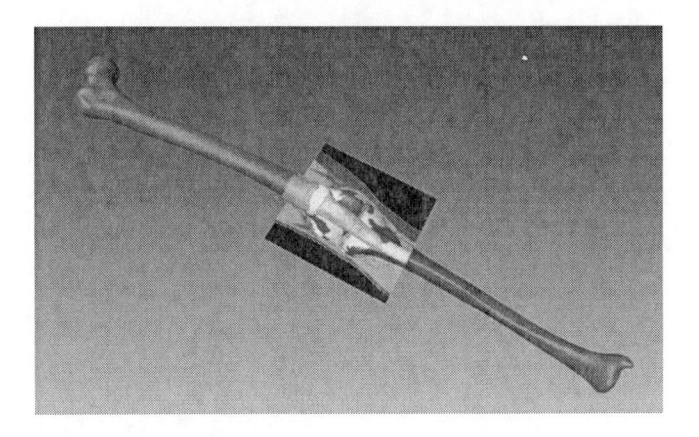

Figure 1. Knee, femur and tibia geometries.

sense, we still need to improve our knowledge about the constitutive behavior of some of the most common biological tissues such as ligaments, tendons, and cartilage. Both magnetic resonance imaging (MRI) and computed tomography (CT) were used to acquire the joint geometry. MRI provides detailed imaging of soft tissue while CT provides excellent images bony anatomy surrounding the joint [32]. Extraction of the geometry of ligaments from CT or MRI data is performed by first segmenting the boundary of the structure. For that purpose, it is usually still necessary to perform manual (or semi-automatic) segmentation of the boundaries. Once the contour of interest is segmented in the 3D image dataset, it is necessary to generate the FE mesh [28]. For accurate solutions, it is recommended the use of hexahedral elements, but the mesh generation in hexahedral elements is not always necessary.

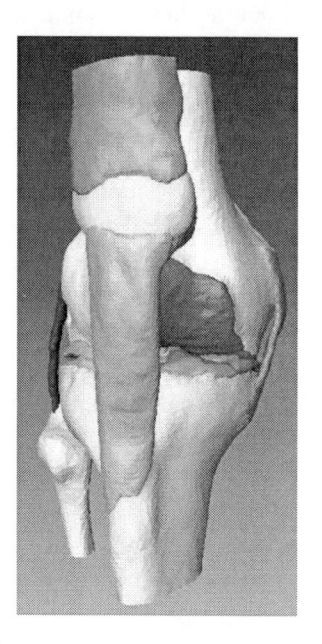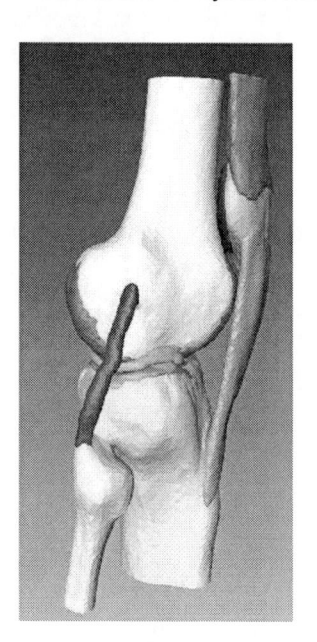

Figure 2. Knee joint geometry.

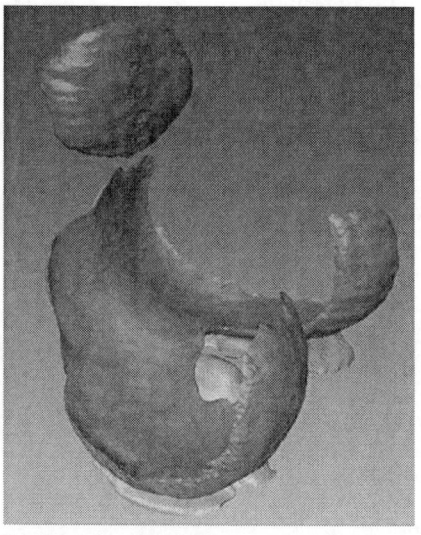

Figure 3. Patella and Articular Cartilage geometry.

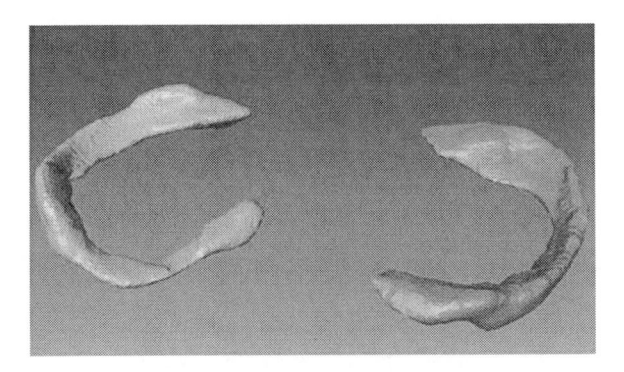

Figure 4. Menisci geometry.

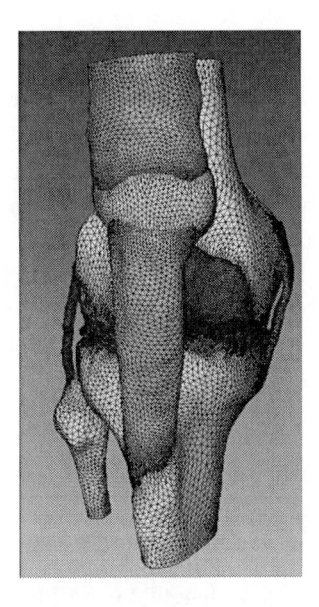

Figure 5. Knee joint finite element mesh.

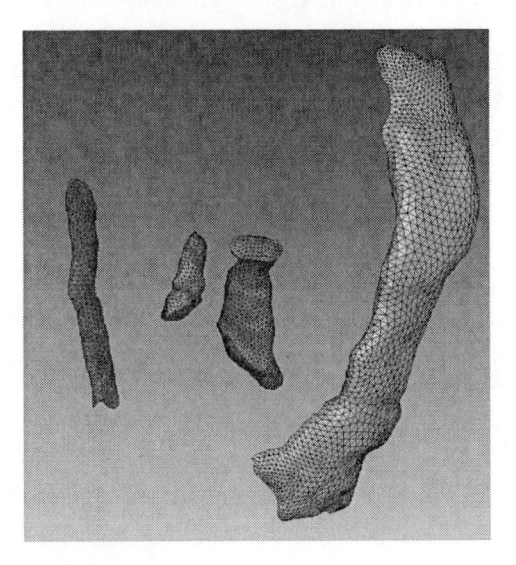

Figure 6. Ligaments finite element meshes.

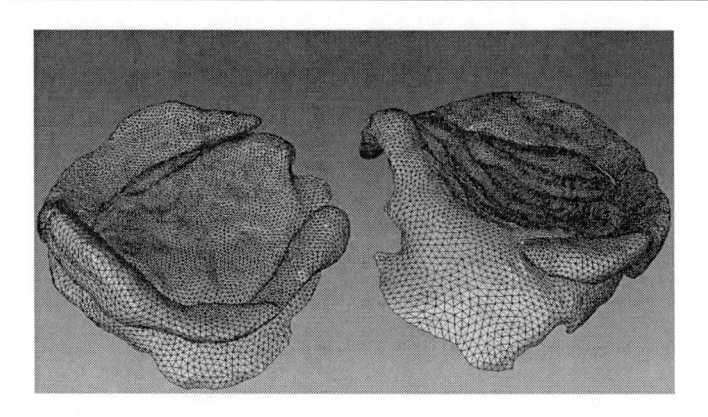

Figure 7. Tibial cartilage and Menisci finite element meshes.

The geometric data of the model developed herein were obtained by NMR (Nuclear Magnetic Resonance) for soft tissues and CT (Computerized Tomography) for bone, with images taken from a normal adult male volunteer by Zuse-Institut Berlin (ZIB). The contours of the femur, tibia, articular cartilage, menisci and ligaments (patellar tendon, anterior cruciate, posterior cruciate, medial collateral and lateral collateral) were identified using AMIRA software developed by ZIB [39]. Tetrahedral meshes of bones, ligaments, menisci and articular cartilage were constructed using the same software (AMIRA). A total of 450000 elements were used to mesh all tissue components of the knee (Figs. 2, 3, 4, 5, 6 and 7). In all cases, we used tri-linear tetrahedral elements with a full geometrically nonlinear formulation of ABAQUS [38].

2.2. Behavior of Biological Tissues

Since bone stiffness is much higher than that of soft tissues and its influence in this study was minimal, bones were assumed to be rigid. Each bony structure (femur, tibia, fibula and patella) was therefore represented by a primary node located at its center of rotation at full extension. In the case of the femur this point was located at the midpoint of the transepicondylar line [29]. These nodes, with six degrees of freedom, controlled the whole kinematics of each bone as rigid body.

Menisci and cartilage are hydrated tissues. However, considering that the loading time of interest corresponded to that of a single leg stance and the viscoelastic time constant of cartilage approaches 1500 seconds [26], articular cartilage was considered to behave as a single-phase linear elastic and isotropic material with an elastic modulus of $E = 5$ MPa and a Poisson ratio of $v = 0.46$ [13]. This is accurate enough to predict short term cartilage response as demonstrated by Donzelli et al. [30], who proved that there are no significant changes in the cartilage contact response shortly after loading. For the same reason, menisci were also assumed to be a single-phase linear elastic and isotropic material with the following average properties: elastic modulus of $E = 59$ MPa and Poisson ratio of $v = 0.49$ [31].

For ligament modeling, two important assumptions were made. First, no difference in the material behavior between the ligament body and its insertion were considered. Second, material characteristics dependent on time such as viscoelasticity, creep and relaxation were neglected [15] due to the high ratio between the viscoelastic time constant of the material and the loading time of interest in this study. We therefore used a transversely isotropic hyperelastic model including the effect of one family of fibers, usually applied to ligaments [32]. The initial direction of the fibers at each point was defined by a unit vector field $\mathbf{a}_0(\mathbf{X})$. Fibers move with the material points of the continuum body. The fiber direction at each time is described by the unit vector field $\mathbf{a}(\mathbf{x}, t)$. Its stretch λ, defined as the ratio between the length of the fiber in the deformed and reference configurations, can be expressed as $\lambda^2 = \mathbf{a}_0 \cdot \mathbf{C} \cdot \mathbf{a}_0$ with $\mathbf{C}$ representing the Cauchy-Green strain measure $\mathbf{C} = \mathbf{F}^T\mathbf{F}$. $\mathbf{F}$ represents the deformation gradient $\mathbf{F} = \frac{\partial \mathbf{x}}{\partial \mathbf{X}}$ with $\mathbf{x}, \mathbf{X}$ representing the coordinates of each point in the current and initial configurations respectively [33].

Due to the well-known difficulties that appear in displacement-based finite elements in the analysis of nearly incompressible materials, a multiplicative decomposition of $\mathbf{F}$ into *volume-changing (dilational)* and *volume-preserving (distortional)* parts was established as $\mathbf{F} = J^{\frac{1}{3}}\overline{\mathbf{F}}$. With the same objective, we postulated the existence of a unique decoupled representation of the strain-energy density function Ψ as:

$$\Psi = \Psi_{vol}(J) + \Psi_{iso}(\overline{\mathbf{C}}, \mathbf{a}_0 \otimes \mathbf{a}_0 \tag{1}$$

where $\Psi_{vol}(J)$ and $\Psi_{iso}(\overline{\mathbf{C}}, \mathbf{a}_0 \otimes \mathbf{a}_0)$ are given scalar-valued functions of the Jacobian $J = det\,\mathbf{F}$ and the modified Cauchy-Green tensor $\overline{\mathbf{C}} = J^{-\frac{2}{3}}\mathbf{C}$ that respectively describe the volumetric and the isochoric responses of the material. The isochoric part Ψiso of the strain energy function was divided into an isotropic part (F_1) that corresponds to a Neo-Hookean model and a second part dependent on collagen fibers (F_2). The volumetric part Ψvol was considered in a standard manner for quasi-incompressible materials as a penalty function of the Jacobian [33]. We had in turn developed:

$$\Psi = \frac{1}{2D} ln(J) + C_1(\overline{I}_1 - 3) + F_2(\lambda) \tag{2}$$

where C_1 is the Neo-Hookean constant and D the inverse of the bulk modulus $k = \frac{1}{D}$, which was chosen for all the ligaments as $\frac{k}{C_1} = 1000$ [35].

Following physical observations in human ligaments, we assumed that collagen fibers do not support compressive loads. Secondly, the stress-strain relation curves for ligaments have two well-defined parts: an initial curve with increasing stiffness (toe region) and a secondary portion with stiffness almost constant (linear region). We used the free-energy function (3) earlier proposed by Weiss et al. [35]:

$$\lambda \frac{\partial F_2}{\partial \lambda} = 0 \quad \lambda < 1$$

$$\lambda \frac{\partial F_2}{\partial \lambda} = C_3(e^{C_4(\lambda-1)} - 1) \quad \lambda < \lambda^*$$

$$\lambda \frac{\partial F_2}{\partial \lambda} = C_5\lambda + C_6 \quad \lambda > \lambda^* \tag{3}$$

where $\bar{I}_1 = tr(\bar{\mathbf{C}})$ is the first invariant of $\bar{\mathbf{C}}$, λ^* is the stretch at which collagen fibers start to be straightened, changing Ψ from exponential to linear, C_3 scales the exponential stress, C_4 is related to the rate of collagen uncrimping and C_5 is the elastic modulus of the straightened collagen fibers. We used the average constants obtained by Gardiner et al. [17] for the MCL in their experimental data. The LCL constants were assumed to be identical to those of the MCL. We fitted the uni-axial stress-strain curves obtained by Butler et al. [34] for ACL, PCL and PT (patellar tendon) with those obtained by Weiss, getting the associated constants that have been included in Table 1.

The local fiber orientation ($\mathbf{a}_0$) was specified according to the local element geometry (see Figure 8). The true Cauchy stress tensor, $\boldsymbol{\sigma}$, and the elasticity tensor in the spatial description were obtained in a standard manner for compressible hyperelastic materials [33,35].

In order to investigate the effect of the variation of some of the model parameters on the predicted contact pressures, maximal compression and shear stresses, several values of E and ν for articular cartilage, menisci and the ligament constants cited above were analyzed.

2.3. Enforcement of Initial Strains

Biological soft tissues are usually exposed to a complex distribution of in vivo residual stresses as a consequence of the continuous growth, remodeling, damage and viscoelastic strain that they suffer during their lifetime. These stresses can be relieved by selective cutting of living tissue to remove internal constraint.

Table 1. Material parameters for the ligament stress-free state [*MPa*]

	C_1	C_2	C_3	C_4	C_5	λ^*	D
MCL	1.44	0.0	0.57	48.0	467.1	1.063	0.00126
LCL	1.44	0.0	0.57	48.0	467.1	1.063	0.00126
ACL	1.95	0.0	0.0139	116.22	535.039	1.046	0.00683
PCL	3.25	0.0	0.1196	87.178	431.063	1.035	0.0041
PT	2.75	0.0	0.065	115.89	777.56	1.042	0.00484

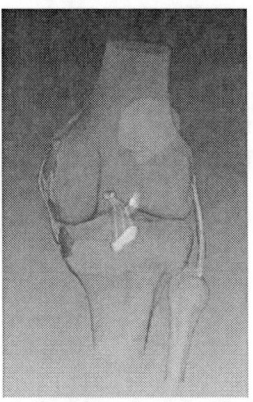

(a) Fiber principal directions in the main knee ligaments.

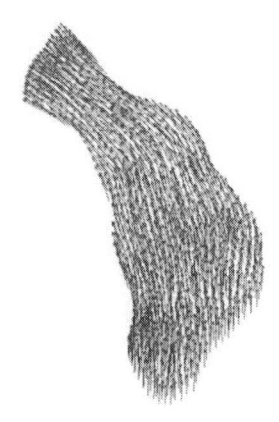

(b) Fiber principal directions in the main knee ligaments.

Figure 8. Local fibers orientation for each ligament.

In order to describe the current deformation state, we followed the methodology initially proposed by Weiss et al. [36] to enforce initial strains in hyperelastic soft tissues. This methodology was later generalized by Peña et al. [37]. Three different configurations are defined: a) the stress-free state (Ω_{fs}), b) the reference state in which the material undergoes initial strains only (Ω_0), and c) the current deformed state (Ω). It is assumed that the total deformation gradient tensor corresponding to the current state $\mathbf{F}$ admits a multiplicative decomposition $\mathbf{F}=\mathbf{F}_r\mathbf{F}_0$, where $\mathbf{F}_0$ represents the deformation gradient corresponding to the initial strains and a subsequent unloaded equilibrium step. $\mathbf{F}_r$ is the deformation gradient that results from applying the external loads to the initial configuration Ω_0.

The initial stress in the reference state, σ_0, is defined for hyperelastic materials in the standard form from the strain-energy density function $\mathbf{\Psi}_{\Omega_{fs}}$ referred to the stress-free state $\mathbf{\Psi}_{fs}$. We assumed that this strain-energy function is modified in the reference state due to the non-linear behaviour of the material and the variation in the fiber direction. The new strain-energy function referred to the unloaded configuration is denoted by $\mathbf{\Psi}_{\Omega_0}$.

To introduce initial strains it is necessary to specify the initial strains and obtain $\mathbf{F}_0$ pointwise within the finite element mesh. The total stress corresponding to the current state, σ, is then computed by

$$\sigma = \frac{2}{J}\mathbf{F}_r[\frac{\sigma_0}{2} + \frac{\partial\mathbf{\Psi}_{\Omega_0}(\mathbf{C})}{\partial\mathbf{C}}]\mathbf{F}_r^T$$

and the elasticity tensor derived in the standard form from the new strain-energy function $\mathbf{\Psi}_{\Omega_0}$.

In the case of ligaments and tendons, Gardiner et al. [17] proposed a relatively easy form to measure length variations along the fiber direction at different points. The concomitant contraction in the perpendicular plane was dictated by the usual incompressibility assumption in biological soft tissues. This information was used to calculate $\mathbf{F}_0$. Initial strains in our model were defined from data available in literature [1, 13, 16], and have been included in Table 2 with the following terminology: a: anterior part of ligament; p: posterior part of

Table 2. % Ligament initial strains at full extension

aAC	pAC	aPC	pPC	aLC	mLC	pLC	aMC	mMC	pMC
0.06	0.1	0.0	0.0	0.0	0.0	0.08	0.04	0.04	0.03

ligament; m: medial part of ligament. We used the initial strain distribution obtained by optimization techniques by [1,13].

Initial strains should provoke an autoequilibrated state. However, the initially prescribed values were obtained by optimization techniques from experimental data and do not produce this autobalanced state [37]. For this reason, it is necessary to enforce an equilibrium step. Obviously, the initial strains obtained after that equilibrium step are not exactly the prescribed ones, but are very close [6].

This constitutive model was implemented into the commercial FE code ABAQUS v.6.2 through a Fortran user subroutine. The resulting numerical model was validated with analytical solutions for different states of homogeneous deformation with excellent agreement.

2.4. Boundary Conditions

One of the most important features of the model presented here is the presence of contacts. In particular, we have defined the following interactions:

- Femoral cartilage with the patella cartilage
- Femoral cartilage with tibial cartilage
- Femoral cartilage with internal and external menisci
- Tibial cartilage with internal and external menisci.

For all cases a zero friction coefficient is considered, which leads to neglected tangential component of the frictional force [8]. To define these contacts the finite sliding option is chosen [38], allowing large relative displacements between the contacting regions.

Ligaments and bones meshes are considered as coincident at the insertion sites, thus leading to important computational saving over the use of connectors, contacts, multi-point constraints (MPCs) and other joining techniques for incompatible meshes. This also leads to more uniform stress distribution at the insertions. In the case of the menisci, the insertion of the horns on the tibial plateau was modeled by means of multi-point constraints. On the contrary, ligaments and bone, outer periphery of the medial meniscus is attached node to node with the internal lateral ligament. The same strategy is applied to the cartilage of the femur, tibia and fibula.

As mentioned before, three different loading conditions were analyzed:

- Flexion of 60 degrees of the femur (simplified model)
  In this first case, rotation of 60 degrees on the femur is imposed while considering the intercondylar line as the axis of rotation with complete restraint of the tibia and fibula (see Fig. 9). Since the bones are considered as rigid bodies, their movements

are governed by the 6 degrees of freedom of the corresponding reference node. In this first model, consisting only of ligaments and bones, the objective was to qualitatively discuss the role of the ligaments during flexion. It is therefore a first approximation to the actual load that develops during this movement.

- Static compression load of 1150 N of the tibia (full model)
  In this case, all degrees of freedom of the tibia were restricted and a compressive vertical load (1150 N) was applied on the reference node of the femur (located at the midpoint of the femoral intercondylar line (Fig. 9)).
- Flexion of 10 degrees of the tibia (full model)
  The last case corresponded to flexion on the complete model. Rotation of 10 degrees to the tibia around the femoral intercondylar line was imposed while the femur remained fully restrained (Fig. 9). The same surface contacts defined in the second load case were also included.

3. RESULTS

CASE I: Flexion of 60 Degrees of the Femur (Simplified Model)

In the absence of the quadriceps tendon, ligaments are subject to a state of excessive load since the important contribution of the tendon against bending is ignored.

Consequently, the results should be treated with caution and interpreted only in a qualitative manner. The appearance of high maximum principal stresses was particularly important at the posterior aspect of the anterior cruciate ligament (50 MPa), (see Fig. 10, 11, 12 and 13).

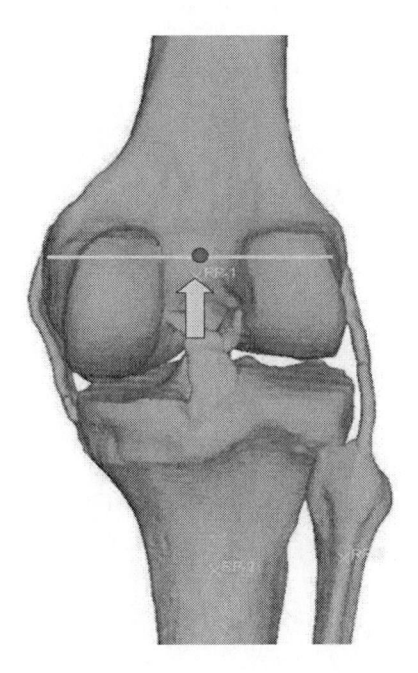

Figure 9. The intercondylar line and its midpoint.

The medial collateral ligament supported combined tension and lateral flexion, which brought the stress value near the 15 *MPa* at its center (see Fig. 13).

CASE II: Static Compression of the Tibia of 1150 *N* (Full Model)

The compressive load applied to the tibia was a static load appropriately weighted to include the effect of impact and take into account the force exerted by an adult on one leg for support. The result was compression in both menisci and the articular cartilage of the femur and tibia. As a result of the cartilage-cartilage in the femur and tibia, the minimum principal stress reached similar values around 6 *MPa*. These values were higher than those in the menisci, which were slightly below 2 *MPa*. It is also relevant to note that the region of cartilage-cartilage contact was somewhat higher than expected (see Fig. 14, 15 and 16).

CASE III: Flexion of 10 Degree of the Complete Model

For the angle considered, the stresses due to contact between cartilage and menisci were practically negligible. Similarly, ligament tension was very low (< 3 *MPa*), which made clear the important contribution of the quadriceps tendon in flexion. Also, high tension begins to appear in the insertion of the anterior cruciate ligament and is accompanied by the contact of the medial meniscus with the medial collateral ligament (see Fig. 17).

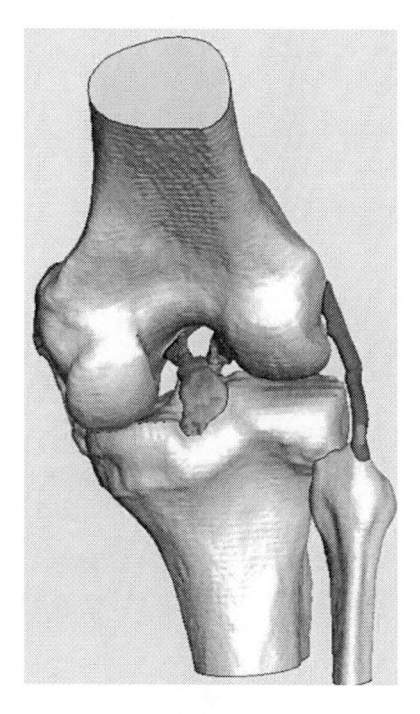

Figure 10. Ligaments maximum principal stresses for flexation of 60 degrees of the femur.

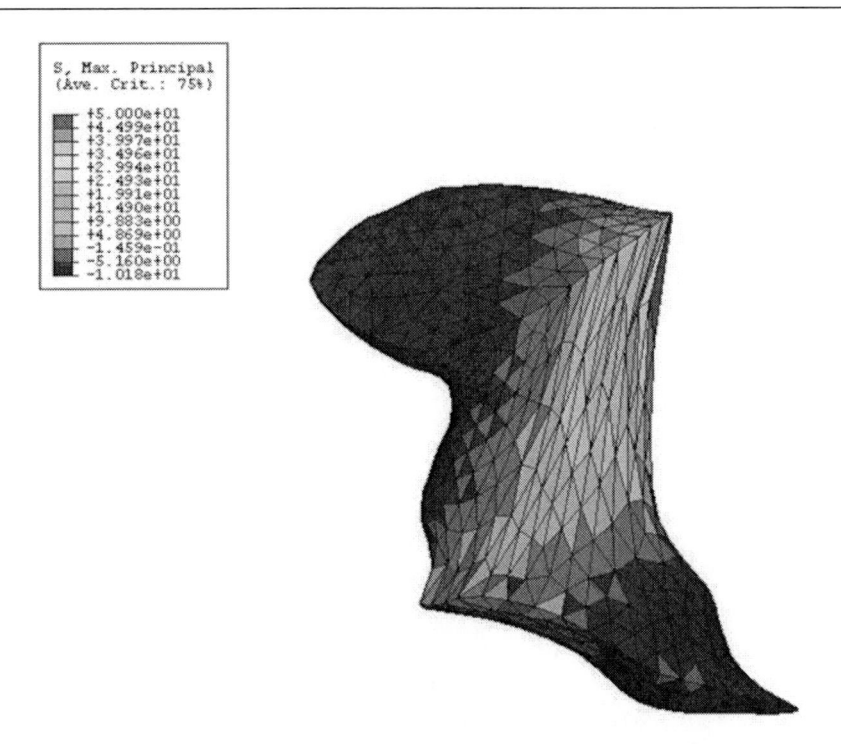

Figure 11. Maximum principal stresses of the Anterior Cruciate Ligament for flexion of 60 degrees of the femur.

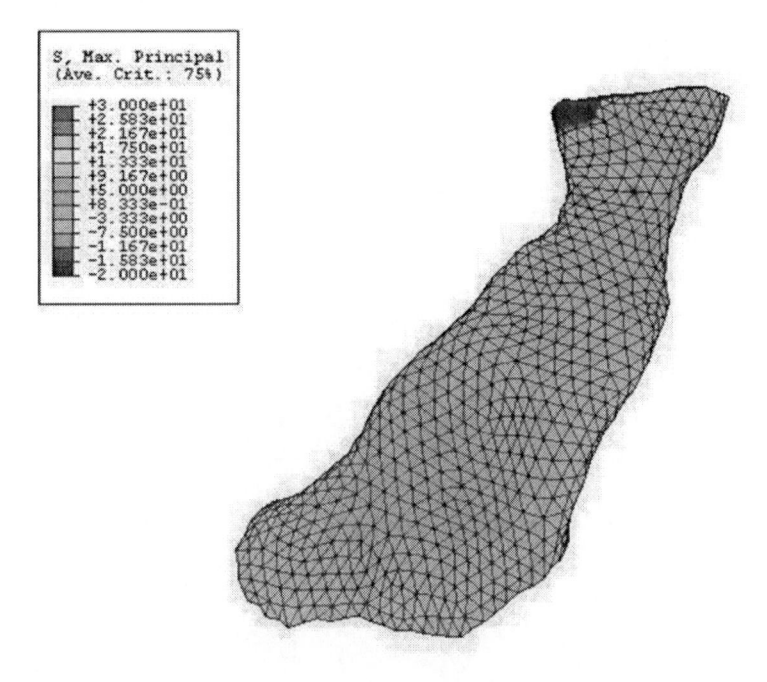

Figure 12. Maximum principal stresses of the Posterior Cruciate Ligament for flexion of 60 degrees of the femur.

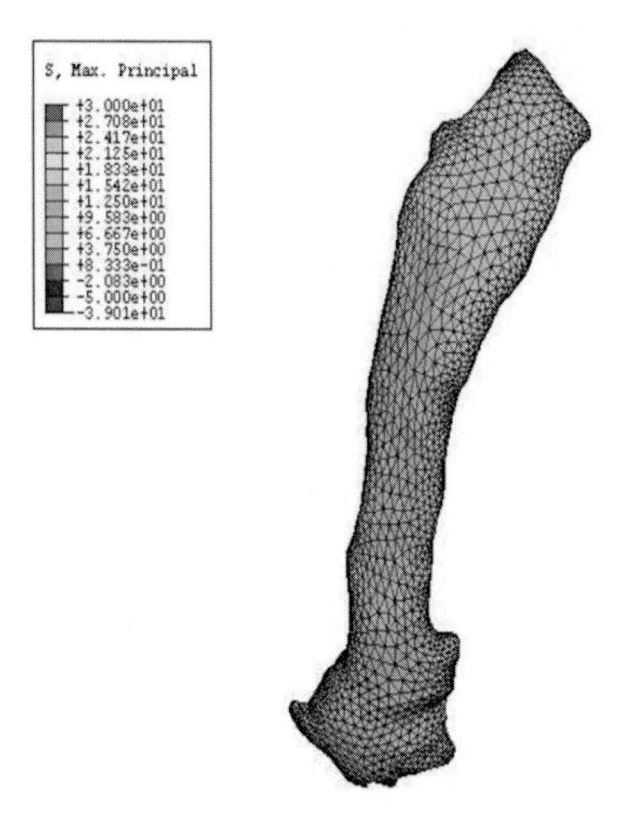

Figure 13. Maximum principal stresses of the Medial Collateral Ligament for flexion of 60 degrees of the femur.

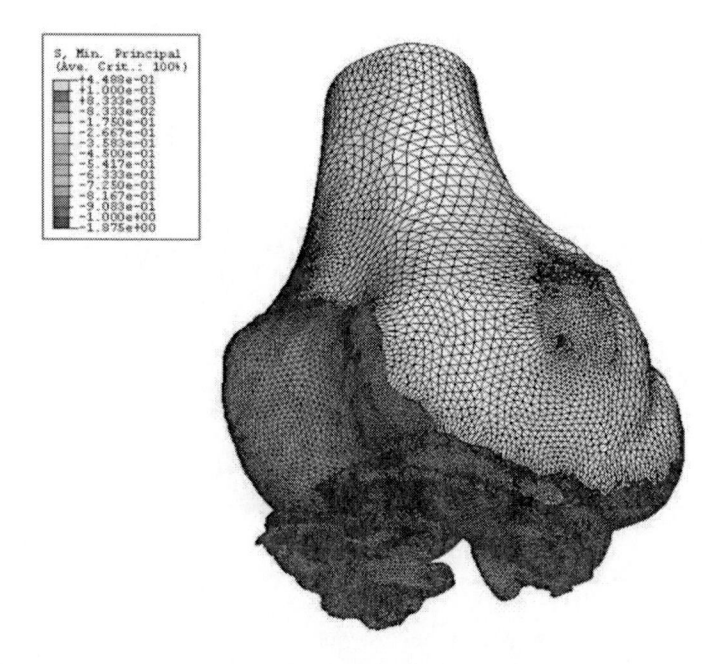

Figure 14. Minimum principal stresses of femoral cartilage and menisci.

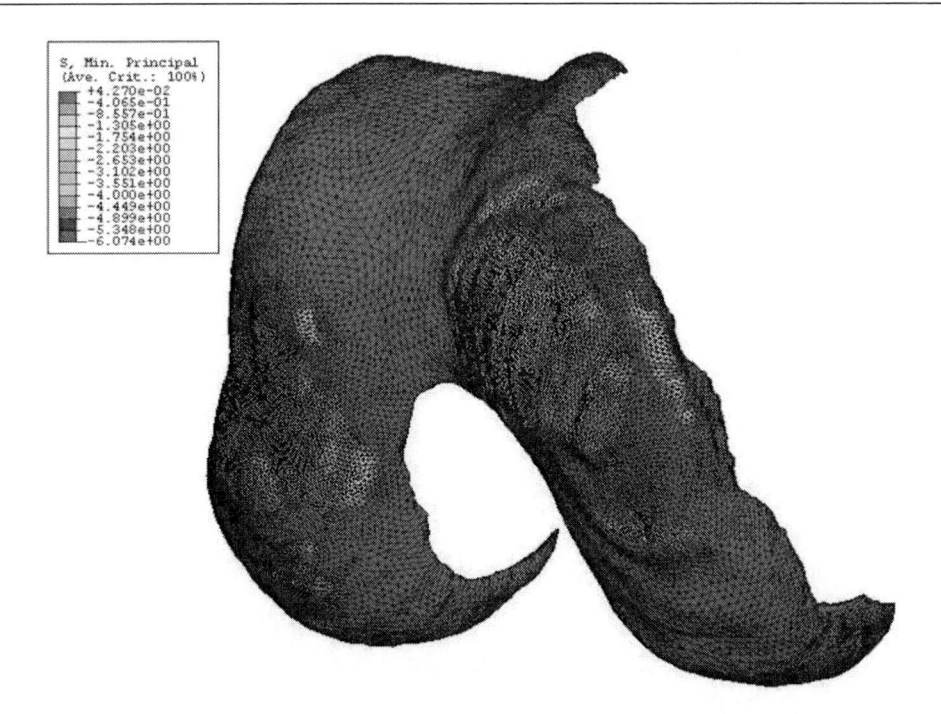

Figure 15. Minimum principal stresses of the femoral cartilage.

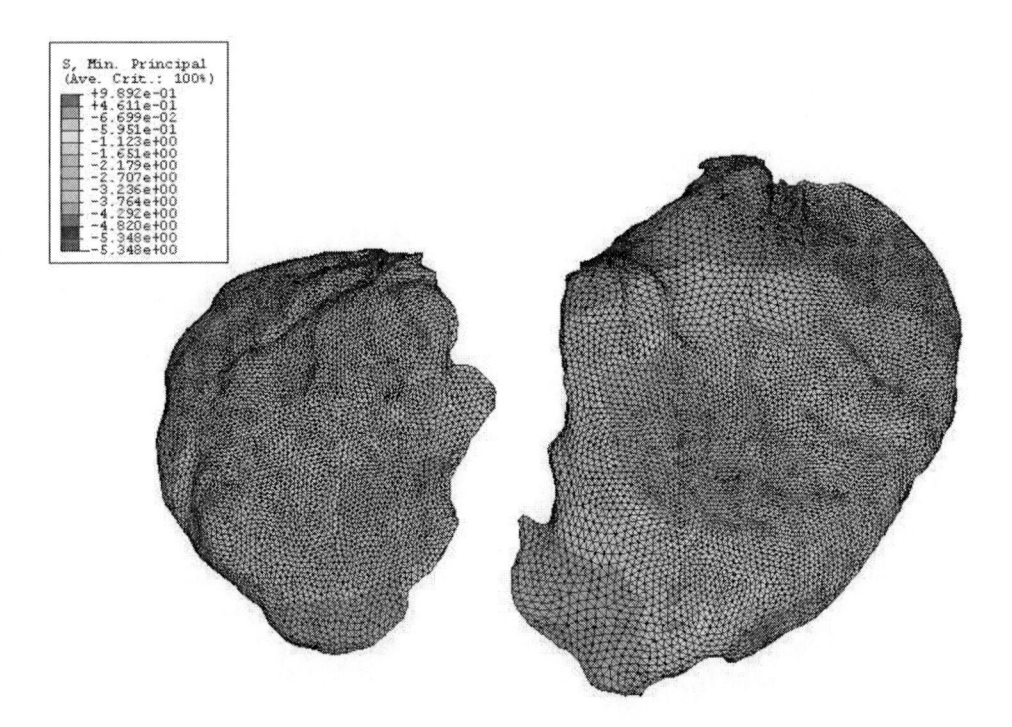

Figure 16. Minimum principal stresses of the tibial cartilage.

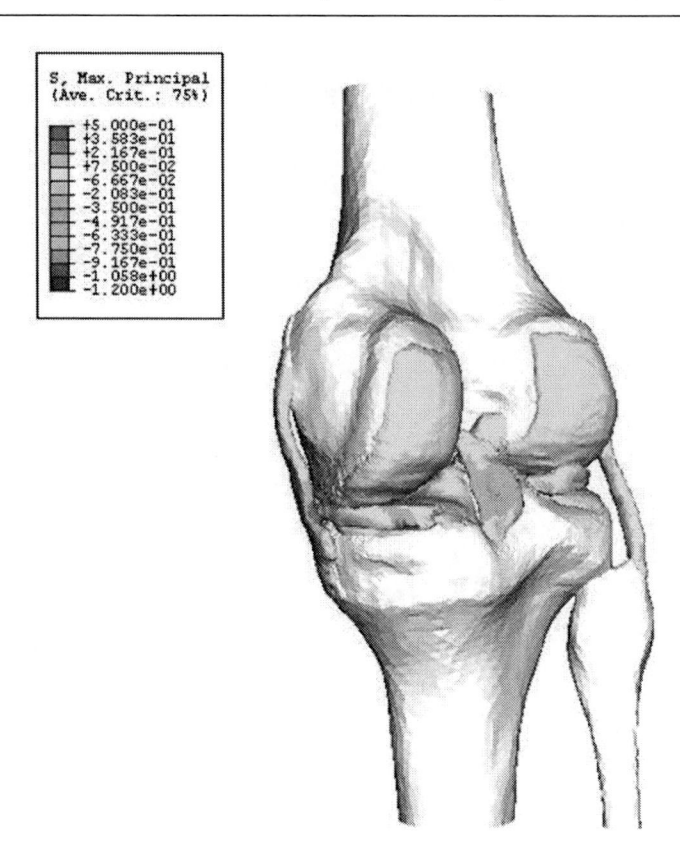

Figure 17. Maximum principal stresses for flexion of 10 degrees of the tibia.

CONCLUSION

Our main goal in this study was to determine the role of menisci and ligaments in the stability of the knee and load distribution. For this, we developed a three dimensional computational model of the tibiofemoral joint in a healthy male adult.

This expanded on the study carried out by Peña et al. [6] by taking advantage of the availability of more accurate baseline data (geometry and mesh) to analyze several loading conditions.

The model includes all components considered relevant to study the biomechanical behavior of the knee (bone, menisci, cartilage, tendons and ligaments), with special emphasis on describing the hyperelastic behavior of ligaments. The femur and tibia were considered to be rigid, while articular cartilage and menisci were assumed to be linearly elastic, isotropic and homogeneous. Ligaments were modeled as hyperelastic and transversely isotropic. Initial strain in all ligaments were considered. This model was validated using experimental and numerical results obtained by Fox et al. [25], Fukubayashi et al. [24], Bendjaballah et al. [20] and Donahue et al. [14].

We analyzed three different loading conditions: (a) Flexion of 60 degrees on a simplified model consisting of bones and ligaments; (b) Vertical compression applied to the tibia to define contact between the tibial and femoral and the menisci; and (c) Flexion of 10 degrees in the full model with the same definition of tibiofemoral contact as in the second case.

The results obtained in ligaments showed high stress at full flexion (60 degrees). This was essentially due to the large sagittal plane rotation of the femoral insertion of the ACL. This was also observed experimentally by Yamamoto et al. [43] when they used photoelasticity to track strains at the ACL surface. Our results also showed high tensile stress on the posterior aspect of the ACL, with moderate tensile stress on the anterior portion.

Anterior load produced a stress distribution in the MCL similar to shear, with tension in the anterior-distal and posterior-proximal portions. Similar results were obtained by Hull et al. [42] in their work, where they measured the strain distribution in the MCL to determine the single and combined external loads most likely to cause injury. Due to the location of the tibial insertion of the PCL, anterior displacement of the knee causes the tibia to push the PCL and provoke bending. This implies that some regions of the PCL relax. Since the initial strain of the PCL considered by Blankevoort and Huiskes [1] was null, the above relaxation implies low compression in the PCL. This could mean that the initial strain distribution of the PCL obtained by Blankevoort and Huiskes [1] is not completely correct and initial tension may have been encountered in the model. Under an axial compressive load of 1150 N, the contact area at the medial plateau of the knee was 359 $mm2$.

Finally, our model was used to study the role of the ligaments and menisci in the stability of the human joint under rotatory loads. Different studies have showed that the MCL provides a primary restraint to valgus rotation and a secondary restraint to external rotation and anterior and posterior translations [13]. Our work supports this conclusion. Maximum principal stress took place in the MCL near the femoral insertion with valgus rotation. Clinical observations of injury patterns confirm that this region is the most common location of injuries in the MCL [41]. Previous experimental [32,40,42] and computational [17] studies also supported this result.

Several limitations of our model must be considered. First of all, the menisci were assumed to be composed of a single-phase linear elastic and isotropic material. Several authors have found that the meniscus is much stiffer circumferentially, which could have some influence in the results [4,44,45]. Second, much of the proposed model is dependent upon data from other papers that do not correspond to a specific subject. For this reason, the results should be considered with caution. In addition, our results depend on load values of 1150 N. This 1150 N load corresponds to the maximal force in the gait cycle obtained by Sathasivam and Walker [46] at full extension. Obviously, the contact area, pressure, and kinematics of the knee would probably change under different loads. Finally, the viscoelastic properties of ligaments and meniscus were not considered. In spite of these limitations, our results demonstrate that subject specific FE models can predict the complex, non-uniform stress and strain fields that occur in biological soft tissues as they relate to knee kinematics. Our model also makes clear the importance of the combined role of menisci and ligaments in the stability of the joint as primary and secondary restraints.

ACKNOWLEDGMENTS

The authors gratefully acknowledge the financial support from the Instituto de Salud Carlos III through the CIBER initiative. The authors are also grateful to Zuse Institute Berlin for providing MRIs and the segmentation of the knee structures.

REFERENCES

[1]   L. Blankevoort, R. Huiskes, Ligament-bone interaction in a three dimensional model of the knee, *ASME Journal of Biomechanical Engineering,* 113 (1991) 263–269.

[2]   V. Vedi, A. Williams, S.J. Tennant, El. Spouse, Meniscal movement, *Journal of Bone and Joint Surgery,* 81-B (1999) 37–41.

[3]   P.S. Walker, M.J. Erkman, The role of the menisci in force transmission across the knee, *Clinical Orthopaedics and Related Research,* 109 (1975) 184–192.

[4]   D.C. Fithian, M.A. Kelly, V.C. Mow, Material properties and structure-function relationship in the menisci, *Clinical Orthopaedic Related Research,* 252 (1990) 19–31.

[5]   M.F. Macnicol, N.P. Thomas, The knee after meniscectomy, *Journal of Bone and Joint Surgery,* 82-B (2000) 157–159.

[6]   E. Peña, B. Calvo, M.A. Martinez, M. Doblaré, A three dimensional analysis of the combined behavior of ligaments and menisci in the healthy human knee joint, *Journal of Biomechanics,* 39 (2006) 1686–1701.

[7]   M.H. Doweidar, B. Calvo, I. Alfaro, P. Groenenboom, M. Doblaré, A comparison of implicit and explicit natural element methods in large strains problems: Application to soft biological tissues modeling, *Computer Methods in Applied Mechanics and Engineering,* 199 (2010) 691–1700.

[8]   T. Murakami, The lubrication in natural synovial joints and joint prostheses, *JSME International Journal,* 33 (1990) 465–474.

[9]   P. G. Fairbank, Knee joints changes after meniseçtomy, *Journal Bone Joint Surgery,* 52 (1948) 564.

[10] C. V. Mow, S. C. Kuei, W. M. Lai, C. G. Amstrong, Biphasic creep and stress relaxation of articular cartilage in compression: theory and experiments, *ASME J. Biomechanical Engineering,* 102 (1980) 73–84.

[11] M. Z. Bendjaballah, A. Shirazi-adl, D. J. Zukor, Biomechanical response of the passive human knee joint under anterior-posterior forces, *Clinical Biomechabics,* 13 (1998) 625–633.

[12] B. Beynnon, J Yu, D. Huston, B. Fleming, R. Johnson, L. Haugh, M. Pope, A sagittal plane model of the Knee and cruciate ligaments with application of a sensitivity analysis, *ASME J. Biomechanical Engineering,* 118 (1996) 227–239.

[13] G. Li, J. Gil, A. Kanamori, S. L. Y. Woo, A sagittal plane model of the Knee and cruciate ligaments with application of a sensitivity analysis, *ASME J. Biomechanical Engineering,* 121 (1999) 657–662.

[14] T. L. Haut Donahue, M. L. Hull, M. M. Rashid, R. C. Jacobs, A Finite Element Model of the human knee joint for the study of tibio-femoral contact, *ASME J. Biomechanical Engineering,* 124 (2002) 273–280.

[15] S. Hirokawa, R. Tsuruno, Three-dimensional deformation and stress distribution in an analytical/computational model of the anterior cruciate ligament, *Journal Biomechanics,* 33 (2000) 1069–1077.

[16] Y. Song, R. E. Debski, V. Musahl, M. Thomas, S. L. Y. Woo, A three-dimensional finite element model of the human anterior cruciate ligament: a computational analysis with experimental validation, *Journal Biomechanics,* 37 (2004) 383–390.

[17] J. C. Gardiner, J. A. Weiss, Subjet-specific finite element analysis of the human medial collateral ligament during valgus knee loading, *Journal Orthopaedic Research*, 21 (2003) 1098–1106.

[18] E. Abdel-Rahman, M. S. Hefzy, A two-dimensional dynamic anatomical model of the human knee joint, *ASME J. Biomechanical Engineering*, 115 (1993) 357–365.

[19] J. Heegard, P. F. Leyvraz, A. Curnier, L. Rakotomana, R. Huiskes, The biomechanics of the human patella during passive knee flexion, *Journal Biomechanics*, 28 (1993) 1265–1279.

[20] M. Z. Bendjaballah, A. Shirazi-adl, D. J. Zukor, Biomechanics of the human knee joint in compression: reconstruction, mesh generation and finite element analysis, *Knee*, 2 (1995) 69–79.

[21] A. Jalani, A. Shirazi-adl, M. Z. Bendjaballah, Biomechanics of human tibio-femoral joint in axial rotation, Knee 4 (1997) 203–213.

[22] D. Périé, M. C. Hobatho, In vivo determination of contact areas and pressure of the femorotibial joint using non-linear finite element analysis, *Clinical Biomechanics.* 13 (1998) 394–402.

[23] B. Beynnon, J Yu, D. Huston, B. Fleming, R. Johnson, L. Haugh, M. Pope, In vivo determination of contact areas and pressure of the femorotibial joint using non-linear finite element analysis, *ASME J. Biomechanical Engineering.* 118 (1996) 227–239.

[24] T. Fukubayashi, H. Kurosawa, The contact area and pressure distribution pattern of the knee, *Acta Orthop. Scand.* 51 (1980) 871–879.

[25] R. J. Fox, C. D. Harner, M. Sakane, G. J. Carlin, S. L. Y. Woo, Determination of the in situ forces in the human posterior cruciate ligament using robotic technology, *Am. J. Spors Med.* 26 (1998) 395–401.

[26] C. G. Armstrong,W. M. Lai, V. C. Mow, An Analisysis of the unconfined compression of articular cartilage, *ASME J. Biomechanical Engineering.* 106 (1984) 165–173.

[27] A. M. Ahmed, D. L. Burke, A. Hydero, Force analysis of the patellar mechanicsy, *J. Orthopaedic Research.* 5 (1987) 69–85.

[28] E. Peña, A. Pérez del Palomar, B. Calvo, M. A. Martínez, M. Doblaré, Computational modelling of diarthrodial joints. Physiological, pathological and pos-surgery simulations, *Arch. Comput. Method Eng.* 14 (2007) 47–91.

[29] D. M. Daniels, Knee Ligaments: Structure, function, injury and repair, New York (1990).

[30] P. S. Donzelli, R. S. Spilker, G. A. Ateshian, V. C. Mow, Contact analysis of biphasic transversely isotropic cartilage layers and correlation with tissue failure, *Journal Biomechanics.* 32 (1999) 1037–1047.

[31] M. A. LeRoux, L. A. Setton, Experimental and biphasic FEM determinations of the material properties and hydraulic permeability of the meniscus in tension, *ASME J. Biomechanical Engineering.* 124 (2002) 315–321.

[32] J. A. Weiss, J. C. Gardiner, Computational modelling of ligament mechanics, *Critical Reviews Biomedical Engineering.* 29 (2001) 1–70.

[33] G. A. Holzapfel, *Nonlinear Solid Mechanics,* Wiley, New York (2000).

[34] D. L. Butler, Y. Guan, M. Kay, J. Cummings, S. Feder, M. Levy, Location-dependent variations in the material properties of the anterior cruciate ligament, *Journal Biomechanics.* 25 (1992) 511–518.

[35] J. A.Weiss, B. N. Maker, S.Govindjee, Finite element implementation of incompressible, transversely isotropic hyperelasticity, *Comput. Methods Appl. Mech. Engrg.* 135 (1996) 107–128.

[36] J. A. Weiss, B. N. Maker, D. A. Schauer, Treatment of initial stress in hyperelastic finite element models of soft tissues, *ASME Summer Bioengineering Conference.* (1995) Beaver Creek, CO.

[37] E. Peña, M. A. Martinez, B. Calvo, M. Doblaré, On the numerical treatment of initial strains in soft biological tissues, *Int. J. Numer Meth. Engng.* 68 (2006) 836–860.

[38] Hibbit, Karlsson and Sorensen, Inc., Abaqus user's guide, v. 6.8, HKS inc. *Pawtucket, RI, USA.,* (1999).

[39] Konrad-Zuse-Zentrum Fur informationstechnik Berlin (ZIB). Germany.

[40] S. Arms, J. Boyle, R. Johnson, M. Pope, Strain in the medial collateral ligament of the human knee: an autopsy study, *Journal of Biomechanics.* 29 (1995) 199–206.

[41] T. Kawada, T. Abe, K. Yamamoto, S. Hirokawa, T. Soejima, N. Tanaka, A. Inoue, Analysis of strain distribution in the medial collateral ligament using a photoelastic coating method, *Medical Engineering and Physics,* 21 (1999) 279–291.

[42] M.L. Hull, G. Berns, H. Varma, A. Patterson, Strain in the medial collateral ligament of the human knee under single and combined loads, *Journal of Biomechanics,* 29 (1995) 199–206.

[43] K. Yamamoto, S. Hirokawa, T. Kawada, Strain distribution in the ligament using photoelasticity. A direct application to the human ACL, *Medical Engineering and Physics,* 20 (1998) 161–168.

[44] R.L. Spilker, P.D. Donzelli, V.C. Mow, A transversely isotropic biphasic finite element model of the meniscus, *Journal of Biomechanics,* 25 (1992) 1027–1045.

[45] C.S. Proctor, M.B. Schmidt, M.A. Kelly, V.C. Mow, Material properties of the normal medial bovine meniscus, *Journal of Orthopaedics Research,* 7 (1989) 771–782.

[46] S. Sathasivam, P.S. Walker, A computer model with surface friction for the prediction of total knee kinematics, *Journal of Biomechanics,* 30 (1997) 177–184.

In: The Knee
Editor: Randy Mascarenhas

Chapter III

EFFECT OF A LOWER LIMB INJURY PREVENTION PROGRAM ON LANDING POSITION IN FEMALE BASKETBALL ATHLETES

Yasuharu Nagano[1], Kiyomi Tsuda[2] and Toru Fukubayashi[3]

[1] Department of Health and Sports,
Niigata University of Health and Welfare, Niigata, Japan
[2] Japan Basketball League Association, Tokyo, Japan
[3] Faculty of Sport Sciences, Waseda University, Saitama, Japan

ABSTRACT

Objective: To determine the effect of a lower limb injury prevention program on athletes with greater knee valgus angles during landing at high risk for ACL injury, who have greater knee valgus angle during landing, and on players with a low risk for ACL injury.

Methods: Forty-two female collegiate basketball athletes (84 limbs) participated in this study. Before and after the prevention program, which lasted four months, the peak knee valgus and peak knee flexion angles during the continuous jump test and the Star Excursion Balance Test (SEBT) scores were recorded. According to the average peak knee valgus angle of the continuous jump test, the subjects were divided into either a high- or a low-risk group. A 2-way ANOVA model (risk(2) × training(2)) was used to examine the main and interaction effects (risk/training/risk × training).

Results: In the high-risk group, the post-training knee valgus angle decreased compared to the pre-training angle ($p < 0.01$). In the low-risk group, the post-training SEBT score was greater than the pre-training score ($p < 0.01$).

Conclusions: The injury prevention program was effective in decreasing the risk of ACL injury in high-risk athletes with greater knee valgus angles during landing. Accordingly, screening for high-risk players and recommending a prevention program for them may allow for more effective prevention of ACL injuries. In low-risk players who did not have a valgus angle exceeding the cut-off value during landing, the prevention program resulted in improved balance ability, which may also lead to a decreased risk of lower limb injury. Based on these results, we conclude that enrolling all athletes in injury prevention programs may help reduce the risk of lower limb injury in sport.

Keywords: ACL injury, knee valgus, balance, injury prevention

INTRODUCTION

Anterior cruciate ligament (ACL) injuries commonly occur in non-contact situations such as landing and cutting [1], with female athletes have an increased risk of injury with an injury rate 3 to 5 times that of male athletes [2, 3]. Hewett et al. [4] reported that greater knee abduction during landing was a risk factor for ACL injury, with increased knee abduction also seen at the moment of injury [5].

Recently, many studies have focused on the prevention of ACL injury [6-8]. These studies have required all athletes to complete an injury prevention program. Since greater knee abduction during landing is one of the risk factors for ACL injury (4), those who demonstrate greater knee abduction angles during landing can be regarded as high-risk athletes. Measuring the effects of an injury prevention program on these high-risk athletes alone may be effective with respect to time and labour, but the differences in outcome of a prevention program in high- and low-risk players are unknown.

In this chapter, athletes who demonstrated greater knee abduction during landing were regarded to be at a high risk for lower extremity injury during sport and were placed in an injury prevention program along with low risk athletes. The hypothesis was that upon completion of the prevention program, high-risk athletes would show a decrease in knee valgus angle during landing and improved balance ability.

METHODS

Study Population

Forty-two female collegiate basketball athletes (84 limbs) participated in the study. The inclusion criteria were the absence of: (1) current lower extremity injury, (2) neuromuscular disorders, and (3) any history that would indicate decreased ability to perform a jump or balance test. The mean (SD) age, height, and weight of the subjects were 19.4 (1.2) years, 168.7 (7.2) cm, and 62.3 (6.4) kg, respectively.

Continuous Jump Testing

Before and after participation in the prevention program, all subjects performed a continuous jump test that consisted of five repeated vertical jumps using both legs with maximal effort [9, 10]. Participants were instructed to place their hands on the lower torso, stand with feet apart at shoulder width, and face a video camera to allow for proper recording of movements. A research assistant first demonstrated the jumps. The subjects were verbally instructed to minimise their foot contact time and to jump as high as possible. They

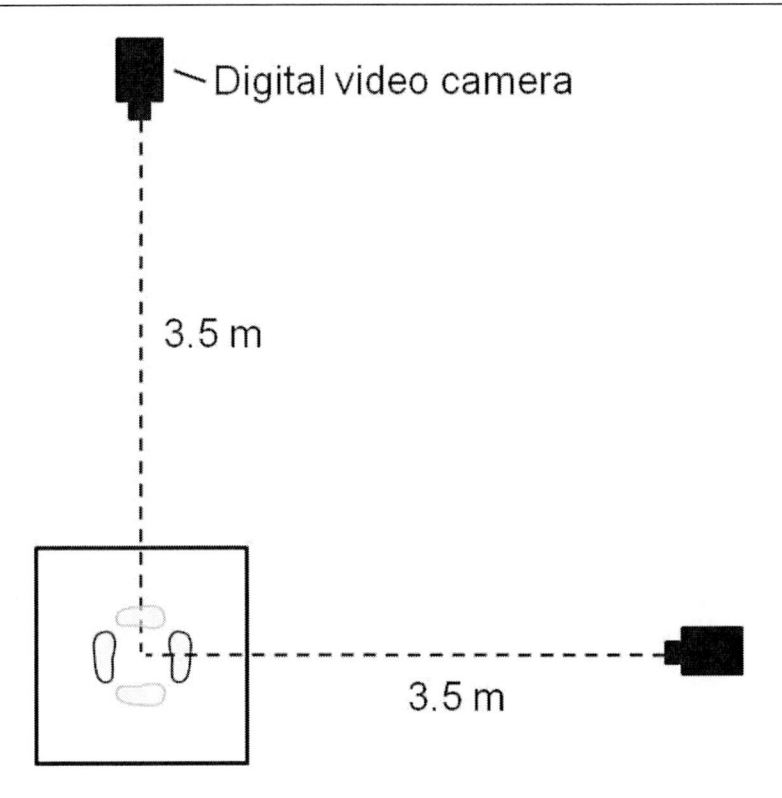

Figure 1. Set-up for continuous jump test. The trial was recorded using digital video cameras from the frontal and sagittal planes. Each digital camera was placed 3.5 m from the landing point at the height of the knee joint.

performed several preparatory trials. Measurements were continued until successful trials had been obtained for both legs. The frontal and right sagittal views of both legs of the subject were filmed using digital video cameras (30 Hz; Panasonic Inc., Japan), with the filming repeated after a 90-degree turn to obtain four views. The trial was excluded if a subject moved out of view of the camera or if the landing position deviated from the start position. The frontal plane camera was placed at a distance of 3.5 meters from both feet and the sagittal plane camera was placed 3.5 meters from the midpoint of the line between both lateral malleoli (Fig. 1). Each video camera was placed at the height of the knee joint.

For each subject, twelve 1.8 cm × 1.8 cm plastic tape markers were secured to the lower limbs. The markers were placed bilaterally on the anterior superior iliac spines (ASIS), the midpoints of the patellae, the midpoints of the medial and lateral malleoli (on the shoes), the greater trochanters, the lateral knee joint lines, and lateral malleoli. The captured images were imported into a digitizing software program (Dartfish Software; Dartfish Co. Ltd., Japan). On the frontal view, the angles formed by lines from the ASIS to the midpoint of the patella and from the midpoint of the patella to the midpoint of the medial and lateral malleoli was recorded as the knee valgus angle. On the sagittal view, the angle between the lines from the greater trochanter to the lateral knee joint, and from the lateral knee joint to the lateral malleolus was recorded as the knee flexion angle. Average peak knee valgus and flexion angles (relative to static standing position) during the second to the fourth landings were recorded for analyses. The average peak knee valgus angle was corrected using a linear regression equation [10]. Because this equation was not applicable to the knee varus, the data obtained when subjects exhibited knee varus during landings were excluded.

From the results of the average peak knee valgus angle of the continuous jump test, we divided the subjects into either a high- or low-risk group. Because a cut-off point for peak knee valgus has not been reported, a receiver operating characteristic (ROC) curve analysis was used to identify such a point for the continuous jump test. From the regression equation and measured data of the 3D knee abduction angle and 2D valgus angle [10], a cut-off point for the corrected 2D knee valgus angle was calculated. Referring to the previous study of Hewett et al. [4], which stated that the average knee abduction angle during the drop jump landing was 9 degrees in athletes with ACL injury, we regarded a 3D knee abduction angle of greater than 9 degrees as a positive risk factor for ACL injury. ROC curve analysis yielded a cut-off point of 6.23 degrees for the 2D corrected knee valgus angle for the continuous jump test, and this cut-off point had a sensitivity of 80% and a specificity of 50%. Therefore, those subjects who demonstrated an average peak knee valgus angle of more than 6.23 degrees during the continuous jump test were placed in the high-risk group.

Balance Ability Testing

Before and after completion of the prevention programme, all subjects performed the Star Excursion Balance Test (SEBT) procedure as described by Plisky et al. [11] using a custom-made device [9]. The participants stood on one leg on a footplate with the most distal aspect of the big toe on the baseline. While maintaining the single-leg stance, the participants were asked to reach with the free leg in the anterior, postero-medial, and postero-lateral directions in relation to the stance foot. The maximum reach distance was measured from the point of the big toe on the baseline to the most distant point of the extended foot. The trials were discarded and repeated if the participants (1) failed to maintain a unilateral stance, (2) lifted or moved the stance foot from the grid, (3) touched down with the reach foot, or (4) failed to return the reach foot to the starting position. The participants practised three trials on each leg in each of the three directions. Formal testing of three trials on each leg in each of the three reach directions was then conducted, and the highest value for each direction from the 3 trials was recorded. The greatest reach distance in each direction was averaged to yield a composite reach distance for analysis of overall test performance. The length of each leg was measured in a standing position from the ASIS to the top of the medial malleolus by using a cloth tape measure, and the length data were normalized for each leg.

Prevention Program

All subjects performed a lower limb injury prevention program that consisted of four training components (strength, balance, jump, and skill/coordination) and three levels (basic, standard, and advanced) (Table 1). Each training component was performed more than twice a week under the supervision of an athletic trainer and the subjects were instructed to perform exercises in a neutral position and to avoid lumbar lordosis, rear axial weight bearing, hip adduction, and knee valgus.

Table 1. Women's Japan Basketball League (WJBL) injury prevention program

		Basic		Standard		Advanced	
Strength	Core1	Bench	for 20-30 sec	Bench with leg lift	for 20-30 sec	Bench with arm & leg lift	for 20-30 sec
	Core2	Sideways bench	for 20-30 sec	Sideways bench with arm & leg lift	for 20-30 sec	Sideways bench with leg swing	10reps
	Lower extremities	Squat / Lunge (Forward, Side)	10reps / 10reps each	Walking lunge	10reps	Twist wakling lunge	10reps
	Core / lower	Bridge	5sec x 10reps	Single leg bridge	5sec x 10reps	Nordic hamstrings	5reps
Balance	Single leg standing	Single leg standing	for 30sec each	Single leg with ball pass	10reps for each pass	Single leg stance side to side pushing	for 10 sec
				Single leg on a balance disc	for 20-30 sec		
	Single leg squat position	Single leg squat position	for 30sec	Single leg with figure of eight ball pass	10reps for each	Single leg squattig stance side to side	for 10 sec
						Single leg squatting on a	for 20-30 sec
Jump	Squat jump	Squat jump	10reps	180 degrees jump	10reps	Signle leg 180 degrees jump	5reps
	Side kick	Single leg squat	10reps	Lateral hop	10reps	Side kick	10reps
	Line jump	Double leg jump	10reps each	Single leg forward / backward hop	5reps	High knee jump	5reps
	X-hop	X-hop	one pass each	Single leg & x-hop	one pass each	High knee & x-hop	one pass each
Skill & coordination	Step / turn	Twisting	20reps	Zigzag run	1-2 reps	Cross back step	10reps
		Twist jump	10reps	Front / back turn	10reps	Backward run & turn	2-3reps
	Running jump	Running jump	5reps	Running jump with half turn	5reps	Running jump footworks	5reps
	Contact	Contact	for 20sec	Contact jump	5resp each	Running contact jump	5reps each

Statistical Analysis

Before and after the completion of the prevention program, the Star Excursion Balance Test (SEBT) score and peak knee valgus and peak knee flexion angles during the continuous jump test were recorded. A 2-way ANOVA model (risk(2) × training(2)) was used to analyse the main effects and interaction effects (risk/training/risk × training). To determine each significant difference, Bonferroni multiple comparison tests were performed as post-hoc tests. Significance was set at $p < 0.05$.

RESULTS

Results were calculated for 33 of the 42 subjects, for a total of 60 limbs. This occurred due to exclusion secondary to some subjects not completing the prevention program and some video data during the continuous jump test having errors. Twenty-three limbs were included for analysis in the high risk group, with 37 limbs included in the low-risk group.

Table 2. The results of continuous jump test and balance test

		Valgus [a]	Flexion [b]	SEBT [c]
High risk group	Pre-training	7.8 (1.3)‡**	46.5 (9.6)	97.3 (6.1)
	Post-training	5.7 (1.8)‡*	45.1 (8.7)	97.7 (4.3)
Low risk group	Pre-training	4.0 (1.3)**	47.2 (6.8)‡	95.2 (7.2)‡
	Post-training	4.5 (2.4)*	42.0 (10.8)‡	99.9 (5.2)‡
All	Pre-training	5.5 (2.3)	46.9 (7.9)	96.0 (6.8)
	Post-training	4.9 (2.2)	43.2 (10.1)	99.1 (4.9)
Main effects (Risk)		$p < 0.01$	n. s.	n. s.
Main effects (Training)		$p < 0.01$	$p < 0.05$	$p < 0.01$
Interaction (Risk x Training)		$p < 0.01$	n. s.	$p < 0.01$

a: Knee valgus during continuous jump (deg), b: Knee flexion during
continuous jump (deg), c: Star Excursion Balance Test Score
*: $p < 0.05$ between high risk group and low risk group
**: $p < 0.01$ between high risk group and low risk group
‡: $p < 0.01$ between Pre-training and Post-Training

Table 2 presents pre- and post-training results of the continuous jump test and SEBT scores. With respect to the knee valgus angle during the continuous jump test, a significant interaction was observed ($p < 0.01$). In the high-risk group, the post-training knee valgus angle decreased compared to the pre-training angle $(p < 0.01)$. Training was also found to have a significant effect on knee flexion angle (p < 0.05). In the low-risk group, the post-training knee flexion angle decreased compared to the pre-training angle (p < 0.01). With regards to the SEBT score, a significant interaction was observed (p < 0.01). In the low risk group, the post-training SEBT score was higher than the pre-training score (p < 0.01).

DISCUSSION

To our knowledge, this is the first study to measure the effect of an injury prevention program on knee valgus landing angles in high-risk athletes. Furthermore, few previous studies have utilised the risk category to analyse effects. In addition to the effect on knee valgus angle during landing, we also evaluated balance ability using the SEBT as a means to predict risk of lower limb injury [11]. The results presented in this chapter aim to indicate whether an injury prevention program should be conducted for all athletes or only for those with a specific risk factors.

The results of this study supported our hypothesis that upon completion of a lower limb injury prevention program, high-risk players showed a decrease in knee valgus angle during landing. The results of this chapter concur with those seen in previous studies [12-14] and suggest that identifying athletes who have greater knee valgus angles and recommending an appropriate prevention programme for them, can produce more effective ACL injury prevention.

Contradictory to our hypothesis, the low-risk group increased their SEBT scores after completion of the prevention program, but the high-risk group showed no change in their SEBT scores. Balance ability has been shown to predict lower limb injury [11]. In the low-risk group, which was identified by the results of the continuous jump test, the prevention program improved balance ability (which may have decreased their risk for lower limb injury) while having no effect on landing posture. Although the low-risk group were at low risk for ACL injury, the risk of sustaining other lower limb injuries in this group was not known. In order to prevent all lower limb injuries, we suggest that all athletes should participate in injury prevention programs. In future studies, the long-term effects on the balance ability of the high-risk group should also be investigated.

This study had several limitations. Firstly, we used two-dimensional methods to measure knee motion during landing. Although there is moderate correlation between two-dimensional knee valgus and three-dimensional knee abduction [10], accurate measurement of knee abduction during landing requires three-dimensional analysis. However, two-dimensional analysis is easier to conduct on large populations. Secondly, we did not select a control group that did not participate in the prevention program. The effect of the prevention program could have been more clearly defined by comparison with the results seen in a control group.

CONCLUSION

The prevention program was effective in decreasing the risk of ACL injury in high-risk athletes with greater knee valgus angles during landing. Screening for high-risk athletes and recommending a prevention program for them can lead to more effective prevention of ACL injury. In low-risk athletes who did not have a valgus angle exceeding the cut-off value during landing, the prevention program resulted in improved balance ability, which can lead to decreased risk of lower limb injury. Therefore, if we intend to reduce the incidence of lower limb injuries in sport, all the players should participate in prevention programs.

ACKNOWLEDGMENTS

We gratefully acknowledge Yoshio Nakamura, Professor, Faculty of Sports Sciences, Waseda University, who participated in the design and coordination of this chapter, and Hideyuki Miki, Japan Basketball League Association, who provided the prevention program. We received generous support from Kumiko Ohshima, Toshihiro Ohtaka, Naho Nakagawa and Shiho Moriya who helped in data collection.

REFERENCES

[1]   Boden, BP; Dean, GS; Feagin, JA, Jr.; Garrett, WE, Jr. Mechanisms of anterior cruciate ligament injury. *Orthopedics.* 2000 Jun 23(6), 573-8.

[2]   Agel, J; Arendt, EA; Bershadsky, B. Anterior cruciate ligament injury in national collegiate athletic association basketball and soccer: a 13-year review. *Am. J. Sports Med.* 2005 Apr 33(4), 524-30.

[3]   Arendt, E; Dick, R. Knee injury patterns among men and women in collegiate basketball and soccer. NCAA data and review of literature. *Am. J. Sports Med.* 1995 Nov–Dec 23(6), 694-701.

[4]   Hewett, TE; Myer, GD; Ford, KR; Heidt, RS, Jr.; Colosimo, AJ; McLean, SG; et al. Biomechanical measures of neuromuscular control and valgus loading of the knee predict anterior cruciate ligament injury risk in female athletes. *Am. J. Sports Med.* 2005 Apr 33(4), 492-501.

[5]   Hewett, TE; Torg, JS; Boden, BP. Video analysis of trunk and knee motion during non-contact anterior cruciate ligament injury in female athletes: lateral trunk and knee abduction motion are combined components of the injury mechanism. *Br. J. Sports Med.* 2009 Jun 43(6), 417-22.

[6]   Gilchrist, J; Mandelbaum, BR; Melancon, H; Ryan, GW; Silvers, HJ; Griffin, LY; et al. A randomized controlled trial to prevent noncontact anterior cruciate ligament injury in female collegiate soccer players. *Am. J. Sports Med.* 2008 Aug 36(8), 1476-83.

[7]   Mandelbaum, BR; Silvers, HJ; Watanabe, DS; Knarr, JF; Thomas, SD; Griffin, LY; et al. Effectiveness of a neuromuscular and proprioceptive training program in preventing anterior cruciate ligament injuries in female athletes: 2-year follow-up. *Am. J. Sports Med.* 2005 Jul 33(7), 1003-10.

[8]   Myklebust, G; Engebretsen, L; Braekken, IH; Skjolberg, A; Olsen, OE; Bahr, R. Prevention of anterior cruciate ligament injuries in female team handball players: a prospective intervention study over three seasons. *Clin. J. Sport Med.* 2003 Mar 13(2), 71-8.

[9]   Nagano, Y; Fukano, M; Itagaki, K; Li, S; Miyakawa, S; Fukubayashi, T. Influence of lower limb clinical physical measurements of female athletes on knee motion during continuous jump testing. *The Open Sports Medicine Journal.* 2011 January 4, 127-32.

[10]   Nagano, Y; Sakagami, M; Ida, H; Akai, M; Fukubayashi, T. Statistical modelling of knee valgus during a continuous jump test. *Sports biomechanics/International Society of Biomechanics in Sports.* 2008 Sep 7(3), 342-50.

[11]   Plisky, PJ; Rauh, MJ; Kaminski, TW; Underwood, FB. Star Excursion Balance Test as a predictor of lower extremity injury in high school basketball players. *The Journal of Orthopaedic and Sports Physical Therapy.* 2006 Dec 36(12), 911-9.

[12]   Lim, BO; Lee, YS; Kim, JG; An, KO; Yoo, J; Kwon, YH. Effects of sports injury prevention training on the biomechanical risk factors of anterior cruciate ligament injury in high school female basketball players. *Am. J. Sports Med.* 2009 Sep 37(9), 1728-34.

[13]   Chappell, JD; Limpisvasti, O. Effect of a neuromuscular training program on the kinetics and kinematics of jumping tasks. *Am. J. Sports Med.* 2008 Jun 36(6),1081-6.

[14]   Noyes, FR; Barber-Westin, SD; Fleckenstein, C; Walsh, C; West, J. The drop-jump screening test: difference in lower limb control by gender and effect of neuromuscular training in female athletes. *Am. J. Sports Med.* 2005 Feb 33(2), 197-207.

In: The Knee

Editor: Randy Mascarenhas

Chapter IV

DELETORIOUS EFFECTS OF FATIGUE ON KNEE JOINT PROPRIOCEPTION IN SOCCER PLAYERS

Fernando Ribeiro,[1,2] Andreia Morato,[1] Jerónimo Francisco[2] and José Oliveira[2]

[1] CESPU, Polytechnic Health Institute of the North,
Physiotherapy Department, R. Central de Gandra,
Gandra PRD, Portugal

[2] University of Porto, Faculty of Sport, Research Centre in Physical Activity,
Health and Leisure, Rua Dr. Plácido Costa, Porto, Portugal

ABSTRACT

Proprioception alterations induced by intense physical exercise may be associated with increased risk of injury. In this sense, the main purpose of the present chapter was to assess the effect of fatigue induced by a soccer match on knee joint position sense in elite soccer players. The second aim of this chapter was to identify possible gender differences in proprioceptive response to fatigue. Twenty soccer players (age: 18.4±1.1 years) were recruited. Knee joint position sense was evaluated using an open kinetic chain technique and active knee positioning, and was reported using absolute and relative angular errors. Knee angles were determined by computer analysis of videotape images of the knee joint using a two-dimensional automatic digitizing module. Joint position sense measures were obtained at rest and immediately after a soccer match. The perceived exertion or exercise intensity was assessed at the end of the match using Borg's rating of perceived exertion (RPE) scale. Of the 20 players, only 17 completed the soccer match reaching or exceeding the score of 15 on the RPE scale. This left 17 players (10 female) for the statistical analysis. After the soccer match a significant increase in absolute (2.1±1.1° to 4.0±2.3°, P=.001) and relative (0.7±2.0° to 3.5±3.1°, P<.001) angular errors was observed. When comparing genders, no differences at rest were observed in absolute (female, 1.8±1.0° vs. male, 2.5±1.2° P>.05) and relative (female, 0.5±1.7° vs. male, 0.8±2.6°, P>.05) errors. However, the absolute error after the match increased to 4.9±3.2° (P=.038) in males and to 3.3±1.2° (P=.014) in females. Additionally, the relative error post-match increased to 3.6±4.8° (P=.049) in males and to 3.3±1.2° (P=.004) in females. No gender differences were detected in the magnitude of the increase in both relative (male, 2.4±2.4° vs. female, 1.6±1.7°; P>.05) and absolute (male, 2.8±3.0° vs. female, 2.8±2.3°; P>.05) angular errors. In conclusion, our results indicate that fatigue induced by a soccer match has a marked deleterious effect on knee joint position sense in elite soccer players irrespective of gender.

Keywords: Soccer, Proprioception, Knee, Fatigue, Gender

INTRODUCTION

Proprioception has been defined as the cumulative neural input to the central nervous system from specialized nerve endings called mechanoreceptors located in joints, capsules, ligaments, muscles, tendons, and skin [1-4]. Proprioception is generally divided into senses of tension, movement, and joint position. Joint position sense represents the ability to perceive a presented joint angle and then actively or passively reproduce the same joint angle following movement of the limb. Proprioception seems to be of vital importance in safely performing a wide range of sporting activities due to its contribution to automatic control of movement, balance, and joint stability [4]. Athletes often suffer injuries in the last third of practice sessions or matches and this may be associated with alterations of lower limb neuromuscular control due to fatigue [5-7].

Soccer exhibits a high prevalence of lower limb injuries, namely knee and ankle sprains [7, 8]. It is a high demanding sporting activity in which muscles are under prolonged and intense stress during matches, which may potentially lead to proprioceptive deficits. This decrease in proprioception may in turn disturb skills accuracy [9] and increase injury risk [10].

Several studies [2,11-14] involving different populations have demonstrated joint position sense deficits as a result of exercise-induced fatigue. These studies were rarely conducted in athletes and the great majority assessed the impact of fatigue induced using laboratory protocols on proprioception. The majority of the laboratory exercise protocols were performed in an isokinetic dynamometer and involved isolated joint movements and muscle groups that did not mimic the specific demands of sporting activities. Additionally, to our knowledge, only two studies [14, 15] have previously assessed changes in proprioception induced by sporting activities. Thus, the main purpose of the present chapter was to assess the effect of fatigue induced by an official soccer match on the knee joint position sense of elite soccer players. It was also our aim to identify possible gender differences in the proprioceptive response to fatigue.

METHODS

Subjects and Study Design

A convenience sample consisting of 20 elite soccer players (age 18.6 ± 1.1 years, height 1.72 ± 0.22 cm, weight 64.4 ± 5.06 kg) with normal knee function was recruited from two soccer teams competing in the Portuguese national championship. One male (n=10, age 18.1

± 0.4 years, height 177 ± 6.5 cm, weight 70.5 ± 4.6 kg) and one female (n=10, age 18.9 ± 1.3 years, height 167 ± 4.0 cm, weight 58.3 ± 5.56 kg) team with an average of 10.6 ± 1.3 years of soccer experience took part in this investigation. Inclusion criteria were: normal knee range of motion, position players (goalkeepers were excluded), completion of a 90-minute soccer match, a rate of perceived exertion (RPE) of 15 or above after the soccer match, and practice of soccer for a minimum of eight years with a frequency of at least three times per week. Participants were excluded according to the following criteria: lower limb or lower back injury in the six months previous to the study, history of knee surgery, use of medication that influenced motor control and/or attention, and vestibular / neuromuscular disorders. The subjects were appropriately familiarized with the experimental protocol and apparatus prior to beginning the study. The knee of the dominant limb, defined as the limb used to kick a ball, was tested. Appropriate ethical approval from our institutional board was granted prior to the commencement of the study. All participants provided written informed consent, and all procedures were conducted according to the Helsinki Declaration of 1975.

In brief, the study design was as follows: recruitment and selection of study subjects was performed one month before data collection. RPE and knee joint position sense were measured at rest and immediately after a competitive soccer match of 90 minutes duration. Due to the time required to accurately assess the acute effects of the match on joint position sense, only two players were evaluated in each match. Additionally, the time to procure data before the match was very small, so a total of ten (five matches of each gender competition) competitive matches were used to collect data from 20 players.

Assessment of Rate of Perceived Exertion

The Borg's rating of perceived exertion scale (scale of 6 to 20 points) was used to assess the RPE at rest and immediately after the soccer match. The aim of using the RPE scale was to ensure that the demands of the game were sufficiently intense to induce fatigue. According to previous studies [12, 14, 16], players were considered to be fatigued if they reported an RPE of 15 or above. It was reported that a score of 15 on a scale of 6 to 20 is strongly correlated with metabolic responses of fatigue including respiratory exchange, heart rate, absolute oxygen consumption, and blood lactate concentration [17].

Assessment of Knee Joint Position Sense

Knee joint position sense (JPS) of the dominant limb was obtained prior to and immediately after the soccer match during open kinetic chain exercises using a technique of ipsilateral active knee matching responses (without visual input) of a passively determined target position.

Prior to JPS assessment, four reflective markers were fixed with double-sided adhesive tape to the apex of the greater trochanter, iliotibial tract level with the posterior crease of the knee flexed to 80°, neck of the fibula, and prominence of the lateral malleolus. Each pair of markers represented the axis of the thigh and lower leg, respectively. Markers were removed after the baseline evaluation and their place was marked on the skin to avoid differences between evaluations. Knee joint positions in the sagittal plane were recorded with a video camera mounted on a tripod at a distance of five meters from the athlete. The camera was manually focused on the field of view, and natural vertical and horizontal lines in the videotaped environment were aligned parallel to the horizontal and vertical edges of the viewfinder to minimize camera tilt. The athletes were then seated in a comfortable position with the legs hanging freely. The starting position was 90° of knee flexion and the knees were then repositioned into extension.

After positioning of the subject and placement of the markers, one test position at a midrange of knee range of motion (between 40° and 60° of knee flexion) was investigated via the following sequence. The examiner (at approximately 10°/s) moved the knee from the starting position of 90° of flexion to a knee angle between 40° and 60° of flexion. The subject then maintained the target position actively (isometrically) for five seconds in order to identify that position. The knee was then moved by the examiner (at approximately 10°/s) to the starting position. Finally, the subject actively reproduced the target angle to the best of their ability and held it for three seconds. Each subject performed three consecutive trials.

Knee angles were determined by computer analysis of the videotape images of the knee joint using the two-dimensional automatic digitizing module of the Ariel Performance Analysis System software (Ariel Dynamics, CA, USA). Each target or matching position was determined as the average of seven consecutive knee angles digitized at 50 Hz from the videotape view of each position.

Knee joint position sense was reported as: (i) absolute angular error defined as the absolute difference between the test position and the position reproduced by the subject, which represents accuracy without directional bias, and (ii) relative angular error defined as the signed arithmetic difference between a test and response position, which represents accuracy with directional bias.

A previous study [18] reported that the intraclass correlation coefficient (ICC) of this method of knee position sense assessment was 0.82 for absolute angular error and 0.85 for relative angular error. The authors also computed the standard error of measurement (SEM) [19] and the smallest real difference (SRD) [20]. They indicated that the SEM was 0.34° and 0.55° and the SRD was 0.94° and 1.52°, respectively, for absolute and relative angular error.

DATA ANALYSIS

All data was analyzed using SPSS for windows (SPSS, version 17.0; SPSS, Inc., Chicago, Illinois). Variables were tested for normal distribution with the Shapiro–Wilk test. All data was expressed as mean ± SD. Paired t-tests were performed to compare the mean differences between joint position sense prior to and after the soccer match. Independent t-tests were used to compare joint position sense among genders at rest and to compare the magnitude of the change in joint position sense. $P<0.05$ was considered statistically significant.

RESULTS

From the twenty athletes that began the study, three male athletes were excluded. This left seventeen athletes (age 18.6 ± 1.1 years) for statistical analysis [10 female and 7 male (age 18.1 ± 0.4 years, height 178 ± 6.9 cm, weight 70.9 ± 3.8 kg)]. Three athletes were excluded due to replacement secondary to physical complaints or coach's decision during the match in which they were assessed. All participants that completed the soccer match (90 minutes duration) reached or exceeded 15 on the RPE scale. Significant increases in absolute and relative angular errors were observed after the soccer match when compared to pre-match data (Table 1).

Table 1. Effects of the soccer match on knee position sense in both genders

Variable	Gender	Rest	After match	P-value
AAE	Female	1.8 ± 1.0°	3.3 ± 1.2°	0.014
	Male	2.5 ± 1.3°	4.9 ± 3.2°	0.038
	Total	2.1 ± 1.1°	4.0 ± 2.3°	0.001
RAE	Female	0.5 ± 1.7°	3.3 ± 1.2°	0.004
	Male	0.8 ± 2.6°	3.6 ± 4.8°	0.049
	Total	0.7 ± 2.1°	3.5 ± 3.1°	<0.001

P-values given reflect changes over time (rest vs. after match). AAE, absolute angular error; RAE, relative angular error.

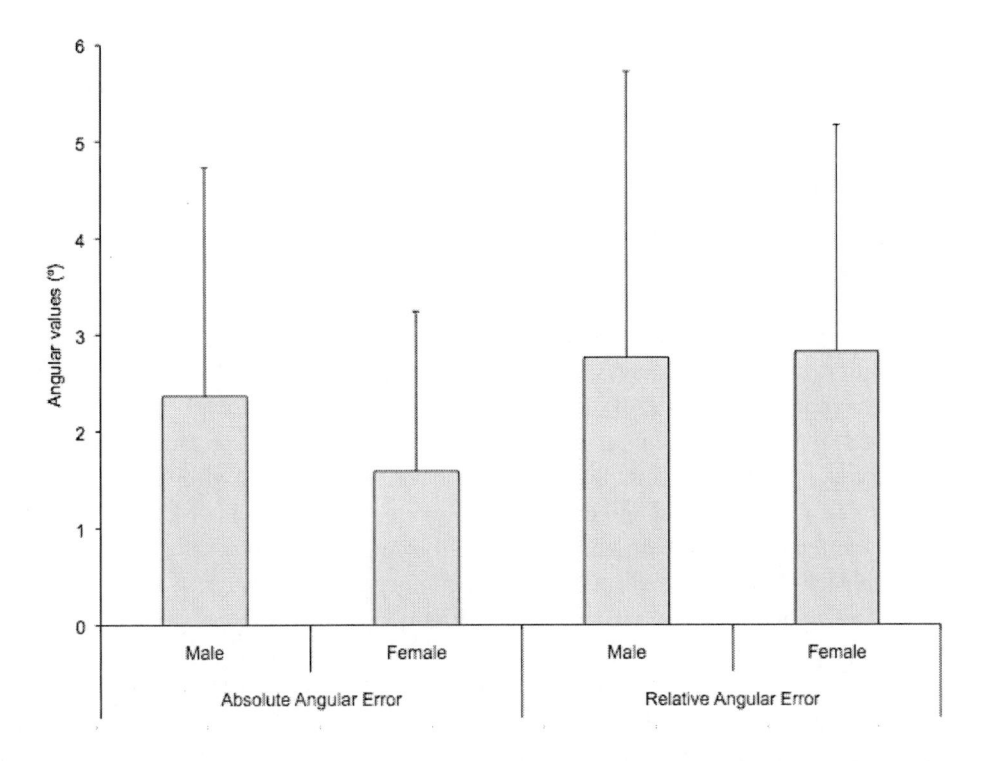

Figure 1. Magnitude of joint position sense increase [in degrees (°)] induced by the soccer match.

When comparing genders, no differences were observed in absolute and relative (female, 0.5 ± 1.7° vs. male, 0.8 ± 2.6°, P>.05) angular errors at rest.

The relative error showed directional bias in movement to extension. Both before and immediately after the match, the players overestimated the target position determined by the examiner (i.e. players reproduced lower knee flexion angles than the pre-determined flexion angle). Match-induced fatigue markedly exacerbated the overestimation of the target position.

After the match, both the absolute and relative angular errors increased significantly. No gender differences were detected in the magnitude of the increase in relative (male, 2.4 ± 2.4° vs. female, 1.6 ± 1.7°; P>.05) and absolute (male, 2.8 ± 3.0° vs. female, 2.8 ± 2.3°; P>.05) angular errors (Figure 1).

DISCUSSION

The main findings of the present chapter indicate that knee joint position sense is decreased as consequence of fatigue induced by prolonged intermittent exercise sustained during a soccer match.

One major difference between our study and others is that fatigue was not induced by a laboratory protocol in our study, but rather by participation in a professional soccer match. In this sense, the results of the present investigation can appropriately be transferred to the athletic setting. It is important to mention that active testing was selected instead of passive testing due to its accuracy [21, 22], functionality, and maximization of the input of muscle spindles. Additionally, one test position was selected between 40° and 60°, as this is the range where the input of muscle receptors are the main source of feedback for knee joint position sense [23].

The evaluation of RPE was performed to ensure that the match intensity was adjusted to fulfill its goals of inducing fatigue on soccer players. The values of perceived exertion were not surprising at the conclusion of the match since it has already been described that soccer players experience reduced performance in the later stages of a match [24]. In soccer, fatigue seems to affect physical performance during the match with players experiencing reduced exercise intensity and sprint performance in the later stages of a match [24]. This impaired exercise ability in the last stages of a match has been attributed to low glycogen concentrations in muscle fibers [24], dehydration, and hyperthermia [25].

The effect of fatiguing exercise on proprioception has been investigated using different exercise protocols, which limits the comparison of our results with previous studies. Nonetheless, our findings are in agreement with previous studies [2, 11, 14, 26, 27] that have examined the effects of fatigue on knee joint position sense. Ribeiro et al. assessed the effect of fatigue induced by a volleyball match on knee joint position sense in 17 (age 18.9 ± 4.2 years) elite volleyball players and reported a significant increase in absolute (2.1°) and relative (1.7°) angular errors after the match [14].

Fatigue may impair proprioceptive acuity by increasing the threshold of muscle spindle discharge and disrupting afferent feedback. A mechanism to explain the decrease in proprioception observed following exercise has been though to lie in the increased intramuscular concentrations of several metabolites and inflammatory substances. This finding has been thought to have a direct impact on the discharge pattern of muscle spindles and alpha–gamma coactivation [28, 29]. In fatigued muscles, nociceptors could thus be activated by the end metabolic products (including bradykinin, arachidonic acid, prostaglandin E2, potassium, and lactic acid) produced during a soccer match. These metabolites and/or inflammatory substances modify the proprioceptive input by increasing the threshold for muscle spindle discharge [29-31], leading to an increase in error in position matching tasks. It has also been proposed that changes in alpha/gamma co-activation or alpha motoneuron activation induced by fatigue could alter muscle spindle excitability through stretch [32]. The observed decrease in joint position sense acuity may also be explained, at least partially, by alterations in the central processing of proprioceptive signals. It has been reported that central fatigue may reduce the accuracy of motor control and interrupt voluntary muscle-stabilizing activity to resist imparted joint forces [27].

Some study limitations should be recognized. These lie mainly in the lack of assessment of maximum voluntary muscle strength, which could had enabled us to provide a direct measure of muscle function to determine the changes related to exercise-induced fatigue. This question remains to be answered in future studies, along with the length of time that the deleterious effect of match-induced fatigue on joint position sense might last.

CONCLUSION

The findings presented in this chapter suggest that fatigue induced by a soccer match diminishes the knee joint position sense acuity of elite soccer players irrespective of gender.

REFERENCES

[1]   Carpenter, JE; Blasier, RB; Pellizzon, GG. The effects of muscle fatigue on shoulder joint position sense. *Am. J. Sports Med.* 1998 26(2),262-5.

[2]   Ribeiro, F; Mota, J; Oliveira, J. Effect of exercise-induced fatigue on position sense of the knee in the elderly. *Eur. J. Appl. Physiol.* 2007 99(4),379-85.

[3]   Voight, ML; Hardin, JA; Blackburn, TA; Tippett, S; Canner, GC. The effects of muscle fatigue on and the relationship of arm dominance to shoulder proprioception. *J. Orthop. Sports Phys. Ther.* 1996 23(6),348-52.

[4]   Riemann, BL; Lephart, SM. The Sensorimotor System, Part I: The Physiologic Basis of Functional Joint Stability. *J. Athl. Train.* 2002 37(1),71-9.

[5]   Barrack, RL; Skinner, HB; Buckley, SL. Proprioception in the anterior cruciate deficient knee. *Am. J. Sports Med.* 1989 17(1),1-6.

[6]   Hiemstra, LA; Lo, IK; Fowler, PJ. Effect of fatigue on knee proprioception: implications for dynamic stabilization. *J. Orthop. Sports Phys. Ther.* 2001 31(10),598-605.

[7]   Rahnama, N; Reilly, T; Lees, A. Injury risk associated with playing actions during competitive soccer. *Br. J. Sports Med.* 2002 36(5),354-9.

[8]   Walden, M; Hagglund, M; Ekstrand, J. UEFA Champions League study: a prospective study of injuries in professional football during the 2001-2002 season. *Br. J. Sports Med.* 2005 39(8),542-6.

[9]   Ribeiro, F; Oliveira, J. Aging effects on joint proprioception: the role of physical activity in proprioception preservation. *Eur. Rev. Aging Phys Act.* 2007 4,71-6.

[10]   Thacker, SB; Stroup, DF; Branche, CM; Gilchrist, J; Goodman, RA; Porter Kelling, E. Prevention of knee injuries in sports. A systematic review of the literature. *J. Sports Med. Phys. Fitness.* 2003 43(2),165-79.

[11]   Lattanzio, PJ; Petrella, RJ; Sproule, JR; Fowler, PJ. Effects of fatigue on knee proprioception. *Clin. J. Sport Med.* 1997 7(1),22-7.

[12]   Tripp, BL; Boswell, L; Gansneder, BM; Shultz, SJ. Functional Fatigue Decreases 3-Dimensional Multijoint Position Reproduction Acuity in the Overhead-Throwing Athlete. *J. Athl. Train.* 2004 39(4),316-20.

[13]   Lee, HM; Liau, JJ; Cheng, CK; Tan, CM; Shih, JT. Evaluation of shoulder proprioception following muscle fatigue. *Clin. Biomech. (Bristol, Avon).* 2003 18(9),843-7.

[14]   Ribeiro, F; Santos, F; Gonçalves, P; Oliveira, J. Effects of volleyball matchinduced fatigue on knee joint position sense. *Eur. J. Sport Sci.* 2008 8(6),397-402.

[15]   Brown, JP; Bowyer, GW. Effects of fatigue on ankle stability and proprioception in university sportspeople. *Br. J. Sports Med.* 2002 36(4),310.

[16]   Pandolf, KB; Billings, DS; Drolet, LL; Pimental, NA; Sawka, MN. Differential ratings of perceived exertion and various physiological responses during prolonged upper and lower body exercise. *Eur. J. Appl. Physiol. Occup. Physiol.* 1984 53(1),5-11.

[17]   Edwards, RH; Melcher, A; Hesser, CM; Wigertz, O; Ekelund, LG. Physiological correlates of perceived exertion in continuous and intermittent exercise with the same average power output. *Eur. J. Clin. Invest.* 1972 2(2),108-14.

[18]   Magalhaes, T; Ribeiro, F; Pinheiro, A; Oliveira, J. Warming-up before sporting activity improves knee position sense. *Phys. Ther. Sport.* 2010 11(3),86-90.

[19]   Weir, JP. Quantifying test-retest reliability using the intraclass correlation coefficient and the SEM. *J. Strength Cond. Res.* 2005 19(1),231-40.

[20]   Beckerman, H; Roebroeck, ME; Lankhorst, GJ; Becher, JG; Bezemer, PD; Verbeek, AL. Smallest real difference, a link between reproducibility and responsiveness. *Qual. Life Res.* 2001 10(7),571-8.

[21]   Pickard, CM; Sullivan, PE; Allison, GT; Singer, KP. Is there a difference in hip joint position sense between young and older groups? *J. Gerontol. A Biol. Sci. Med. Sci.* 2003 58(7),631-5.

[22]   Proske, U; Wise, AK; Gregory, JE. The role of muscle receptors in the detection of movements. *Prog. Neurobiol.* 2000 60(1),85-96.

[23]   Olsson, L; Lund, H; Henriksen, M; Rogind, H; Bliddal, H; Danneskiold-Samsoe, B. Test-retest reliability of a knee joint position sense measurement method in sitting and prone position. *Adv. Physiother.* 2004 6(1),37-47.

[24]   Mohr, M; Krustrup, P; Bangsbo, J. Fatigue in soccer: a brief review. *J. Sports Sci.* 2005 23(6),593-9.

[25]   Reilly, T. Energetics of high-intensity exercise (soccer) with particular reference to fatigue. *J. Sports Sci.* 1997 15(3),257-63.

[26]   Skinner, HB; Wyatt, MP; Hodgdon, JA; Conard, DW; Barrack, RL. Effect of fatigue on joint position sense of the knee. *J. Orthop. Res.* 1986 4(1),112-8.

[27]   Miura, K; Ishibashi, Y; Tsuda, E; Okamura, Y; Otsuka, H; Toh, S. The effect of local and general fatigue on knee proprioception. *Arthroscopy.* 2004 20(4),414-8.

[28] Pedersen, J; Lonn, J; Hellstrom, F; Djupsjobacka, M; Johansson, H. Localized muscle fatigue decreases the acuity of the movement sense in the human shoulder. *Med. Sci. Sports Exerc.* 1999 31(7),1047-52.

[29] Pedersen, J; Sjolander, P; Wenngren, BI; Johansson, H. Increased intramuscular concentration of bradykinin increases the static fusimotor drive to muscle spindles in neck muscles of the cat. *Pain.* 1997 70(1),83-91.

[30] Djupsjobacka, M; Johansson, H; Bergenheim, M. Influences on the gamma-muscle-spindle system from muscle afferents stimulated by increased intramuscular concentrations of arachidonic acid. *Brain Res.* 1994 663(2),293-302.

[31] Djupsjobacka, M; Johansson, H; Bergenheim, M; Wenngren, BI. Influences on the gamma-muscle spindle system from muscle afferents stimulated by increased intramuscular concentrations of bradykinin and 5-HT. *Neurosci. Res.* 1995 22(3),325-33.

[32] Marks, R; Quinney, HA. Effect of fatiguing maximal isokinetic quadriceps contractions on ability to estimate knee-position. *Percept. Mot. Skills.* 1993 77(3 Pt 2),1195-202.

In: The Knee
Editor: Randy Mascarenhas

ISBN: 978-1-61942-268-1
© 2012 Nova Science Publishers, Inc.

Chapter V

KNEE JOINT KINEMATICS IN HEALTHY CHILDREN AND CHILDREN WITH HYPERMOBILITY SYNDROME

Francis Fatoye[1] and Marietta van der Linden[2]

[1] Department of Health Professions, Manchester Metropolitan University,
Manchester, UK
[2] Physiotherapy Subject Area, Queen Margaret University,
Musselburgh, UK

INTRODUCTION

Gait analysis is a broad term that can refer to many different methods of evaluating an individual's walking pattern [1]. One of the main purposes of the rehabilitative process is to help patients achieve a high level of functional independence within the limits of their particular impairments. Human gait is one of the basic components of independent functioning that is commonly affected by either disease processes or injury.

In children, gait may be affected by age [2], walking speed [3, 4, 5], pathological conditions and the ability of clinicians to accurately measure gait parameters in a repeatable manner. Abnormal gait kinematics has been reported in children with rheumatological conditions such as juvenile idiopathic arthritis [6] and hypermobility syndrome [7, 8]. It is believed that a combination of pain, generalized joint laxity, reduced joint proprioception, muscle weakness and reduced stamina may affect the gait of a child with hypermobility syndrome [9].

Gait analysis may be used to identify the mechanisms causing gait pattern dysfunction in children [10]. It can also be used to classify the severity of disability, predict patient prognosis, and describe the differences between a patient's performance and normal gait [11, 12]. Gait analysis has also been shown to be effective in guiding the management of children with Cerebral Palsy [13].

Gait kinematics analysis is an important component of gait analysis, as it enables clinicians to identify any gait impairments and document any changes following treatment interventions [14, 15]. Despite this, the ability of clinicians to perform gait analysis may vary over time.

This chapter will discuss the effect of age and walking speed on knee joint kinematics in children using data in healthy children. Reproducibility of knee kinematics assessment in healthy children and children with hypermobility syndrome is also discussed. The chapter will also examine how knee joint kinematics are affected in children with hypermobility syndrome compared to their healthy counterparts.

FACTORS INFLUENCING KNEE KINEMATICS IN CHILDREN

Kinematics is the study of movements in the absence of the forces producing them [2]. The influence of age and walking speed on knee kinematics will be discussed in section.

INFLUENCE OF AGE

Knowledge of the influence of age on gait kinematics is important for diagnosis and development of appropriate treatment interventions for children with gait pathology. There is limited information on the influence of age on gait kinematics in children. It is a generally believed that kinematics patterns in children differ from adults [2], but start to look similar to adults by 3 to 4 years of age [16,17]. Additionally, minimal differences in knee joint angles during walking have been observed in children aged 1 to 7 years [17].

Ganley and Powers [18] examined knee gait kinematics in fifteen 7-year old children using a six-camera Vicon motion analysis system. All children were screened to rule out any neurological or musculoskeletal problems that would affect gait. The authors found no significant differences in knee joint kinematics between the 7-year olds and adults. Similarly, Oberg et al. [19] reported only minor changes in knee kinematics with age when they compared adults with children. They reported differences measuring less than one degree when comparing knee kinematics in participants 10-19 years of age with those 20-29 years old.

INFLUENCE OF GAIT SPEED

Dimensionless walking speed has been found to be an important determinant of gait in healthy children [3, 4, 5]. In a five year longitudinal study by Stansfied et al. [3], the authors found that gait kinematics were significantly influenced by gait speed. In a follow-up study, Stansfield et al. [4] reported that gait kinematics were strongly influenced by walking speed in a 5-year longitudinal study of twenty six 5-year-old healthy children using a three dimensional motion analysis system.

Van der Linden et al. [5] examined gait kinematic characteristics of healthy children walking at a range of clinically relevant walking speeds. Thirty-six healthy children with a mean age of nine participated in the study. Knee kinematics were measured at five different dimensionless speeds for each child using the Vicon camera system. The authors observed that knee kinematics varied with speed and that the effect of speed on knee kinematics was not linear [5]. For example, the peak knee flexion in swing did not vary much between the three fastest speeds, but decreased for the two slowest speeds.

REPEATABILITY OF GAIT KINEMATICS

Repeatability is the extent to which an instrument can consistently measure the same parameter under specified conditions [20]. A repeatable measurement tool measures a variable consistently on multiple occasions with accuracy, predictability, and without variation [20].

Accurate assessment of gait can aid diagnosis by helping to identify subtle gait abnormalities in children with conditions such as hypermobility syndrome (HMS). It also enables the clinician to evaluate progress or regression and to modify any treatment interventions [21].

Research in physiotherapy focuses on alleviating impairments and evaluating the efficacy of treatment interventions [22]. Abnormal gait kinematics may be found in children with HMS [8] and it has been suggested that gait analysis be added to clinical examination to complement anthropometric, clinical and laboratory data [23]. Furthermore, abnormal joint kinematics, pain and neuromuscular deficits are all co-existent in children with HMS [7]. This is important to remember when considering the mechanisms, prevention and assessment of orthopaedic conditions [24].

The primary goals of providing physiotherapy to children with musculoskeletal complaints are to alleviate their impairments, improve their functional status, and improve their overall quality of life [22]. Computerized three dimensional motion analysis systems have been used to assess gait kinematics and to identify gait abnormalities in children with various musculoskeletal conditions. In order for an assessment method to obtain widespread clinical acceptance as a useful clinical tool, the repeatability of its measurement is a fundamental requirement that must be sufficiently established [25]. Although repeatability of measurement of knee kinematics in healthy children and children with Cerebral Palsy have been assessed in previously[26], repeatability of measurement of knee kinematics has not been reported in children with HMS. Gait kinematics in children and the ability to examine them may vary over time. Therefore, it is important to ascertain the repeatability of gait kinematics in healthy children and those with HMS using 3D motion analysis.

ASSESSMENT OF TEST-RETEST REPEATABILITY OF GAIT KINEMATICS

Test-retest repeatability of an instrument is the consistency with which it measures the same parameter on multiple occasions under the same conditions [27]. This is assessed by taking repeated measurements across the range of values expected to be found in actual use of the instrument [27].

Twenty children (10 healthy and 10 with HMS) aged 8 – 15 years participated in this investigation. The healthy group was recruited from local schools in Edinburgh and consisted of five boys and five girls. The HMS cohort was recruited from the Royal Hospital for Sick

Children in Edinburgh and was made up of two boys and eight girls diagnosed with HMS. None of the subjects enrolled in the study had history of trauma to either knee joint. No subject had visual impairment and none suffered from any systemic or vestibular-system disorders. Written informed consent was obtained from the participants and their parents/guardians before participation in the study. This study was approved by QMU Ethics Committee, the Education Department of the City of Edinburgh Council and the NHS Lothian Local Research Ethics committee. Participants were tested twice (one week apart).

A brief explanation of the procedure was given to each subject before the testing. Subjects wore lycra shorts and their physical characteristics were assessed. Height was measured using a standiometer and body mass was measured with a weighing scale. Leg length was determined in the supine position as the distance between the most prominent point of the anterior superior iliac spine (ASIS) to the most prominent point of the ipsilateral medial malleolus using a measuring tape [28]. Lower limb dominance was also established as the leg used by the subject to kick a soccer ball [28, 29]. The test limb (knee) of the healthy children was determined using computer randomization on SPSS. The more symptomatic (painful) knee of the HMS subjects was tested.

Knee joint kinematics were assessed using the Vicon 612 3-D motion analysis system (Vicon Oxford Metrics Ltd., Oxford, England). Eight M8 Vicon cameras (Oxford Metrics Ltd, Oxford, England) were used, operating at a 100 Hz sampling rate. Fifteen (14 mm diameter) infra-red reflective markers were attached to the following anatomical locations: the sacral marker was placed at the mid-point of the line connecting the posterior superior iliac spines, bilateral pelvic markers on both anterior superior iliac spines, and thigh wand markers on the midpoint of the line connecting the greater trochanter and femoral condyle. Knee markers were placed on the lateral femoral condyles, shank wand markers were placed on the mid point of the line between the knee joint line and the lateral malleoli, and ankle markers were placed on the lateral malleoli. Toe markers were placed between the second and third metatarsal head and heel markers on the calcaneum in vertical alignment with the toe markers. All measurements were carried out by a single rater.

Each subject was instructed to walk barefoot six times at a self-selected pace along a seven meter walkway. The first two meters allowed for acceleration and normal ambulation, the last two meters allowed for deceleration, and the middle three meters were used for data capturing. Subjects performed at least six trials [30] and the average knee joint angles during the six walks normalized for one full gait cycle were calculated for the subjects using Polygon® software.

The test-retest repeatability of the data collected during the two sessions in both healthy children and children with HMS were analyzed using measures of repeatability calculated for each group: Intraclass correlation coefficient (ICC) and 95% limits of agreement [31, 32]. ICC values were considered poor when they were below 0.6, good between 0.6 and 8.0 and excellent if 0.8 and above [33, 34].

The mean (Standard Deviation) of knee kinematics measurements, ICC values and the 95% limits of agreement between these sessions (1 and 2) in healthy children and children with HMS are summarized in Tables 1 and 2 respectively. Figures 3 and 4 show the mean knee joint angle measurements during walking in healthy children and HMS children.

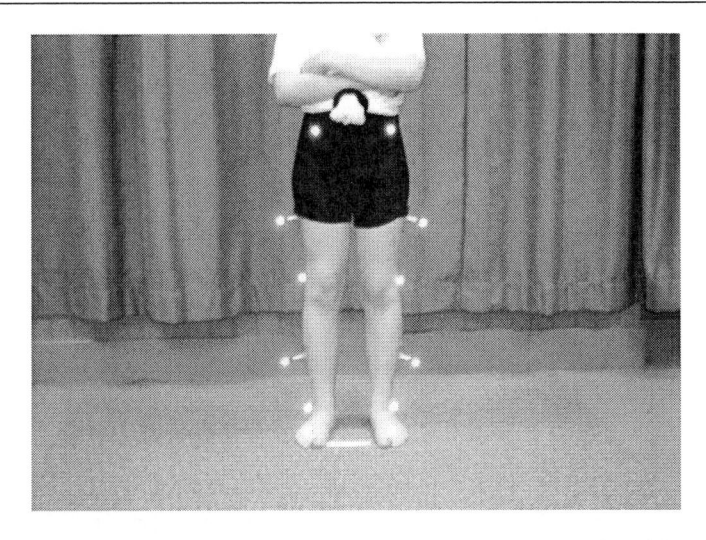

Figure 1. Marker placement on anatomical landmarks (anterior view) – reproduced from Fatoye (2008).

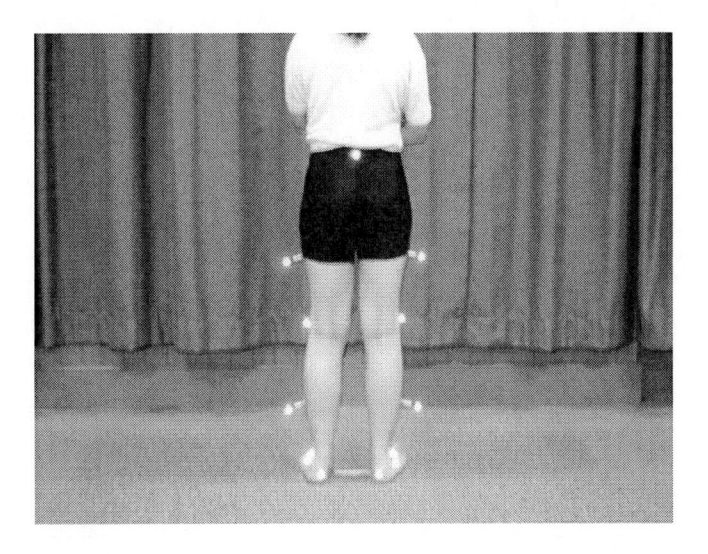

Figure 2. Marker placement on anatomical landmarks (posterior view) – reproduced from Fatoye (2008).

Table 1. Results of test-retest repeatability in healthy children

Variable	Day 1 Mean (SD)	Day 2 Mean (SD)	ICC	95% Limits of Agreement between measurements
Peak Knee Extension Mid Stance (0)	4.7 (5.9)	3.9 (3.6)	0.74	-7.75 to 10.28
Knee Flexion During Loading Response (0)	19.6 (9.4)	18.2 (6.3)	0.84	-6.15 to 7.59
Maximum Knee Flexion (0)	61.9 (8.0)	59.4 (6.9)	0.48	-12.91 to 17.42

ICC = Intraclass correlation coefficient; SD = Standard deviation.

Table 2. Results of test-retest repeatability in children with HMS

Variable	Day 1 Mean (SD)	Day 2 Mean (SD)	ICC	95% Limits of Agreement between measurements
Peak Knee Extension in Mid Stance (0)	-0.73 (3.93)	-1.54 (4.19)	0.68	-5.74 to 7.38
Knee Flexion During Loading Response (0)	12.86 (4.77)	12.63 (3.38)	0.48	-8.50 to 8.95
Maximum Knee Flexion (0)	52.98 (3.55)	52.58 (3.41)	0.81	-4.07 to 4.86

ICC = Intraclass correlation coefficient; SD = Standard deviation. A negative value for extension signifies flexion.

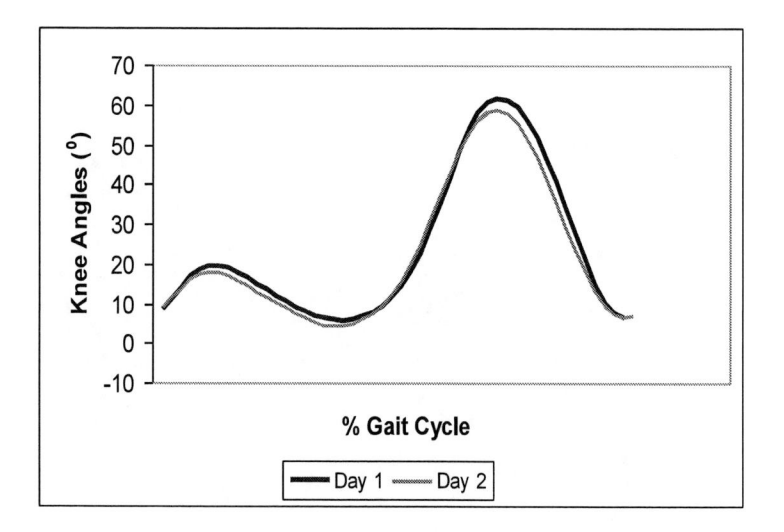

Figure 3. Repeated measurements of sagittal knee motion during walking in healthy children.

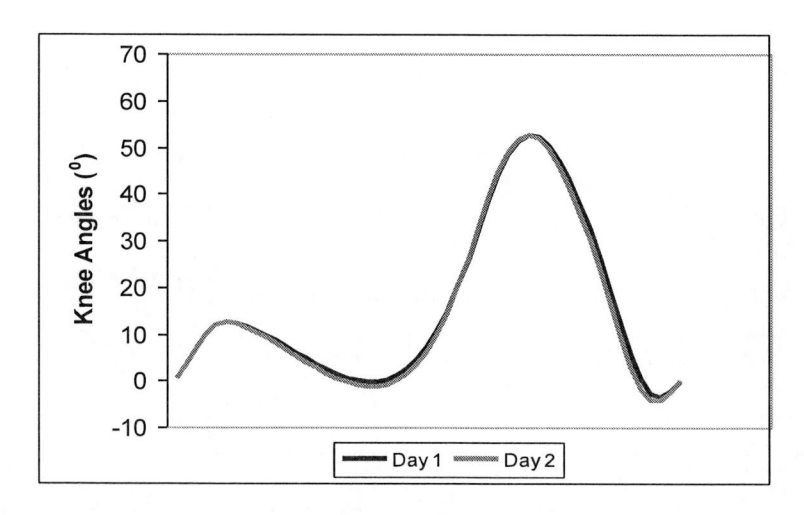

Figure 4. Repeated measurements of sagittal knee motion during walking in children with HMS.

The results of repeatability based on ICC show that knee flexion during the loading response and maximum knee flexion were measured with excellent repeatability in healthy children (ICC = 0.84) and those with HMS (ICC = 0.81) respectively. However, 95% limits of agreement LOA showed a small amount of measurement error between days for functional ROM in healthy children, with the exception of maximum knee flexion. In addition, LOA demonstrated minimal variation during repeated measurements of knee kinematics in children with HMS, indicating excellent repeatability with the exception of maximum knee flexion during swing in healthy children.

These findings are in agreement with those of Gorton et al. [35]. They reported low between-days repeatability of knee joint kinematics in healthy children using the VICON system. Marker placement was carried out by the investigator on both days. Despite the extreme care taken in marker placement, it was difficult to repeatedly align the knee joint axis of rotation. Therefore, the results seen for knee joint kinematics may have been influenced by error in determining the axis of the knee joint in children [36]. The results of knee kinematic measures could also have been influenced by skin movement due to reflective marker placement on the skin. Walking patterns in children are affected by speed, mood, and fatigue [37]. All these could have affected the test-retest repeatability of knee kinematics in this study.

Since children with HMS may present with pain, it was anticipated that test-retest repeatability was going to be poorer in children with this condition than the controls. However, it was interesting to observe that based on 95% LOA, the test-retest variation of knee kinematics measurements was lower in the HMS group than in controls. The reasons for these findings are not obvious. It has been observed that younger children had lower test-retest repeatability of knee kinematics measurements than their older counterparts [35]. Therefore, the results of test-retest repeatability of knee kinematics presented in this chapter may be due to the age difference of the participants, as the HMS cohort was on average two years older than the healthy group. These findings suggest that the results of measuring knee kinematics in healthy children and those with HMS should be used with caution.

GAIT KINEMATICS IN CHILDREN WITH HMS

Twenty-nine children with HMS and 37 healthy children participated in this study. The testing procedure was as presented above for the repeatability study. Analyses were performed using the Statistical Package for the Social Sciences (SPSS) version 13 (Chicago, IL). Differences between groups for knee kinematics and gait speed were examined using independent t-test analysis. Statistical significance was set at $p < 0.05$.

Participant characteristics and the mean (standard deviation = SD) values for knee kinematic measurements in healthy children and those with HMS are illustrated in Table 3. The mean knee angles in the sagittal plane in the two groups are shown in Figure 5. The peak knee flexion during loading response and maximum knee flexion were both significantly lower (both $p < 0.001$) in children with HMS than the controls. Children with HMS also demonstrated significantly increased ($p < 0.001$) knee extension in mid-stance compared with the controls. These findings imply that children with HMS ambulate with a gait involving reduced knee flexion and increased knee extension in comparison with the healthy controls. Gait speed was not significantly ($p = 0.496$) different between healthy children and those with HMS.

Table 3. Participants' characteristics and mean (SD) values of gait kinematics

Cohort	Healthy children (n = 37)	Children with HMS (n = 29)	p - values
Age (years)	11.5(2.6)	11.9 (1.8)	0.482
Body Mass (kg)	48.3 (4.3)	51.7 (17.3)	0.386
Height (cm)	153.0 (16.0)	152.0 (15.0)	0.814
Peak Knee Flexion LR (0)	20.0 (6.1)	12.6(4.7)	**<0.001**
Peak Knee Extension	4.2 (5.5)	-1.0 (3.5)	**<0.001**
Peak Knee Flexion Swing	60.4(6.6)	53.5(4.6)	**<0.001**
Gait Speed (m/s)	1.2 (0.4)	1.2 (0.1)	0.496

LR = Loading response; SD = Standard Deviation; Significant p values are indicated in boldface.

In summary, knee extension during walking was significantly higher (p < 0.001) in children with HMS than the controls. Additionally, knee flexion (during loading response and maximum flexion in swing phase) during walking was significantly (p < 0.001) lower in children with HMS than the controls. To date, functional range of motion (ROM) during walking has not been investigated in either children or adults with HMS.

Possible Reason for Reduced Knee Flexion and Increased Extension in Children with HMS

The reasons behind reduced knee flexion and increased knee extension during walking are unclear. Based on ICC and 95% limits of agreement, some of the functional ROM parameters were found to have low between-days repeatability in healthy children and those with HMS (Tables 1 and 2). However, the repeatability of t-tests demonstrated no significant differences (p range = 0.328 to 0.875) between repeated measurements (one week apart) of functional ROM parameters.

It has been demonstrated that knee flexion angle at the end of loading/midstance increases with higher walking speeds [3], and diminished knee flexion during walking has been attributed to reduced walking speed [5]. However, there was no significant difference (p = 0.496) in walking speed between the control and HMS groups.

Another explanation for the results seen in our study may be that joint laxity in children with HMS could have increased knee varus and valgus moments when compared with controls due to laxity of the knee joint. This would possibly prevent normal sagittal motion of the knee joint during walking and may serve as an area for future investigation. It has also been suggested that reduced knee flexion during walking may be due to muscle weakness [38]. Therefore, the increased knee extension and reduced knee flexion during walking may be due to knee muscle weakness that was observed in these children with HMS [39].

Pain perception has also been shown to be significantly higher in children with HMS than their healthy counterparts [40]. Pain may reduce knee flexion during walking as individuals attempt to minimize the shear forces that accompany knee joint motion and to reduce the compressive force from a contracting quadriceps [38]. It is acknowledged that pain with walking was not examined in our study, but paired t-test analysis revealed no statistically significant differences in maximum knee flexion during swing between the more painful and less painful limbs in children with HMS. As a result, it is unlikely that the level of pain in children with HMS could have accounted for the observed findings.

The reduced knee flexion and hyperextension during the loading response may be due to reduced tibial progression, which requires more plantar flexion of the ankle in pre-swing to progress the leg forward [40]. Toe-walking observed in children with HMS [41] may also reduce the need to flex the contralateral knee during swing for clearance of the foot [40].

The observed findings of reduced maximum knee flexion during loading response in swing phase may be the result of impaired knee joint position sense. This finding has been suggested to cause people with HMS to move their joints to positions outside their normal range of motion [42]. This may also be the case in children with HMS, as these children have been found to have impaired joint position sense [39]. The data presented in this chapter has provided reference values of knee kinematic data in these children with which future investigations can be compared. The observed findings of knee kinematics imply that children with HMS walk with a knee hyperextension. Gait kinematics assessment in children diagnosed with HMS may be useful and they may benefit from gait re-education programs to reduce increased knee flexion during stance and decrease knee hyperextension.

CONCLUSION

This chapter has discussed the effects of age on knee kinematics in children. It has also examined the repeatability of measuring knee kinematics in healthy children and children with HMS. Review of the literature suggests that there are only minor changes in knee kinematics in children compared with adults [18, 19]. It has also been shown that gait kinematics vary with gait speed in children. This therefore implies that walking speed, especially dimensionless walking speed which accounts for changes in leg length, is an important factor to be considered when making a clinical decision regarding gait pathology in children. The evidence presented in this chapter indicates that test-retest repeatability of knee joint kinematics assessment in healthy children and children with HMS ranged form poor to excellent.

This chapter has demonstrated that on average, children with HMS had reduced knee flexion in swing and increased knee extension during stance compared with healthy children. It therefore suggests children with HMS may walk with knee hyperextension. Abnormal gait kinematics in children with musculoskeletal disorders such as those with HMS could be due to pain, muscle weakness and impaired joint proprioception. Gait kinematics may be an important component of clinical assessment of children with HMS. Clinicians and physiotherapists should be aware of gait abnormalities in children with HMS as those who experience problematic symptoms during walking may benefit from gait re-education programmes via muscle strengthening exercises and the use of ankle and foot orthotic devices.

REFERENCES

[1] Rose, S. A. Õunpuu S., DeLuca, P. A. 1991. "Strategies for the assessment of pediatric gait in the clinical setting". *Physical Therapy*, vol. 71. no. 12: pp. 961-980.

[2] Sutherland D. H. 2002. "The evolution of clinical gait analysis Part II Kinematics. *Gait and Posture*. Vol. 16; pp. 159–179

[3] Stansfield, B.W., Hillman, S.J., Hazlewood, M.E., Lawson, A.A., Mann, A.M., Loudon, I.R., Robb, J.E., 2001a. "Normalized speed, not age, characterizes ground reaction force patterns in 5- to 12-year-old children walking at self-selected speeds". *Journal of Pediatric Orthopedics*, vol. 21, 395–402.

[4] Stansfield, B. W., Hillman, S. J., Hazlewood, M. E., Lawson, A. A., Mann, A. M., Loudon, I. R., Robb, J. E., 2001b. "Sagittal joint kinematics, moments, and powers are predominantly characterized by speed of progression, not age, in normal children". *Journal of Pediatric Orthopedics*, vol. 21, 403–411.

[5] Van der Linden, M., Kerr, A. M., Hazlewood, M. E., Hillman, S. J., & Robb, J. E. 2002, "Kinematic and kinetic gait characteristics of normal children walking at a range of clinical relevant speeds", *Journal of Pediatric Orthopaedics*, vol. 22, no. 6, pp. 800-806.

[6] Hartmann M, Kreuzpointner F, Haefner R, Michels H, Schwirtz A, Haas J. P. 2010 "Effects of juvenile idiopathic arthritis on kinematics and kinetics of the lower extremities call for consequences in physical activities recommendations". *International Journal of Pediatricsdoi:10.1155/2010/835984*

[7] Fatoye FA, An assessment of neuromuscular performance, functional range of motion and quality of life in children with hypermobility syndrome. Queen Margaret University, Edinburgh, United Kingdom. PhD Thesis. 2008

[8] Fatoye F., Palmer S., Van der Linden M., Rowe P. and Macmillan F. 2011a. "Gait kinematics and passive knee joint range of motion in children with hypermobility syndrome", *Gait and Posture*, vol. 33, no. 3. pp. 447-451

[9] Maillard, S. & Murray, K. J. 2003, "Hypermobility syndrome in children," in Hypermobility syndrome: Recognition and management for physiotherapists, R. Keer & R. Grahame, eds., Butterworth Heinemann, London, pp. 33-50.

[10] Perry J, Burnfield J. 2010 Gait analysis: normal and pathological function. New Jersey, Slack Inc

[11] Muller, R. B. P. 1997, "A critical discussion of intraclass correlation coefficients Statistics in Medicine", *Statistics in Medicine*, vol. 16, no. 7, pp. 281-283.

[12] Von Schroeder, H. P. 1995, "Gait parameters following stroke: A practical assessment", *Journal of Rehabilitation and Research Development*, vol. 32, no. 1, pp. 25 - 31.

[13] Gough, M, Shortland, A. P. 2008. "Can clinical gait analysis guide the management of ambulant children with bilateral spastic cerebral palsy?" *Journal of Pediatric Orthopaedic*, vol. 28, no.8, pp. 879-83.

[14] Damiano, D. L., Kelly, L. E., & Vaughn, C. L. 1995, "Effects of quadriceps femoris strengthening on crouch gait in children with spastic diplegia", *Physical Therapy*, vol. 75, no. 8, pp. 668 – 671.

[15] Selby-Siverstein, L., Farrett, W. D., Maurer, B. T., & Hillstorm, H. J. 1997, "Gait analysis and bivalved serial casting of an athlete with shortened gastrocnemius muscles: A single case design", Journal of Orthopaedic Sports *Physical Therapy*, vol. 25, no. 4, pp. 382 - 288.

[16] Sutherland D. H, Olshen R, Cooper B. A, Woo S. L. Y. 1980. "The development of mature gait". *Journal of Joint and Bone Surgery*. 62-A (3): pp. 336–53.

[17] Sutherland DH, Olshen R, Biden EN, Wyatt MP. 1988. The development of mature walking. London: MacKeith Press.

[18] Ganley K. J. and Powers C. M. 2005. "Gait kinematics and kinetics of 7-year-old children: a comparison to adults using age-specific anthropometric data", *Gait and Posture*, vol. 21, no. 2; pp. 141-145

[19] Oberg T, Karsznia A, 1994. "Oberg K Joint angle parameters in gait: Reference data for normal subjects, 10-79 year of age". *Journal of Rehabilitation Research and Development*, vol. 3; no. 3; pp. 199—213

[20] O'sullivan, S. B. & Schmitz, T. J. 2001, Physical rehabilitation, assessment and treatment, Fourth edn, F.A. Davis Company, Philadelphia.

[21] Thibault, A., Robert, F., & Lambert, J. 1994, "Evaluation of cutaneous and proprioceptive sensation in children: A reliability study", *Developmental Medicine and Child Neurology*, vol. 36, no. 9, pp. 796-812.

[22] Jette, A. M. 1993, "Using Health-Related Quality of life measures in physical therapy outcomes research", *Physical Therapy*, vol. 73, no. 8, pp. 528-537

[23] Bell, M., Bombardier, C., & Tugwell, P. 1990, "Measurement of functional status, quality of life, and utility in rheumatoid arthritis", *Arthritis and Rheumatism*, vol. 33, no. 4, pp. 591-601.

[24] Baker, V., Bennell, K., Stillman, B., Cowan, S., & Crossley, K. 2002, "Abnormal knee joint position sense in individuals with patellofemoral pain syndrome", *Journal of Orthopaedic Research*, vol. 20, no. 2, pp. 208-214.

[25] Brand, R. A. & Crowninshield, R. D. 1981, "Comment on criteria for patient evaluation tools", *Journal of Biomechanics*, vol. 14, p. 655.

[26] Steinwender G, Saraph V, Scheiber S, Zwick EB, Uitz C, Hackl K. 2000. "Intrasubject repeatability of gait analysis data in normal and spastic children". *Clinical Biomechanics*, vol.15, no. 2:pp. 134-9.

[27] Domholdt, E. 2000, Physical Therapy research principles and applications, section ed, W.B. Saunders Company, London.

[28] Wiggin, M., Wilkinson, K., Habatz, S., Chorley, J., & Watson, M. 2006, "Percentile values of isokinetic peak torque in children six through thirteen years old", *Pediatric Physical Therapy*, vol. 18, no. 1, pp. 3-18.

[29] Sadeghi H. Allard, P. & Duhaime, M. 2000, "Contributions of lower-limb muscle power in gait of people without impairments" *Physical Therapy*, vol. 80, no. 12, pp. 1188-1196.

[30] Kadaba, M. P., Ramakrishma, H. K., & Wooten, M. E. 1990, "Measurement of lower extremity kinematics during level walking", *Journal of Orthopaedic Research*, vol. 8, no. 3, pp. 383-392.

[31] Rankin, G. & Stokes, M. 1998, "Reliability of assessment tools in rehabilitation: an illustration of appropriate statistical analyses", *Clinical Rehabilitation*, vol. 12, no. 3, pp. 187-199

[32] Ageberg, E., Flenhagen, J. & Ljung, J. 2007, "Test-retest reliability of knee kineasthesia in healthy adults". BMC Musculoskeletal Disorders, vol. 8, no. 7, pp. 57-63.

[33] Merlini, L., Dell'Accio, D., & Granata, C. 1995, "Reliability of dynamic strength knee muscle testing in children", *Journal of Orthopaedic and Sports Physical Therapy*, vol. 22, no. 2, pp. 73-76.

[34] Tiffreau, V., Ledoux, I., Eymard, B., Thevenon, A., & Hogrel, J.-Y. 2007, "Isokinetic muscle testing for weak patients suffering for neuromuscular disorders: A reliability study", *Neuromuscular Disorders*, vol. 17, no. 7, pp. 524-531.

[35] Gorton, G. E., Stevens, C. M., Masso, P. D., & Vannah, W. M. "Repeatability of the working patterns of normal children", *Gait and Posture*, vol. 5, no. 2, 155-156. 1997.

[36] Leardini, A., Capozzo, A., Catani, F., Toksvig-Larsen, S., Petitto, A.,Sforza, V., Cassanelli, G., Giannini, S., 1999. "Validation of a functional method for the estimation of hip joint centre location". *Journal of Biomechanics*, vol. 32, pp. 99–103.

[37] Beck, R. J., Andraicchi, T. P., Kuo, K. N., Fermier, R. W., & Galante, J. O. 1981, "Changes in the gait patterns of growing children", *Journal of Bone and Joint Surgery*, vol. 63A, no.9, pp. 1452-1456.

[38] Perry, J. (1992). Gait Analysis: Normal and Pathological Function. Thorofare, New Jersey, Slack, Inc.

[39] Fatoye F., Palmer S., Macmillan F., Rowe P., Van der Linden M. 2009. "Proprioception and muscle torque deficits in children with hypermobility syndrome" *Rheumatology*, vol.48 no.2, pp.152-157

[40] Fatoye F., Palmer S., Macmillan F., Van der Linden M. 2011b. "Pain and quality of life in children with hypermobility syndrome", *Rheumatology International* DOI: 10.1007/s00296-010-1729-2

[41] Engelbert R. H. H, Uiterweal C. S. P. M, van der Putte E, Helders P. J. M, Sakkers, R. J. B, van der Tintelen P, Bank R. A. "Pediatric joint hypermobility and musculoskeletal complaints: A new entity? Clinical, biomechanical, and osseal characteristics", *Pediatrics*, 2004; vol. 113: 714-19

[42] Mallik, A. K., Ferrell, W. R., McDonald, A. G., & Sturrock, R. D. 1994, "Impaired proprioceptive acuity at the proximal interphalangeal joint in patients with the hypermobility syndrome", *British Journal of Rheumatology*, vol. 33, no. 7, pp. 631-637.

In: The Knee
Editor: Randy Mascarenhas

ISBN: 978-1-61942-268-1
© 2012 Nova Science Publishers, Inc.

Chapter VI

THE MATURE SHEEP AS AN ANIMAL MODEL FOR BIO-ENHANCED ANTERIOR CRUCIATE LIGAMENT REPAIR AND RECONSTRUCTION

B. Proffen, P. Vavken, R. Palmer, B. C. Fleming and M. M. Murray

Department of Orthopaedic Surgery, Children's Hospital Boston,
Boston, MA, US
Colorado State University–VTH, Fort Collins, CO, US
Department of Orthopaedics, Warren Alpert Medical School of Brown University,
Rhode Island Hospital, Coro West, Providence RI, US

ABSTRACT

Anterior cruciate ligament (ACL) injuries are increasingly common and ACL reconstruction, the gold standard of treatment, can result in relatively high rates of graft rupture in adolescent patients[1]. Additionally, up to 80% of patients undergoing ACL reconstruction may develop some degree of osteoarthritis in the long term[2]. Development of improved techniques in ACL reconstruction is thus of great clinical interest. The development of such techniques would be aided with the use of a large animal model to simulate ACL injury and treatment. While prior studies focusing on bio-enhanced primary ACL repair (where a suture repair was supplemented with a bioactive scaffold designed to stimulate ACL healing) have used an immature porcine model with promising results, study of this procedure in an adult animal model would be desirable.

To study bio-enhanced ACL repair in adult animals, we selected an ovine model that has been previously used in studies focusing on ACL reconstruction and repair. The ovine model has anatomic and biomechanical similarities to the human knee. Prior studies have described the gross anatomy, histology, and biomechanics of the ACL in the healthy ovine knee. Additionally, there have been several studies investigating the biomechanical and histological outcomes of various ACL reconstruction techniques in an ovine model. Our group recently completed a study in adult sheep evaluating the efficacy of this model in studying bio-enhanced ACL repair.

In our experiment, eight skeletally mature sheep underwent unilateral ACL transection and bio-enhanced repair. Four animals each were euthanized after three and six months of healing, and AP laxity of the knee and structural properties of the repaired ACL were evaluated. Unpaired t-tests were used to compare the three and six month values. The average yield load, maximum load, and stiffness of the healing ligaments increased significantly from three to six months from 108 N to 320 N (p = 0.023), 121 N to 343 N (p = 0.034), and 28 N/mm to 58 N/mm (p = 0.035), respectively. All these values remained significantly lower than the contralateral control ACLs, but were comparable with results in the literature for ACL reconstruction in the ovine model. AP laxity was not significantly different between three and six months.

In summary, the mature sheep has proven to be a reliable model for ACL reconstruction and bio-enhanced ACL repair. Bio-enhanced ACL repair in the mature sheep model resulted in progressively increasing yield load, maximum load and linear stiffness of the repair from three to six months of healing. Values obtained at six months validated the hypothesis that the functional outcomes of this new technique are comparable with those found in this model for ACL reconstruction. These promising results suggest that further work may result in a new and innovative strategy for the treatment of human ACL injuries, and that the mature ovine model is well-suited to development of new ACL treatment methods.

INTRODUCTION

Anterior cruciate ligament (ACL) injuries are amongst the most common ligament injuries in the knee and affect an estimated 400,000 US patients[3], including a significant number of children and adolescents[4]. The ACL plays a crucial role in knee motion and stability. Loss of the ACL results in joint instability and secondary damage to the menisci and articular cartilage, leading ultimately to early-onset osteoarthritis[5]. Surgery is thus often recommended as a treatment option following ACL rupture. The current gold standard for surgical treatment is ACL reconstruction, where the torn ACL is replaced with autologous or allogeneic tendon graft. This procedure restores gross knee stability, but does not replace the geometry or proprioceptive function of the ACL[6, 7] and fails to re-establish normal knee kinematics[8]. Systematic long-term follow-up studies of ACL reconstruction suggest that this loss of normal knee kinematics may explain long-term joint degeneration following ACL injury[9]. In addition to the long term complication of osteoarthritis, ACL reconstruction also has a relatively high failure rate (as high as 30%) in young, active patients[10]. Additionally, transphyseal drilling of ACL tunnels in skeletally immature patients is a potential risk factor for subsequent physeal arrest and angular deformities[11]. Thus, new treatment options are of interest. One option would be to repair rather than replace the ACL, which may restore native knee kinematics by potentially maintaining the complex architecture, insertion sites, and proprioceptive nerve receptors of the intact ACL[12].

HISTORY OF ACL REPAIR

The ACL is unique in its inability to heal spontaneously. This is in stark contrast to the collateral ligaments of the knee, which generally heal without surgical interventiont[13-15]. A simple suture repair was first suggested as a treatment for ACL rupture in the late 19th century[16]. However, the long-term outcome study by Feagin and Curl[17] in 1976 reported a failure rate of 90% and showed that suture repair alone had no benefit over conservative treatment[18]. Although suture repair was more or less abandoned after these poor results, the etiology of failure following suture repair remained unknown. Researchers attempted to find an explanation for failure of ACL healing at the cellular and tissue levels by comparing the cellular migration, proliferation, and biosynthesis rates of the collateral ligament to those of the ACL. This led to ruling out any contribution of these factors in inhibition of ACL healing[19, 20]. However, an important finding from these studies was the absence of a wound-filling clot between the ruptured ends of the ACL as compared to the healing response seen in the collateral ligaments. The ACL wound site was thus missing a scaffold into which surrounding cells could migrate and remodel into healing tissue[14]. One reason for the clot deficiency may be high levels of an enzyme that quickly degraded fibrin clot in the synovial fluid of the knee following injury[21, 22]. It was hypothesized that if premature loss of the provisional scaffold provided by the clot was the reason for the failure of ACL healing, engineering a replacement scaffold designed to resist the enzymatic and fluid environment of the knee could be a solution for ACL repair. Tissue engineering of a provisional scaffold substitute is therefore a promising new approach in reviving research in the abandoned field of ACL repair.

DEVELOPMENT OF BIO-ENHANCED ACL-REPAIR

To foster functional ACL healing, it was necessary to develop a suitable substitute scaffold that would not be prematurely degraded in the synovial environment. A promising material was type 1 collagen, which is a major extracellular matrix component of the native and has demonstrated biocompatibility and safety in numerous tissue engineering applications. It comes in forms ranging from an injectable gel to a sturdy sponge, which allows for flexibility in operative delivery[23]. In addition, another advantage of type 1 collagen was the ability of ACL fibroblasts to migrate and proliferate within the scaffold itself[24].

Apart from providing structural support into which cells could migrate and remodel into within the ACL wound site, the physiological fibrin clot also provides a large number of growth factors and extracellular matrix proteins. These elements all play an important role in stimulating and regulating the process of wound healing and remodeling[25]. This biologic function is likely critical in emulating the productive environment of a viable healing wound, as seen in a healing collateral ligament of the knee. The application of individual exogenous growth factors has yielded poor results[26, 27], suggesting that a more complex replication of the wound healing process may be required. Platelets are embedded in fibrin clot and initiate the wound healing growth factor cascade. Thus, these cells may serve as a reasonable biologic delivery system for the multiple growth factors required for successful wound healing. With this in mind, a collagen-platelet composite (CPC) was developed in vitro and then tested in vivo. Interestingly, implantation of an engineered collagen-platelet construct in an ACL wound site fostered a physiologic bioactive scaffold in which growth factor expression patterns were similar to the wound site of an injured collateral ligament (which successfully heals)[28]. This suggested that the placement of an engineered scaffold capable of persisting in the joint and gently activating the platelets within it could result in a biologically productive wound site for the ACL[29]. Additional experimentation demonstrated stimulation of fibroblast migration, biosynthesis, and proliferation by the applied platelet concentrate[30]. These findings were later verified in a central defect model of a canine ACL that showed increased defect filling and improved biomechanical outcomes when using the CPC. The CPC in the central defect model also produced histological features equivalent to that of a healing medial collateral ligament or patellar tendon[28, 30]. This mechanically stable, central defect model supported the effectiveness of the bio-active scaffold, but did not simulate the actual clinical problem of a complete ACL rupture. Therefore, a complete ACL transection model was developed, where the ligament was transected completely and then repaired with a sutures and the bio-active collagen-platelet scaffold as described below.

SURGICAL TECHNIQUE FOR BIO-ENHANCED REPAIR OF THE ACL

Bio-enhanced ACL repair currently combines the enhancement of a collagen-platelet scaffold with temporary mechanical stabilization provided by a femoro-tibial stent suture[31]. This is accomplished by loading an Endobutton device (Smith and Nephew, Andover, MA) with three sutures, so that six suture limbs are trailing from the Endobutton. A small drill hole (4.5 mm) is made through the femoral footprint of the native ACL to the proximal lateral femoral cortex. The loaded Endobutton is then passed through this tunnel, flipped and engaged on the proximal femoral cortex. Of the six suture ends now exiting the femoral tunnel, four are guided through the collagen scaffold, through a 2.5mm tibial tunnel, and then tied over an extracortical button on the medial tibial cortex. These femoro-tibial stent sutures provide initial anterior-posterior stability of the knee while also anchoring and aligning the collagen scaffold within the ACL wound site in the direction of the original ACL. When absorbable sutures (Vicryl, Ethicon, Somerville, NJ) are used, they lose approximately 25% of their initial strength weekly. This results in the repair tissue being gradually exposed to increasing amounts of mechanical stress and stimulation until the sutures are completely absorbed after 63 days. The remaining two suture limbs from the femoral Endobutton are tied to a whipstitch in the tibial ACL stump to position the ACL stump adjacent to the collagen scaffold. Blood is drawn and used to prepare a platelet solution, which is then used to saturate the collagen scaffold.

LARGE ANIMAL MODELS FOR ACL SURGERY

In order to bring new innovations in ACL treatment through to clinical application, an in vivo model for the human knee joint is critical. As mentioned above, in the first stage of developing the bio-enhanced ACL repair technique, a canine stable central defect model was chosen[28]. Although dogs are well established as large animal models for many types of surgery, ACL procedures that are routinely successful in humans typically fail in dogs because of significant differences in anatomy and biomechanics. These factors make the canine model a less favorable ACL repair model. Knee anatomy and biomechanics in sheep and pigs more closely mimic those of the human knee joint[32], with both being approved as economical animal models for knee surgery and ligament repair. While the majority of the studies looking at the development of a bio-enhanced ACL repair technique were originally conducted in a complete cruciate rupture model in pigs[28, 30, 33-35], the question remains as whether the porcine model is the best available ACL model for human application. Anatomically, neither the porcine or ovine models perfectly mirror the human knee and ACL. While the force trajectory of the porcine ACL is relatively close to that of the human ACL[36], the length of the porcine ACL is proportionally significantly longer than the human ACL[32]. Additionally, the maximal extension of the pig knee to 30^0 coupled with early uncontrolled weight bearing on the operative leg cause a high load on the initial repair tissue. These factors may have played a role in the results of a study comparing ACL repair in pigs of different ages, where adolescent pigs showed a significantly better biomechanical outcome after fifteen weeks when compared to adult pigs[37]. Adolescent pigs showed a higher initial cellularity in the repair tissue[38] and a higher potential for migration, proliferation and biosynthesis of the fibroblasts[37]. Additionally, the greater weight of adult pigs may also have contributed to worse outcomes by overloading their repair construct too early. In contrast to the porcine model, the ACL proportions of the sheep are closer to that of the human ACL. The straight resting position while standing also provides more stability for the initially delicate repair tissue. Additionally, the lower activity level of the sheep makes it less likely to overstrain the early repair construct. Therefore, we decided to use the sheep as the large animal model for testing the bio-enhanced ACL repair in adult subjects.

REVIEW OF SHEEP AS AN ANTERIOR CRUCIATE LIGAMENT MODEL

The ovine model has been extensively used as an adult model for ACL research in the past. Therefore, the biomechanics, molecular aspects[39], vascular[40] and neural anatomy[41, 42], and proprioception[43] of the healthy mature ovine ACL is well described. Almost all ACL reconstructions options have been tested in the adult ovine model. Only a few studies have used immature sheep, namely one conducting transphyseal reconstruction of the ACL with split of the ipsilateral superficial flexor digitorum tendon and gastrocnemius tendon[44] and another comparing PET-augmented versus non-augmented primary ACL repair[45].

The most common free tendon graft (hamstring surrogate in humans) in the ovine model was the superficial flexor digitorum tendon because it is easily to approach and to harvest while providing enough length and strength for ACL reconstruction. Allografts and autograft[49] fixation using absorbable interference screws[46], transcondylar screws[47], and microporous pure β-tricalcium phosphate implants for press-fit fixation[48] have been compared. The superficial flexor digitorum tendon grafts had failure loads of up to 808N after 6 months[48] and up to 685 N for reconstructions after one year[46, 49], which are values still less than half that of the ACL-intact controls (1500N). Fresh-frozen allografts and autografts of the superficial digital flexor tendon were compared in a long-term study, resulting in a significantly stronger performance of the autografts after one year (yielding 632 N compared to 307 N for the flexor tendon frozen allografts)[49].

Less common was the use of split Achilles tendon[50, 51] or semitendinosus tendon grafts, which in sheep are too short and thin to work as a suitable grafts[27]. These graft choices resulted in initial loads to failure of 337 N[50] to 685 N after 52 weeks[51] for the Achilles tendon graft and 300 N after 12 weeks[27] for the semitendinosus graft. Fascia lata grafts resulted in the poorest biomechanical outcomes, with failure loads of 300N after 48 weeks[52]. Preliminary studies using a double DLET as a free tendon autograft reconstruction suggests that graft may be even stronger than the superficial flexor digitorum grafts previously reported[53], possibly due in part to the increased time zero strength of the DLET compared to the superficial flexor digitorum graft (see Table 1).

A number of experiments have examined the patellar tendon as a bone-tendon-bone construct for ACL reconstruction. Eighty sheep where studied over a period of 6 months to compare the long term results of patellar tendon versus a DLET graft[47] , but did not find a significant difference between graft types (580 N – 600 N for both grafts). Mayr et al compared Achilles tendon autograft to flexor tendon autograft and found a load to failure of 651 N for the Achilles tendon and 808 N for the flexor tendon graft after 1 year[48]. Another one year study evaluated the biomechanical performance of a patellar tendon graft with or without PDS augmentation, but did not find any significant improvement with using PDS-augmentation[54]. No group regained more than 50% (901 N) of the intact ACL strength (1500 N) after 52 weeks of healing.

Only one study used frozen bone-ACL-bone allografts as a reconstruction method. Their biomechanical results yielded 360 N for the allograft group after 52 weeks, reaching about 30% of the strength of the control group[55].

Primary suture repair has also been conducted in a few ovine studies. However, primary repair of the ACL in sheep showed little, if any, spontaneous healing - similar to the clinical findings in humans. In one study, ACL transection at the femoral insertion site was either repaired with absorbable sutures or augmented with a 2 mm PDS II cord. After 13 weeks, the non-augmented repair bore a maximum load of 252 N compared to 239 N of the augmented repair. Both repair groups had significantly lower load values than the control groups[56]. In another study of partial ACL injury, transection of the medial portion of the ACL was immediately repaired by primary suture followed by augmentation with an absorbable poly-lactic acid device. After 48 weeks, the maximum load of this construct was only 175 N[52].

BIO-ENHANCED PRIMARY REPAIR IN ANADULT OVINE MODEL

A recent study in our laboratory using the immature porcine model demonstrated no significant difference between ACL reconstruction and bio-enhanced ACL repair in biomechanical outcomes after 15 weeks of healing[57]. The hypothesis of a subsequent study was that similar efficacy could be demonstrated in a mature ovine model. Eight skeletally mature sheep were used in this follow-up study. All sheep underwent unilateral ACL transection and non-absorbable sutures were used to tether and align the collagen-platelet composites and adjacently position the tibial stump of the ACL as described earlier. In brief, after sterile preparation and draping, the ACL was exposed through an infra-patellar incision. The ACL was transected at the junction of the middle and proximal thirds. A femoro-tibial

Table 1. Biomechanical data for different reconstruction methods (intact=intact ACL of control group; Graft=graft strength separately tested before implantation; F=Femoral; N=Newton; PDS=Polydioxanone; PLLA=Poly-L-Lactide; TCP=Tri Calcium Phophate; T=Tibial)

Reconstruction Technique			Failure Load (N) after months (m)						Reference
Graft Choice		Fixation	Graft	0 m	3 m	6 m	12 m	Intact	
Superior Digital Flexor Tendon (SDF)	Autograft	Endobutton (F) and Sutured bone bridge (T)			392		632	1,671	Scheffler et al, Arthroscopy 08
		Interference Screw (F and T)	1,120		237	314	685	1,513	Hunt et al, Arch Orthop 05
		Microporous β-TCP (F and T)		256	233	808		1,764	Mayr et al, Arthroscopy 09
		Endobutton (F) and Washer (T)			316	523		759	Meller et al, Arthroscopy 08
	Frozen Allograft	Endobutton (F) and Sutured bone bridge (T)			281		307	1,671	Scheffler et al, Arthroscopy 08
Achilles tendon	Autograft (tendon split)	Cross-pin graft fixation (F and T)		337					Zantop et al, Arthroscopy 07
		Interference Screw (F and T)		228					
		Interference Screw (F and T)	1,120	267	237	314	685	1,513	Weiler et al, Arthroscopy 02
Fascia lata	Autograft + PLLA	Richards fixation staples (F and T)			124	296	295	1,425	Laitinen et al, Arch Orthop 93
Double Lateral Digital Extensor (DLET)	Autograft	Endobutton (F) and Interference (T)			580	1,100			Shaw et al, ORS '10
		Transcondylar screw (F) and Interference (T)	1,140	1,033	188	584		723	Milano et al, Arthroscopy 05
	Allograft	Endobutton (F) and Interference (T)			400	600			Shaw et al, ORS '10

Table 1. (Continued)

Reconstruction Technique			Failure Load (N) after months (m)						Reference
Graft Choice		Fixation	Graft	0 m	3 m	6 m	12 m	Intact	
Patellar Tendon (PT)	Autograft (Tendon Split)	Set screw (F) and Interference screw (T)	830	608	185	603		723	Milano et al, Arthroscopy 05
		Microporous β-TCP (F and T)		198	599	714		1,764	Mayr et al, Arthroscopy 09
		Interference (F and T) and PDS augmentation					901	1,516	Holzmueller et al, Unfallch 92
Anterior Cruciate Ligament	Frozen Allograft	Bone-to-Bone and Endobutton (F and T)	1,398	263	267		360	1,398	Jaskulka et al, Unfallch 97

suture stent consisting of #2 Ethibond suture was used to tether and align a collagen scaffold (Children's Hospital Boston, Boston, MA) in the gap of the transected ACL along the original ACL trajectory. The scaffold was saturated with 3 ml of autologous blood prior to tightening the sutures. The tibial stump of the ACL was tethered adjacent to the setting hydrogel. The knee was closed in layers. After three and six months of healing, four animals were euthanized at each time period and AP laxity of the knee was assessed in addition to tensile testing of the repaired ACL. Unpaired t-tests were used to compare the three and six month values.

At three months (n=4), the average yield load of the healing ligaments was 108 +/-40N, a value that increased significantly to 320 +/- 134N by six months (n=4, p=0.023). The maximum load of the healing ACL also increased from 121 +/- 42N at three months to 343+/- 157N at six months (p=0.034). These values all remained significantly lower than the contralateral control ACLs (yield load was 1600N) and lower than most reported results for ACL reconstruction using large autografts (Table 1). However, these preliminary results were comparable with results in the literature for ACL reconstruction using autograft Achilles tendon (Weiler et al 2002) at six months and with SDF allograft at one year (Scheffler 2008). Interestingly, the strength of the repair tissue with bio-enhanced repair increased during the six month healing period, while that of the grafts had not improved from the time zero value after six months of healing. The stiffness also increased, from 28 +/- 10 N/mm at three months to 58 +/- 20 N/mm at six months (p=0.035). AP laxity was not significantly different between three and six months for any of the angles tested (p>0.4 for all comparisons).

CONCLUSION

In summary, the mature sheep is a reliable model for both ACL reconstruction and bio-enhanced ACL repair. Furthermore, bio-enhanced ACL repair in the mature sheep model resulted in progressively increasing yield load, maximum load and stiffness of the repair from three to six months of healing. Values obtained at 6 months validated the hypothesis that the functional outcomes of this new technique are starting to approach those reported in ovine ACL reconstruction. These promising results suggest that further work in the ovine model may result in a new and innovative strategy in the treatment of human ACL injuries.

REFERENCES

[1]   Shelbourne, K. D., Gray, T. Minimum 10-year results after anterior cruciate ligament reconstruction: how the loss of normal knee motion compounds other factors related to the development of osteoarthritis after surgery. *Am. J. Sports Med.* 2009;37: 471-80.

[2]   Von Porat, A., Roos, E. M., Roos, H. High prevalence of osteoarthritis 14 years after an anterior cruciate ligament tear in male soccer players: a study of radiographic and patient relevant outcomes. *Ann. Rheum. Dis.* 2004;63: 269-73.

[3]   Kibler, W. B. Orthopaedic Knowledge Update 4: Sports Medicine. Rosemont IL: *American Academy of Orthopaedic Surgeons.* 2009: 135.

[4]   McIntosh, A. L., Dahm, D. L., Stuart, M. J. Anterior cruciate ligament reconstruction in the skeletally immature patient. *Arthroscopy.* 2006;22: 1325-30.

[5]   Lohmander, L. S., Ostenberg, A., Englund, M., Roos, H. High prevalence of knee osteoarthritis, pain, and functional limitations in female soccer players twelve years after anterior cruciate ligament injury. *Arthritis Rheum.* 2004;50: 3145-52.

[6]   Lanzetta, A., Corradini, C., Verdoia, C., Miani, A., Castano, S., Castano, P. The nervous structures of anterior cruciate ligament of human knee, healthy and lesioned, studied with confocal scanning laser microscopy. *Ital. J. Anat.Embryol.* 2004;109: 167-76.

[7]   Gomez-Barrena, E., Bonsfills, N., Martin, J. G., Ballesteros-Masso, R., Foruria, A., Nunez-Molina, A. Insufficient recovery of neuromuscular activity around the knee after experimental anterior cruciate ligament reconstruction. *Acta. Orthop.* 2008;79: 39-47.

[8]   Tashman, S., Kolowich, P., Collon, D., Anderson, K., Anderst, W. Dynamic function of the ACL-reconstructed knee during running. *Clin. Orthop. Relat. Res.* 2007;454: 66-73.

[9]   Beynnon, B. D., Uh, B. S., Johnson, R. J., Abate, J. A., Nichols, C. E., Fleming, B. C., et al. Rehabilitation after anterior cruciate ligament reconstruction: a prospective, randomized, double-blind comparison of programs administered over 2 different time intervals. *Am. J. Sports Med.* 2005;33: 347-59.

[10]   Mohtadi, N., Grant, J. Managing anterior cruciate ligament deficiency in the skeletally immature individual: a systematic review of the literature. *Clin. J. Sports Med.* 2006;16: 457-64.

[11]   Wester, W., Canale, S. T., Dutkowsky, J. P., Warner, W. C., Beaty, J. H. Prediction of angular deformity and leg-length discrepancy after anterior cruciate ligament reconstruction in skeletally immature patients. *J. Pediatr. Orthop.* 1994;14: 516-21.

[12]   Vavken, P., Murray, M. M. Translational Studies in Anterior Cruciate Ligament Repair. *Tissue Eng.* Part A. 2009.

[13]   Murray, M. M., Spector, M. Fibroblast distribution in the anteromedial bundle of the human anterior cruciate ligament: the presence of alpha-smooth muscle actin-positive cells. *J. Orthop. Res.* 1999;17: 18-27.

[14]   Murray, M. M., Martin, S. D., Martin, T. L., Spector, M. Histological changes in the human anterior cruciate ligament after rupture. *J. Bone Joint Surg. Am.* 2000;82-A: 1387-97.

[15]   Murray, M. M., Bennett, R., Zhang, X., Spector, M. Cell outgrowth from the human ACL in vitro: regional variation and response to TGF-beta1. *J. Orthop. Res.* 2002;20: 875-80.

[16]   Robson, A. W. VI. Ruptured Crucial Ligaments and their Repair by Operation. *Ann. Surg.* 1903;37: 716-8.

[17]   Feagin, J. A., Jr., Curl, W. W. Isolated tear of the anterior cruciate ligament: 5-year follow-up study. *Am. J. Sports Med.* 1976;4: 95-100.

[18]   Sandberg, R., Balkfors, B. Reconstruction of the anterior cruciate ligament. A 5-year follow-up of 89 patients. *Acta. Orthop. Scand.* 1988;59: 288-93.

[19]   Frank, C., Schachar, N., Dittrich, D. Natural history of healing in the repaired medial collateral ligament. *J. Orthop. Res.* 1983;1: 179-88.

[20] Hannafin, J. A., Attia, E. T., Warren, R. F., Bhargava, M. M. Characterization of chemotactic migration and growth kinetics of canine knee ligament fibroblasts. *J. Orthop. Res.* 1999;17: 398-404.

[21] Brommer, E. J., Dooijewaard, G., Dijkmans, B. A., Breedveld, F. C. Plasminogen activators in synovial fluid and plasma from patients with arthritis. *Ann. Rheum. Dis.* 1992;51: 965-8.

[22] Rosc, D., Powierza, W., Zastawna, E., Drewniak, W., Michalski, A., Kotschy, M. Post-traumatic plasminogenesis in intraarticular exudate in the knee joint. *Med. Sci. Monit.* 2002;8: CR371-8.

[23] Lynn, A. K., Yannas, I. V., Bonfield, W. Antigenicity and immunogenicity of collagen. *J. Biomed. Mater. Res. B Appl. Biomater.* 2004;71: 343-54.

[24] Murray, M. M., Martin, S. D., Spector, M. Migration of cells from human anterior cruciate ligament explants into collagen-glycosaminoglycan scaffolds. *J. Orthop. Res.* 2000;18: 557-64.

[25] Weibrich, G., Kleis, W. K., Hafner, G., Hitzler, W. E. Growth factor levels in platelet-rich plasma and correlations with donor age, sex, and platelet count. *J. Craniomaxillofac. Surg.* 2002;30: 97-102.

[26] Weiler, A., Forster, C., Hunt, P., Falk, R., Jung, T., Unterhauser, F. N., et al. The influence of locally applied platelet-derived growth factor-BB on free tendon graft remodeling after anterior cruciate ligament reconstruction. *Am. J. Sports Med.* 2004;32: 881-91.

[27] Yoshikawa, T., Tohyama, H., Katsura, T., Kondo, E., Kotani, Y., Matsumoto, H., et al. Effects of local administration of vascular endothelial growth factor on mechanical characteristics of the semitendinosus tendon graft after anterior cruciate ligament reconstruction in sheep. *Am. J. Sports Med.* 2006;34: 1918-25.

[28] Murray, M. M., Spindler, K. P., Ballard, P., Welch, T. P., Zurakowski,D., Nanney, L. B. Enhanced histologic repair in a central wound in the anterior cruciate ligament with a collagen-platelet-rich plasma scaffold. *J. Orthop. Res.* 2007;25: 1007-17.

[29] Jacobson, M., Fufa, D., Abreu, E. L., Kevy, S., Murray, M. M. Platelets, but not erythrocytes, significantly affect cytokine release and scaffold contraction in a provisional scaffold model. *Wound Repair Regen.* 2008;16: 370-8.

[30] Murray, M. M., Spindler, K. P., Devin, C., Snyder,B. S., Muller, J., Takahashi, M., et al. Use of a collagen-platelet rich plasma scaffold to stimulate healing of a central defect in the canine ACL. *J. Orthop. Res.* 2006;24: 820-30.

[31] Murray, M. M., Magarian, E., Zurakowski, D., Fleming, B. C. Bone-to-bone fixation enhances functional healing of the porcine anterior cruciate ligament using a collagen-platelet composite. *Arthroscopy.* 2010;26: S49-57.

[32] Proffen, B. M., Martha, M., McElfresh, Megan Fleming, Braden, C. Anatomy of the Cruciate Ligaments and Menisci in Seven Species. Transactions Vol. 36, *Long Beach*, CA, 2011. 2011.

[33] Spindler, K. P., Murray, M. M., Carey, J. L., Zurakowski, D., Fleming, B. C. The use of platelets to affect functional healing of an anterior cruciate ligament (ACL) autograft in a caprine ACL reconstruction model. *J. Orthop. Res.* 2009;27: 631-8.

[34] Murray, M. M., Spindler, K. P., Abreu, E., Muller, J. A., Nedder, A., Kelly,M., et al. Collagen-platelet rich plasma hydrogel enhances primary repair of the porcine anterior cruciate ligament. *J. Orthop. Res.* 2007;25: 81-91.

[35] Murray, M. M., Palmer, M., Abreu, E., Spindler, K. P., Zurakowski, D., Fleming, B. C. Platelet-rich plasma alone is not sufficient to enhance suture repair of the ACL in skeletally immature animals: an in vivo study. *J. Orthop. Res.* 2009;27: 639-45.

[36] Xerogeanes, J. W., Fox, R. J., Takeda, Y., Kim, H. S., Ishibashi, Y., Carlin, G. J., et al. A functional comparison of animal anterior cruciate ligament models to the human anterior cruciate ligament. *Ann. Biomed. Eng.* 1998;26: 345-52.

[37] Mastrangelo, A. N., Magarian, E. M., Palmer, M. P., Vavken, P., Murray, M. M. The effect of skeletal maturity on the regenerative function of intrinsic ACL cells. *J. Orthop. Res.* 2010;28: 644-51.

[38] Mastrangelo, A. N., Haus, B. M., Vavken, P., Palmer, M. P., Machan, J. T., Murray, M. M. Immature animals have higher cellular density in the healing anterior cruciate ligament than adolescent or adult animals. *J. Orthop. Res.* 2010;28: 1100-6.

[39] Rumian, A. P., Wallace, A. L., Birch, H. L. Tendons and ligaments are anatomically distinct but overlap in molecular and morphological features--a comparative study in an ovine model. *J. Orthop. Res.* 2007;25: 458-64.

[40] Seitz, H., Hausner, T., Schlenz, I., Lang, S., Eschberger, J. Vascular anatomy of the ovine anterior cruciate ligament. A macroscopic, histological and radiographic study. *Arch. Orthop. Trauma Surg.* 1997;116: 19-21.

[41] Raunest, J., Sager, M., Burgener, E. Proprioception of the cruciate ligaments: receptor mapping in an animal model. Arch. Orthop. *Trauma Surg.* 1998;118: 159-63.

[42] Halata, Z., Wagner, C., Baumann, K. I. Sensory nerve endings in the anterior cruciate ligament (Lig. cruciatum anterius) of sheep. *Anat. Rec.* 1999;254: 13-21.

[43] Raunest, J., Sager, M., Burgener, E. Proprioceptive mechanisms in the cruciate ligaments: an electromyographic study on reflex activity in the thigh muscles. *J. Trauma.* 1996;41: 488-93.

[44] Meller, R., Willbold, E., Hesse, E., Dreymann, B., Fehr, M., Haasper, C., et al. Histologic and biomechanical analysis of anterior cruciate ligament graft to bone healing in skeletally immature sheep. *Arthroscopy.* 2008;24: 1221-31.

[45] Seitz, H., Marlovits, S., Schwendenwein, I., Muller, E., Vecsei, V. Biocompatibility of polyethylene terephthalate (Trevira hochfest) augmentation device in repair of the anterior cruciate ligament. *Biomaterials.* 1998;19: 189-96.

[46] Hunt, P., Scheffler, S. U., Unterhauser, F. N., Weiler, A. A model of soft-tissue graft anterior cruciate ligament reconstruction in sheep. *Arch. Orthop. Trauma Surg.* 2005;125: 238-48.

[47] Milano, G., Mulas, P. D., Sanna-Passino, E., Careddu, G. M., Ziranu, F., Fabbriciani, C. Evaluation of bone plug and soft tissue anterior cruciate ligament graft fixation over time using transverse femoral fixation in a sheep model. *Arthroscopy.* 2005;21: 532-9.

[48] Mayr, H. O., Dietrich, M., Fraedrich, F., Hube, R., Nerlich, A., Von Eisenhart-Rothe, R., et al. Microporous pure beta-tricalcium phosphate implants for press-fit fixation of anterior cruciate ligament grafts: strength and healing in a sheep model. *Arthroscopy.* 2009;25: 996-1005.

[49] Scheffler, S. U., Schmidt, T., Gangey, I., Dustmann, M., Unterhauser, F., Weiler, A. Fresh-frozen free-tendon allografts versus autografts in anterior cruciate ligament reconstruction: delayed remodeling and inferior mechanical function during long-term healing in sheep. *Arthroscopy*. 2008;24: 448-58.

[50] Zantop, T., Weimann, A., Wolle, K., Musahl, V., Langer, M., Petersen, W. Initial and 6 weeks postoperative structural properties of soft tissue anterior cruciate ligament reconstructions with cross-pin or interference screw fixation: an in vivo study in sheep. *Arthroscopy*. 2007;23: 14-20.

[51] Weiler, A., Peine, R., Pashmineh-Azar, A., Abel, C., Sudkamp, N. P., Hoffmann, R. F. Tendon healing in a bone tunnel. Part I: Biomechanical results after biodegradable interference fit fixation in a model of anterior cruciate ligament reconstruction in sheep. *Arthroscopy*. 2002;18: 113-23.

[52] Laitinen, O., Pohjonen, T., Tormala, P., Saarelainen, K., Vasenius, J., Rokkanen, P., et al. Mechanical properties of biodegradable poly-L-lactide ligament augmentation device in experimental anterior cruciate ligament reconstruction. *Arch. Orthop. Trauma Surg.* 1993;112: 270-4.

[53] Shaw, J. C., Renee; Palmer, Ross; Nichols, Anastasia; Turner, Anthony; Boivin, Gregory; Hunter, Shawn. Biomechanical Comparison of Supercritical CO2 Treated and Gamma Irradiated Tendon Allografts with Autograft. *Transactions* Vol. 35, New Orleans, LA, 2010. 2010.

[54] Holzmuller, W., Rehm, K. E., Perren, S. M. [Mechanical properties of PDS-augmented patellar tendon transplants in reconstruction of the anterior cruciate ligament]. *Unfallchirurg*. 1992;95: 306-10.

[55] Jaskulka, R., Ittner, G., Birkner, T. [Replacement of the anterior cruciate ligament by cold preserved bone-cruciate ligament-bone allotransplants. An experimental study in the sheep]. *Unfallchirurg*. 1997;100: 724-36.

[56] Richter, M., Durselen, L., Ignatius, A., Missler, F., Claes, L., Kiefer, H. Acutely repaired proximal anterior cruciate ligament ruptures in sheep - by augmentation improved stability and reduction of cartilage damage. *J.Mater. Sci. Mater. Med.* 1997;8: 855-9.

[57] Joshi, S. M., Mastrangelo, A. N., Magarian, E. M., Fleming, B. C., Murray, M. M. Collagen-platelet composite enhances biomechanical and histologic healing of the porcine anterior cruciate ligament. *Am. J. Sports Med.* 2009;37: 2401-10.

In: The Knee
Editor: Randy Mascarenhas

ISBN: 978-1-61942-268-1
© 2012 Nova Science Publishers, Inc.

Chapter VII

ANATOMIC DOUBLE-BUNDLE ACL RECONSTRUCTION

Kellie K. Middleton, Albert Lin, Paulo Araujo and Freddie H. Fu

Department of Orthopaedic Surgery, University of Pittsburgh Medical Center, Pittsburgh, PA, US

ABSTRACT

Anterior cruciate ligament (ACL) reconstruction ranks among the most commonly performed orthopaedic procedures worldwide. The concepts behind surgical management of ACL deficiency have continued to evolve over the past few decades. Historically, most ACL reconstruction methods have focused on single bundle (SB) reconstruction techniques that may not recreate native anatomy by ignoring the posterolateral (PL) bundle and its importance in rotatory stability. Recent data suggests that non-anatomic ACL reconstruction may lead to altered joint kinematics with concern for long-term joint health. A school of thought has emerged which suggests that a key to optimizing joint function and long term health may rest on an anatomic surgical approach to ACL injury. These approaches have focused on individualized surgery based on patient anatomy and anatomical restoration of the ACL, which consists of the anteromedial (AM) bundle (primary contributor to antero-posterior stability) and the PL bundle (allows rotatory stability). During the past several years, there has been an increasing trend towards double bundle (DB) ACL reconstruction in an attempt to restore anatomy and preserve the individual and synergistic functions of the AM and PL bundles. Recent biomechanical research suggests that anatomic DB ACL reconstruction can better reproduce native knee function when compared to conventional non-anatomic SB reconstruction. Further long-term clinical and biomechanical studies comparing anatomic DB ACL construction to non-anatomic SB reconstruction will more fully elucidate whether restoration of native knee joint kinematics and function have any bearing on future joint health.

INTRODUCTION AND HISTORICAL BACKGROUND

Introduction

Surgical management of anterior cruciate ligament (ACL) deficiency has been a popular discussion in the orthopaedic community over the past few decades. This surge of interest is likely secondary to the advent of minimally invasive arthroscopic techniques, increasing diversity of graft choices, more sophisticated fixation options and advanced rehabilitation protocols.

The primary goals of treatment after ACL injury are the restoration of lost function and the prevention of long-term joint degeneration. Traditional ACL reconstruction techniques involve the arthroscopic reconstruction of the anteromedial (AM) bundle of the ACL with little regard for the posterolateral (PL) bundle, which allows rotation with the knee in a flexed position. For the most part, single-bundle reconstruction techniques meet the goals of ACL reconstruction as most patients have no detectable antero-posterior residual instability following AM based single-bundle ACL reconstruction. In fact, many studies report that success rates for single-bundle ACL reconstruction range from 69 – 90 % [16, 18]. However, long-term joint health and residual rotational instability after ACL injury remain as concerns. During the past few years, there has been an increased trend towards double-bundle ACL reconstruction in an attempt to restore long-term joint health and the rotational stability provided by the PL bundle.

History

In 1938, Palmer was the first to propose double-bundle ACL reconstruction [48]. However, his study did not receive much attention and only many years later would this discussion be resumed. In 1983, Mott described a double-bundle ACL reconstruction technique using semitendinosus autograft through two separate tibial and femoral tunnels [41]. A few years later, Zaricznyj reported a double-bundle ACL reconstruction technique using a single femoral tunnel and two tibial tunnels. He showed good to excellent results in 12 of 14 patients at an average of 3.6 years postoperatively [69]. Radford and Amis studied the biomechanical significance of reconstructing both ACL bundles. They hypothesized that "ACL behavior might be modeled more closely by implants which seek to duplicate its complexity." By comparing single-bundle (SB) to double-bundle reconstruction, the authors found that DB reconstruction was the only construct that reproduced the function of the intact ACL at both 20° and 90° of knee flexion.

Over the past five years, more sophisticated biomechanical studies of double-bundle ACL reconstruction have appeared in the literature, including the biomechanical influence of graft placement and geometry [1, 7, 23, 24, 30, 38, 43, 57, 59, 61 – 64]. Specifically, the ability to elucidate the influence of graft placement on both anterior translation and coupled rotation have greatly advanced the understanding of the PL bundle and its role in both knee kinematics and ACL reconstruction.

Anatomy

The ACL consists of dense connective tissue enveloped in a synovial membrane, which places the ligament in an intra-articular, but extra-synovial position [4, 13]. The ligament originates from a fossa on the posterior aspect of the lateral femoral condyle and runs in an oblique course distally, anteriorly, and medially to insert between the medial and lateral spines of the tibial plateau. It attaches to the femur and the tibia as a collection of fascicles that fan out as they approach their insertion sites [4, 13,22,26,53]. The area of insertion is 3 to 3.5 times larger than the cross-sectional area of the ligament midsubstance [22]. The cross-sectional area of the mid-substance ACL is approximately 36 to 44 mm^2 [2], while the cross-sectional area of the femoral and tibial insertion sites is between 113 and 136 mm^2 [26]. These cross-sectional dimensions produce an anchor-shaped design of the ACL footprint. A relatively broad ACL footprint may serve to minimize stresses on the ligament-bone interface [25].

The ACL consists of 2 functional bundles, the AM and the PL bundles, named for the position of their insertion sites on the tibia (Figure 1).

Embryologic studies have observed ACL formation in fetal development as early as 8 weeks gestation, and the development of 2 distinct bundles of the ACL at 16 weeks gestation [14, 21, 45]. The AM bundle is the main contributor to anterior-posterior stability. Based on preliminary findings in an ongoing study at the University of Pittsburgh, ACL length ranges from 25 – 45 mm with an average length of 35 mm. Primary function of the PL bundle is rotational stability [11, 14, 18, 47], but the PL bundle has been less well studied. Kummer and Yamamoto measured the PL bundle in 50 cadavers and found a mean length of 17.8mm [31]. In general, the AM bundle is larger than and thus comprises a larger area on the tibial and femoral footprints than the PL bundle [26, 59].

ACL Kinematics and Functional Anatomy

Biomechanical studies have demonstrated that ACL bundles are not isometric throughout knee range of movement. Each bundle serves a unique purpose at varying degrees of knee flexion and extension. Furthermore, the biomechanics of the two bundles differ between loaded and unloaded conditions [66].

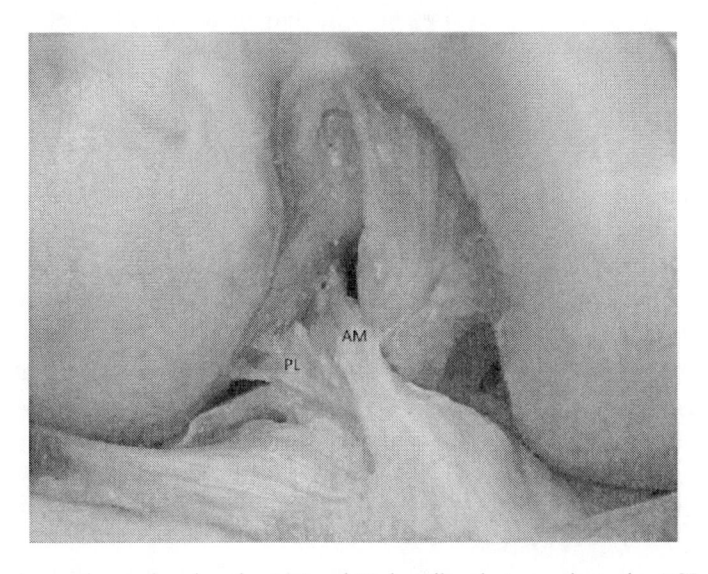

Figure 1. Cadaveric specimen showing the AM and PL bundles that constitute the ACL.

In unloaded conditions, knee flexion results in lengthening of the AM bundle and relaxation of the PL bundle. In knee extension, on the other hand, the PL bundle lengthens and the AM bundle relaxes [32, 49]. An understanding of the relative lengthening behavior of each bundle was more precisely elucidated by Bach et al. via utilization of strain gauges in the AM and PL bundles to measure strain changes during full range of motion [5]. The results supported the current understanding of the length – flexion relationship: the AM bundle was elongated at full extension and full flexion while remaining relatively relaxed between 10° to 90° of knee flexion with changes of less than 1% strain. The PL bundle was maximally elongated in full extension and relaxed when knee flexion exceeded 40° [5].

The two bundles of the ACL function differently when the knee joint is loaded compared to unloaded conditions. Li et al found the AM bundle had a relatively constant length from full extension to 90° of flexion, while the PL bundle decreased in length with flexion [33]. Jordan et al. also found that both the AM and PL bundles were maximally elongated at low flexion angles and shorted significantly with increasing flexion [29]. This difference in elongation patters after loading may be a direct effect of quadriceps muscle contraction during weightbearing conditions. Kurosawa et al. showed that quadriceps contraction significantly stretched both the AM and PL bundles, particularly during 0˚ to 60˚ of flexion [32].

It is especially important to understand the clinical implications of the in vivo length-flexion relationship in loaded circumstances. In fact, several studies have recommended that double-bundle grafts should be fixed at lower flexion angles to prevent excessive tension on each bundle during everyday weight-bearing conditions [29, 36].

Kinematics after Anatomic ACL Reconstruction

Anatomic DB ACL reconstruction has been shown to result in superior biomechanical outcomes, especially under rotatory loads, when compared to traditional non-anatomic single bundle reconstruction [50,61,62]. Yagi et al measured anterior tibial translation after applying a 134-N anterior load and a combined rotatory load to the tibia [61]. They found that anterior tibial translation after anatomic DB reconstruction was significantly less than that after SB reconstruction at full extension and at 30˚ of knee flexion for anterior loading and at both 15˚ and 30˚ of knee flexion for rotatory loading. Their findings that anatomic DB reconstruction more closely replicates native ACL length and tension patterns than SB reconstruction were supported by numerous other studies [6,35,52,60, 65]. For example, Yasuda et al found that the AM graft in-situ forces were highest at full extension, decreased with knee flexion between 0˚ and 30˚, plateaued between 30˚ and 90˚, and gradually increased beyond 90˚. Conversely, PL graft tension was highest at full extension and gradually relaxed with knee flexion from 0˚ to 90˚.

Biomechanical studies including those mentioned above have demonstrated that anatomic DB ACL reconstruction can restore knee function significantly more closely to the native knee when compared with conventional non-anatomic SB reconstruction. However, there is a dearth of research comparing biomechanical outcomes of anatomic double-bundle procedures to anatomic single-bundle procedures.

ACL Injury History, Risk Factors, Physical Exam and Imaging

History

When working up an ACL tear, it is important to conduct a thorough history and physical exam. ACL injuries can occur via both high-energy (e.g. motor vehicle accidents) and low-energy (e.g. contact or noncontact field sports). Seventy percent of ACL patients sustain an ACL tear via non-contact injury, most commonly during an athletic activity [10, 19]. Common sports associated with ACL injuries include skiing, soccer, basketball and tennis. Mechanism of injury usually involves sudden deceleration and change of direction (i.e. cutting) or pivoting in a way that involves rotation or lateral bending (i.e. valgus stress).

Patients often complain of feeling a "pop" in their knee at the time of injury, acute swelling thereafter, and the feeling of an unstable knee that "gives out." A large majority of patients develop an effusion secondary to hemarthrosis, but only 67 – 77 percent of patients presenting with acute traumatic knee hemarthrosis have an ACL injury [37, 44].

After swelling has subsided, patients generally are able to bear weight on the affected leg, but complain of instability. Instability is exacerbated by activities such as squatting, pivoting, lateral movement, and walking down stairs. Possible associated injuries include meniscal tears, articular cartilage damage, subchondral bone bruises, and other ligament injuries [15, 25].

Physical Examination

Physical examination of the knee includes inspection, palpation, testing of mobility, strength, and stability, as well as special tests for ACL integrity. The best time to conduct a Lachman test on a patient is immediately after injury, thus avoiding the resulting hemarthrosis. If a large effusion exists, consider aspiration for pain relief and to inspect the aspirate for any fat globules suggesting a fracture.

Some patients may have laxity that is not pathologic. Thus, it is always important to compare to the contralateral, normal side. Varus/valgus instability testing should be conducted to rule out injury to the collateral ligaments. Furthermore, evaluation of gait will help assess for varus thrust. McMurray's test and palpation for joint line tenderness is beneficial to evaluate for meniscal tears and bone contusions. Sensitivity of the McMurray test ranges from 51-53 % and specificity ranges from 59-97 % [28, 46]. Hence, a negative test does not necessarily exclude a meniscal tear.

Clinical data such as range of motion, Lachman grade, anterior drawer grade, pivot-shift grade, KT-1000 arthrometer measurements, and subjective knee scores such as the International Knee Documentation Committee Subjective Knee Form (IKDC) and Lysholm score are routinely performed and collected for outcome evaluation. A discrepancy between the Lachman and pivot shift maneuvers suggests a partial tear involving either the AM or PL bundles. An isolated positive Lachman test is often more indicative of an AM bundle tear, whereas an isolated positive pivot shit is usually more indicative of a PL bundle tear. A positive KT-1000 test indicates a side-to-side difference in anterior translation. A prominent anterior drawer in the presence of a positive Lachman test may suggest concomitant posteromedial ligament instability or posterior horn meniscal injury.

Imaging

Although an ACL tear can be diagnosed clinically, a complete knee series consisting of weight-bearing antero-posterior, notch, lateral, and patellofemoral merchant views should be obtained. MRI is confirmatory and useful for evaluating other intra- and extra-articular injury. Pre-op ACL measurements on the MRI including insertion site sizes, ACL length, inclination angle, quadriceps and patellar tendon thickness are routinely measured to aid in developing the operative plan (Figure 2).

MRI and radiographs together allow for evaluation of soft tissues, bony anatomy, capsular lesions, physeal growth capability and arthritic changes.

INDICATIONS/CONTRAINDICATIONS

Non-Operative V. Operative Management of ACL Injuries

Acute ACL injuries can be managed operatively or non-operatively. Few patients with ACL injury are capable of returning to sustained, high-level athletic activity without surgical correction. [27]. A recent randomized controlled trial compared early ACL reconstruction with a program of initial rehabilitation [17]. The findings suggested that improvement in Knee Injury and Osteoarthritis Outcome Scores were nearly identical in both groups. As such, the authors concluded that in young, active adults with acute ACL injuries, rehabilitation plus early ACL reconstruction was not superior to a strategy of rehabilitation plus optional delayed ACL reconstruction. In their series, however, patients who were randomized to the initial rehabilitation program showed a higher rate of meniscal injuries after two years follow-up. Bernstein published a decision analysis approach to ACL tear management and concluded that early surgery for ACL injury may be the preferred approach for some patients, particularly active patients who possess a higher likelihood of developing a meniscal tear [8]. Furthermore, Bernstein argues that early surgical repair may be considered to be more cost efficient in treating both ACL and meniscus tears [8].

In conclusion, deciding on operative over non-operative management involves analysis of different factors including age, level of activity, functional demands, and presence of associated injuries.

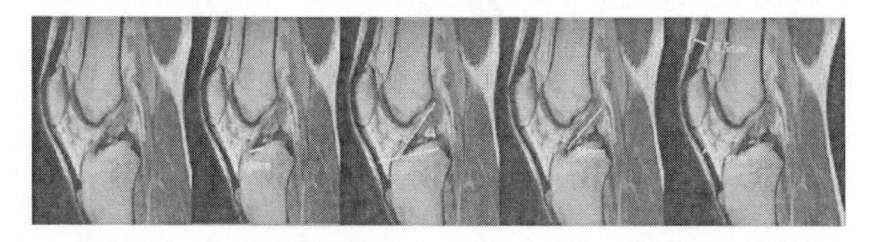

Figure 2. Pre-op ACL measurements on MRI.

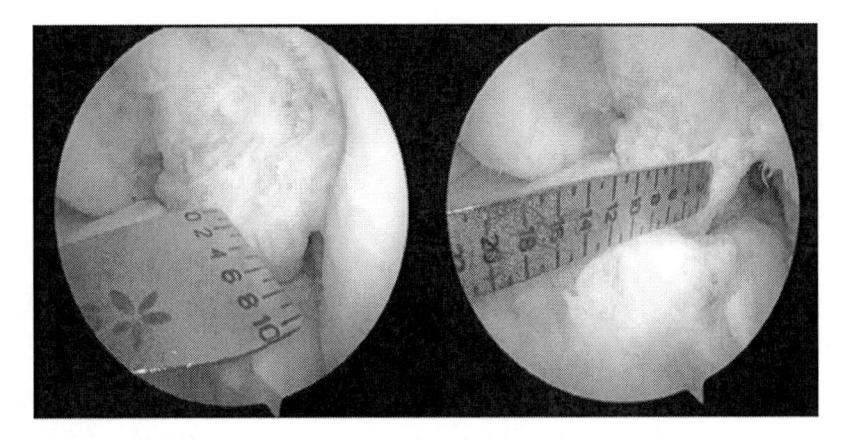

Figure 3. Arthroscopic measurement of the tibial insertion site and notch width showing a possible double bundle reconstruction scenario.

Indications and Contraindications for Anatomic ACL Double Bundle Reconstruction

ACL reconstruction, regardless of technique, is indicated in patients who participate in high-demand sports that involve cutting, jumping, pivoting, and quick deceleration. Patients with heavy labour occupations, those who experience significant knee instability in spite of rehabilitation, and those with associated injuries including meniscus tears or severe injuries to other structures within the knee may all also benefit from surgery.

Anatomic double-bundle ACL reconstruction focuses on restoring the native anatomy and footprints of the ACL by reconstructing both the AM and PL bundles. This is a more technically demanding operation and must be performed by experienced surgeons. Indications for double-bundle reconstruction are similar to those for traditional single-bundle reconstruction.

Anatomic double-bundle ACL reconstruction is our preferred method of ACL reconstruction unless there is a contraindication. Absolute contraindications include acute intra-articular sepsis, advanced degenerative changes of the knee, patients who are not able to comply with the rehabilitative program, and patients with severe bone bruising (particularly of the lateral femoral condyle) [58]. Relative contraindications to anatomic double bundle reconstruction are notch width <12 mm and tibial insertion site <14 mm (Figure 3) and will be discussed in the pre-op planning section. Finally, caution is warranted in patients with open physes and large growth potential.

Timing of Surgery

It is difficult to pinpoint the best time to undergo ACL reconstruction. However, it is well known that the best chances of surgical success occur when patients have minimal swelling, good quadriceps function, and full range of motion of the knee. Premature surgery has been shown to increase the risk of arthrofibrosis [9, 39]. Patients often undergo two to four weeks of pre-habilitation to maximize knee strength and motion prior to surgery.

SURGICAL RECONSTRUCTION

Pre-Operative Planning

Once a comprehensive history, physical exam, and imaging have all been completed and the decision has been made to proceed with ACL reconstruction, pre-operative planning is essential in preparing for anatomic double-bundle reconstruction. Anatomy is the fundamental basis for the surgery and it is thus important to respect individual anatomy when performing ACL reconstruction. Anatomic ACL reconstruction is defined as the functional restoration of the ACL to its native dimensions, collagen orientation, and insertion sites. The goal of anatomic ACL reconstruction is to provide each individual patient with the best potential for a successful outcome. There are four fundamental principles. The first is to appreciate the patient's native anatomy. The second is to tailor each surgery to the patient's individualized anatomy and needs. The third is to restore anatomy by placing the tunnels and grafts in the center of the patient's native footprints. The fourth is to restore function by tensioning the grafts to mimic the native ACL as closely as possible.

To this end, quality pre-operative MRI imaging is invaluable in helping to determine whether a patient might be suitable for an anatomic double versus single-bundle reconstruction. Pre-operative assessment of the tibial insertion site is routinely performed as highlighted in the imaging section. Double-bundle reconstruction is preferable when tibial insertion site is >14mm (Figure 3). Likewise, when the tibial insertion site is <14mm, the possibility of drilling two appropriately sized tunnels without coalescing them and maintaining an appropriate 2mm bone bridge may be technically challenging or impossible [55]. Thus, if pre-operative assessment reveals a tibial insertion site <14mm, single-bundle ACL reconstruction is the best option. In addition, pre-operative MRI assessment of anatomic intra-articular graft length, as well as quadriceps and patellar tendons thickness may aid in graft choice. Measurement of the native sagittal ACL inclination angle on preoperative MRI may help guide future post-operative evaluation of how accurately ACL anatomy has been restored after surgery (Figure 2).

Additionally, pre-operative CT scans with 3D reconstruction are extremely helpful in decision making for revision surgery to determine previous tunnel placement in relationship to native ACL footprints (Figure4). This will aid in determining whether new tunnels can be drilled separately from previous ones, whether a previous tunnel can be accepted, or whether a staged revision with bone grafting is needed to avoid coalescing tunnels in revision scenarios.

The decision for autograft versus allograft as a graft source is multifactorial and includes consideration of patient age, primary versus revision surgery, associated injuries, previous surgeries, and the patient's individualized needs and preferences. The graft source chosen should be able to restore 80 - 90 % of the native insertion site. The complexities of decision-making for graft selection are beyond the scope of this chapter. However, when possible, our preference for double-bundle ACL reconstruction is quadriceps tendon autograft [53]. A preoperative MRI can determine the thickness of the graft –measured 15 mm above the superior pole of the patella (figure 5).

The preferred minimum width is 7 mm to accommodate the tunnel sizes planned for double bundle reconstruction (see below). If the width is <7mm as determined by the preoperative MRI, hamstring autograft with the addition of allograft if necessary, or allograft reconstruction is planned.

Assessing associated injuries such as meniscal and collateral ligament injuries pre-operatively is also critical to pre-operative planning and must be thoroughly investigated via history, physical exam, and imaging prior to formulating a surgical plan.

Surgical Technique (Hamstring Autograft and Soft Tissue Allograft)

The procedure is performed under either general anaesthesia, regional anaesthesia, or both depending on the preference of the patient and anesthesiologist. Once anaesthesia has been induced, a thorough examination under anesthesia is performed. Range of motion, Lachman testing, pivot shift testing, anterior drawer, as well as internal and external rotation at both 30 and 90 degrees are specifically documented and compared to the contralateral extremity. Other associated findings such as varus/valgus stability, posterior drawer, and patellar examinations are also recorded depending on suspected associated injuries.

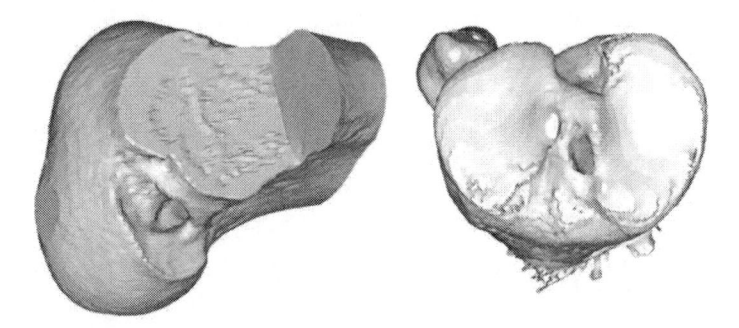

Figure 4. Pre-op planning for a revision case. A 3D CT scan image was obtained and showed a high position of the femoral tunnel and medial position of the tibial tunnel.

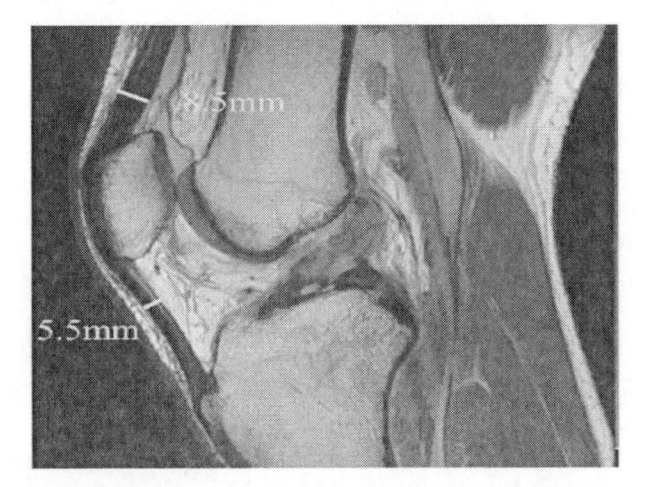

Figure 5. MRI sagittal view showing quadriceps and patellar tendon thickness.

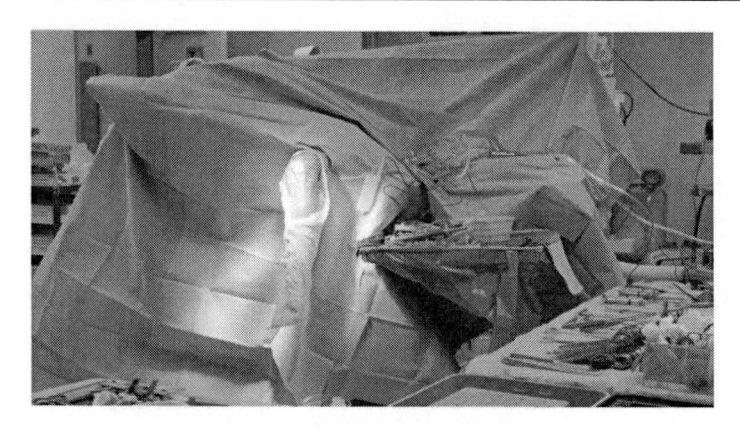

Figure 6. Set up for ACL reconstruction.

Once the exam under anesthesia has been performed, the patient is positioned supine on the operating table with the non-operative leg in a flexed and abducted position away from the operative field (Figure 6). Special care should be taken to pad the non-operative leg to avoid positioning complications such as tourniquet effect and peroneal nerve palsy in the unaffected leg. A pneumatic tourniquet is applied to the upper thigh in the injured limb with the pressure ranging from 300-350 mm Hg, depending on the leg size of the patient. The operative limb is then held in an arthroscopic leg holder to allow varus and valgus stress to be placed on the knee during the arthroscopy while allowing a range of motion from full extension to 120 degrees of flexion.

A three portal technique is used; high anterolateral portal (AL), central anteromedial portal (CP), and accessory anteromedial (AM) portal (Figure 7) [3]. The high AL portal is established first and a diagnostic arthroscopy is performed through this portal. The diagnostic arthroscopy should include a thorough evaluation of menisci and chondral surfaces, as well as the rupture pattern of the ACL. The high AL portal avoids the pre-patellar fat pad and allows an unobstructed view of the tibial footprint. Next, under spinal needle visualization, the CP and accessory AM portals are established. The central portal should be low and just medial or through the medial one-third of the patellar tendon, as well as above the intermeniscal ligament in line with the ACL fibers (Figure 8).

The accessory AM portal is made approximately 2 cm from the medial border of the patellar tendon just above the meniscus. There should be at least 2 mm of clearance from the medial femoral condyle to avoid injury to the medial femoral condyle and cartilage when drilling the ACL femoral tunnels. Special care should be taken to avoid meniscal injury while establishing this portal with a scalpel. The main advantage of these portals is that the accessory AM portal can be used as working portal while the central portal is used as a viewing portal for better visualization of the medial wall of the lateral femoral condyle (Figure 8b).

Before the ACL procedure, meniscal and chondral injuries that require treatment should first be addressed. The fat pad and synovial tissue are removed to improve visualization. To thoroughly evaluate the ACL rupture pattern, a thermal device on the lowest settings is used instead of a more aggressive shaver. At this point, we take several measurements with a ruler to verify that the patient's anatomy can be safely reproduced with a double-bundle reconstruction as well as to confirm tunnel sizes that can be drilled based on the patients anatomy and the size of available grafts.

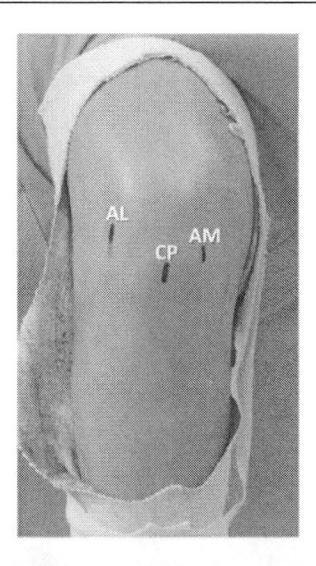

Figure 7. Patient set up showing the three portal technique.

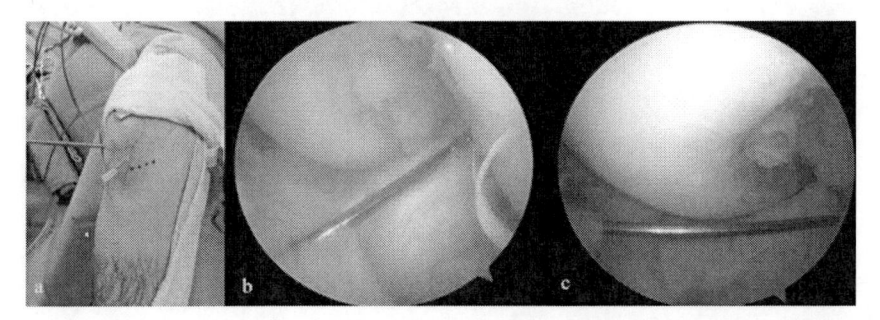

Figure 8. a: High lateral portal as a viewing portal and a spinal needle through the medial third of the patellar tendon to position the central portal. b: A probe showing the good placement of the central portal in the central portion of notch in its lower third and aligned with ACL fibers. c: Spinal needle showing a good position for the accessory medial portal.

These measurements include overall tibial insertion length, AM and PL tibial footprint widths, overall femoral insertion length, AM and PL femoral footprint widths, notch sizes at the base, middle, and apex as well as notch height (Figure 9). At this point, tibial insertion site size is examined to confirm a total insertion size of at least 14 mm. Also, base width of the notch should be at least 12 mm to proceed with double-bundle reconstruction. A single-bundle procedure is chosen if these parameters are not met.

For the anatomic ACL double-bundle reconstruction, the footprints of the tibial AM and PL bundles are marked with the thermal device while viewing with the scope in the AL portal and the thermal device in the CP. The footprints of the femoral AM and PL bundles are marked with the scope in the central portal and the thermal device in the accessory AM portal. These tunnels will be drilled later in the central portion of the native insertion sites to restore normal ACL anatomy. Two bony landmarks on the lateral wall of the intercondylar notch can assist in localizing femoral tunnel placement. The lateral intercondylar ridge, or the "resident's ridge", is the upper limit of the femoral AM and PL bundle insertion sites when the knee is flexed at 90 degrees while the lateral bifurcate ridge separates the femoral AM and PL bundle insertion sites (Figure 10).

a)

b)

c)

d)

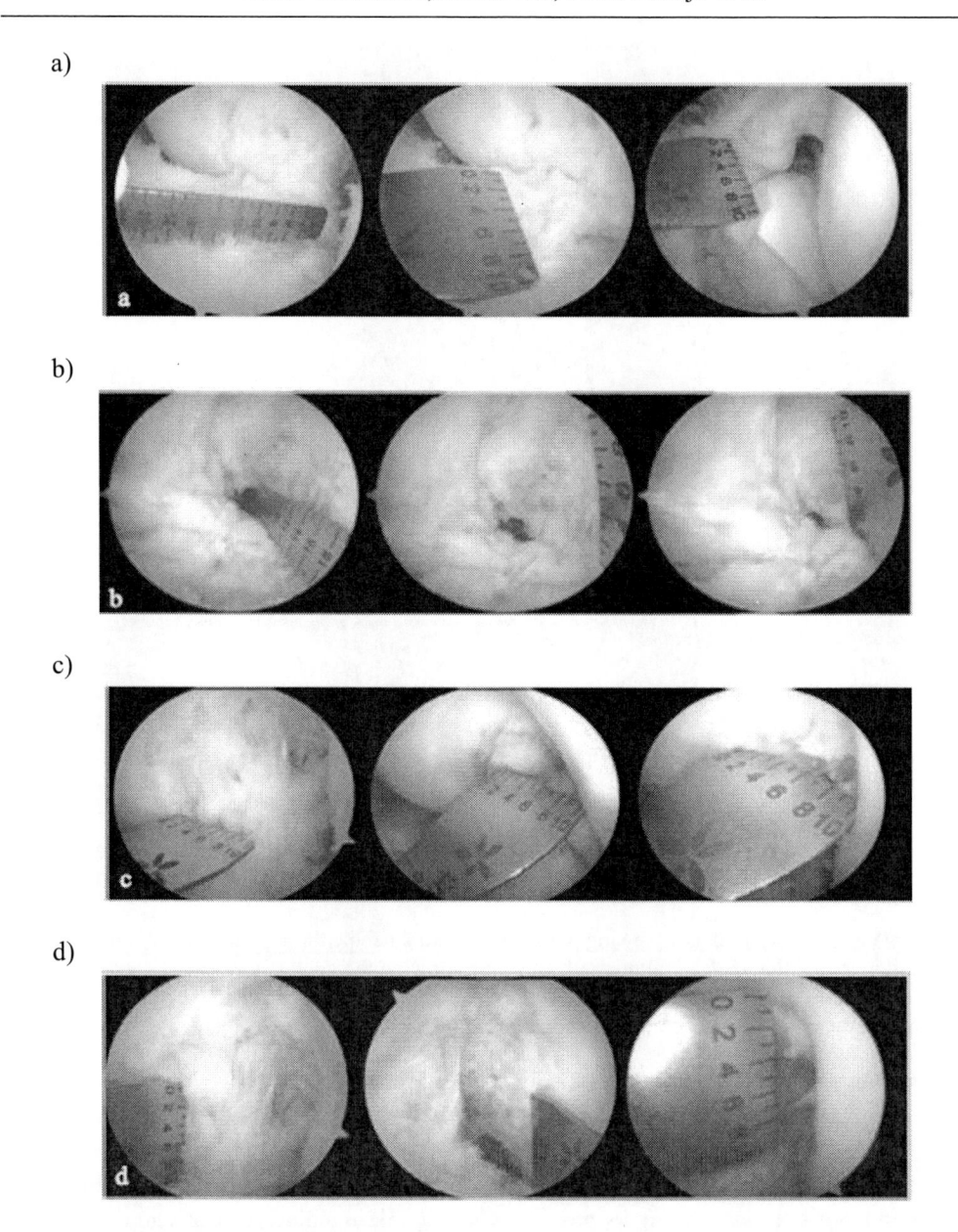

Figure 9. a: Tibial insertion site measurements. Overall length, AM width and PL width. b: Femoral insertion site measurements. Overall length, PL width and AM width. c: Notch width measurements at the bottom, middle and top. d: Notch height measurements at the medial and lateral walls.

Looking from the CP, a Steadman awl through the accessory AM portal is used to mark the center of the femoral insertion sites. These holes will later be used to place the guide wires for the femoral AM and PL footprints prior to drilling the femoral tunnels (Figure 11)

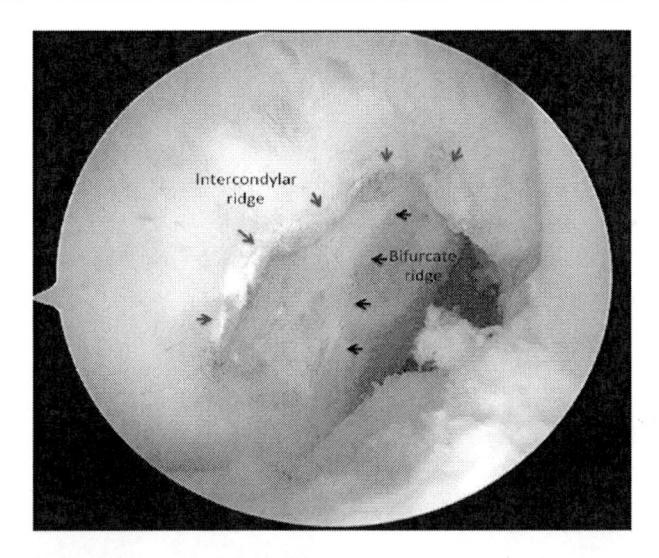

Figure 10. Intercondylar ridge in blue and bifurcate ridge in black.

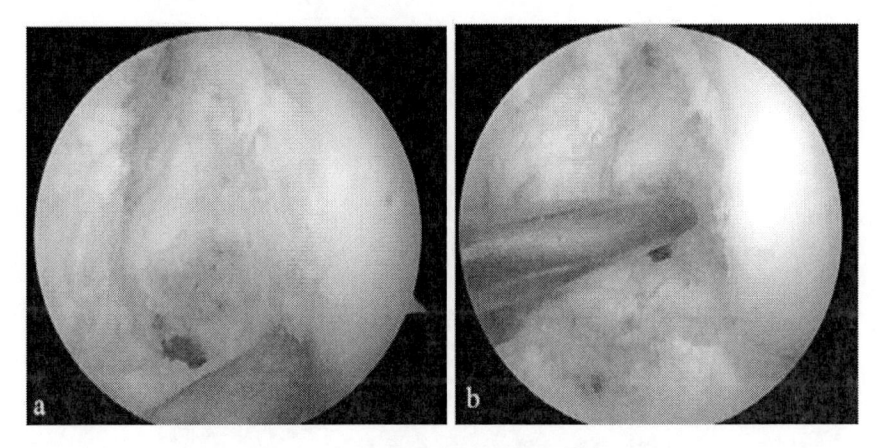

Figure 11. a: Steadman awl marking PL femoral placement. b: AM femoral placement.

The PL femoral tunnel is drilled first with the knee held in 110 degrees of flexion by an assistant. This protects the peroneal nerve and also ensures proper femoral tunnel length. As stated previously, the scope is placed in the CP portal while the PL femoral tunnel is drilled through the accessory AM portal. This position optimizes visualization of the lateral intercondylar notch. A 3.2 mm guide wire is inserted into the PL femoral footprint in the location previously marked by the Steadman awl and thermal device. A 7 mm cannulated acorn drill is inserted over the guide wire to drill the PL femoral tunnel typically to a depth of 25mm. The far cortex is then breached with a 4.5 mm EndoButton drill (Smith and Nephew, Andover, MA). The distance from the entrance of the PL femoral tunnel to the far cortex is measure with a depth gauge – if there is a significant difference in this length to the drilled tunnel length, the PL femoral tunnel length can be increased by drilling with the acorn drill by hand for better control to accommodate more graft within the tunnel.

Attention is then turned to the tibial side. A 3-4 cm vertical incision is made over the anteromedial surface of the tibia at the level of the tibial tubercle so that the AM and PL tunnels can be drilled through this incision. The scope is placed in the high AL portal to view the tibial footprints with a tibial guide placed in either the CP or the accessory AM portal. A tibial drill guide set at 45 degrees is first used to drill the PL tunnel with the tip of the drill guide placed at the center of the PL tunnel marked by the thermal device. The PL tibial insertion site is located within the triangle formed by the AM tibial insertion site, the PCL, and the posterior root of the lateral meniscus (Figure 12).

It is important to visualize the posterior root of the lateral meniscus to avoid damaging and/or detaching the root when drilling the PL tibial tunnel. A 3.2 mm guidewire is then passed for the PL tunnel using the tibial guide. Next, the tibial drill guide is set at 55 degrees for the AM tunnel. The tip of the drill guide is then placed at the center of the AM tunnel marked by the thermal device and in a similar fashion to the PL tibial tunnel, a 3.2 mm guidewire is passed for the AM tunnel using the tibial guide (Figure 13).

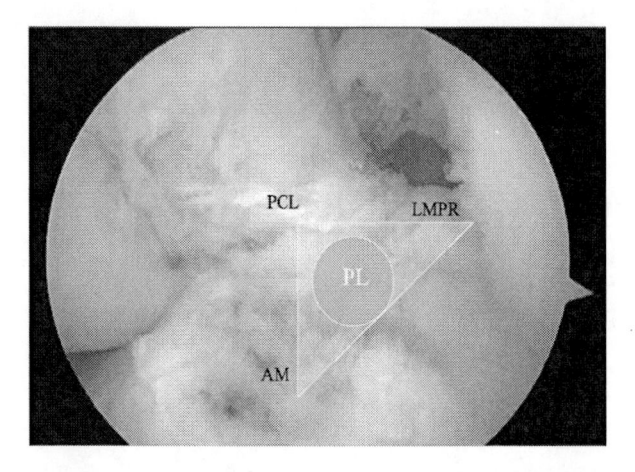

Figure 12. PL insertion site position within the triangle formed by AM insertion site, PCL and lateral meniscal posterior root (LMPR).

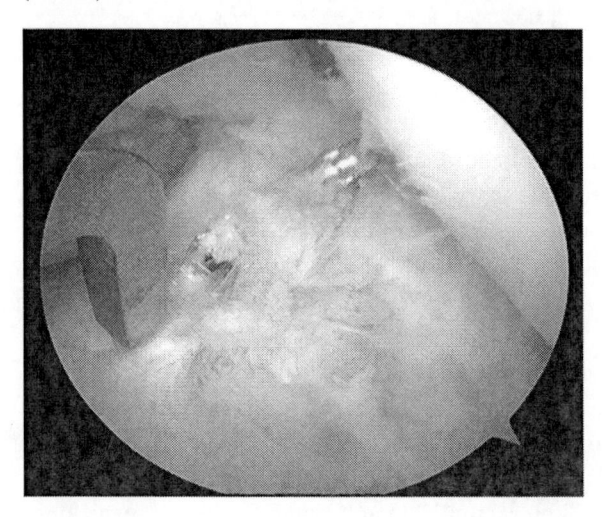

Figure 13. Drill guide positioning the AM guide wire with PL guidewire previously positioned in the same fashion.

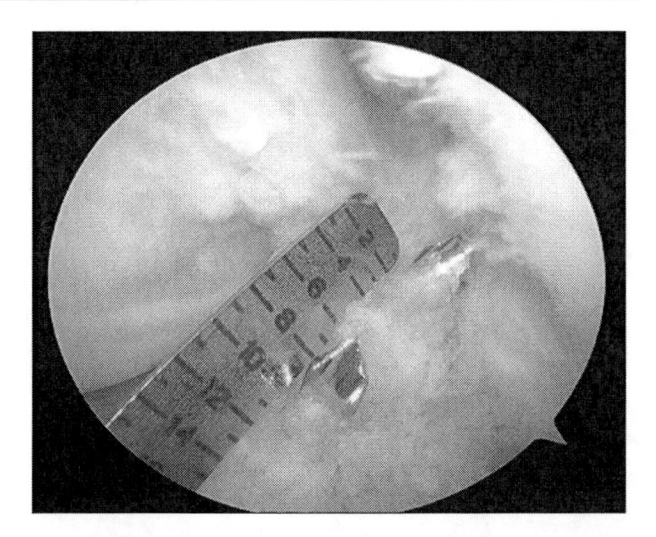

Figure 14. Measurement of the distance between the pins to ensure adequate space for two tibial tunnels during double-bundle ACL reconstruction.

With both guidewires in place, the distance between the pins is measured to confirm the drilling safety and ensure that there will not be any possible tunnel confluence. Distance between tunnels will vary depending on the diameter of the desired tunnels. In smallest insertion site double-bundle scenario (where the desired tunnels are 7 mm for the AM tunnel and 5 mm for the PL tunnel), the distance between the tunnels should be at least 8 mm to accommodate 2 mm of bone bridge (Figure 14).

The AM and PL tibial tunnels are then drilled using a cannulated compaction drill. The initial drill size used on power is typically 1 mm less than the desired size of the tunnels. A curette is placed over the guide wire intraarticularly to protect the femoral chondral surfaces when drilling into the joint. At the anteromedial tibial cortex, the PL tunnel is more medial and just anterior to the superficial medial collateral ligament while the AM tunnel is more anterior and central than the PL tunnel.

There should be at least a 10 mm osseous bridge between the 2 tunnels at their starting points. The tunnels are then usually dilated by hand typically to a 7 mm PL tibial tunnel and an 8 mm AM tibial tunnel (figure 15).

Next, attention is turned to the AM femoral tunnel. Again, the scope is placed in the CP to view the lateral intercondylar notch. Three different approaches may be used to reach the anatomic insertion site of the femoral AM tunnel. Depending on the patient's anatomy, a 3.2 mm guide wire can be placed transtibially through the AM or PL tibial tunnels, or the accessory AM portal can be utilized to reach the femoral AM tunnel. About 10% of the time, the femoral tunnel can be drilled in a transtibial fashion using the AM tibial tunnel, and 50% of the time, using the PL femoral tunnel [55]. The transtibial approach for the AM femoral tunnel is the preferred approach as this allows for more divergent tunnels and a longer tunnel length, but requires a half-moon special drill to avoid tibial PL tunnel enlargement (Figure 16).

If the transtibial approach does not allow us to reach the anatomic femoral AM insertion site, we use the accessory AM portal. In likewise fashion, the tip of the guidewire is inserted into the femoral AM insertion site using the previously marked hole from the Steadman awl and an 8 mm cannulated acorn drill is inserted over the guidewire.

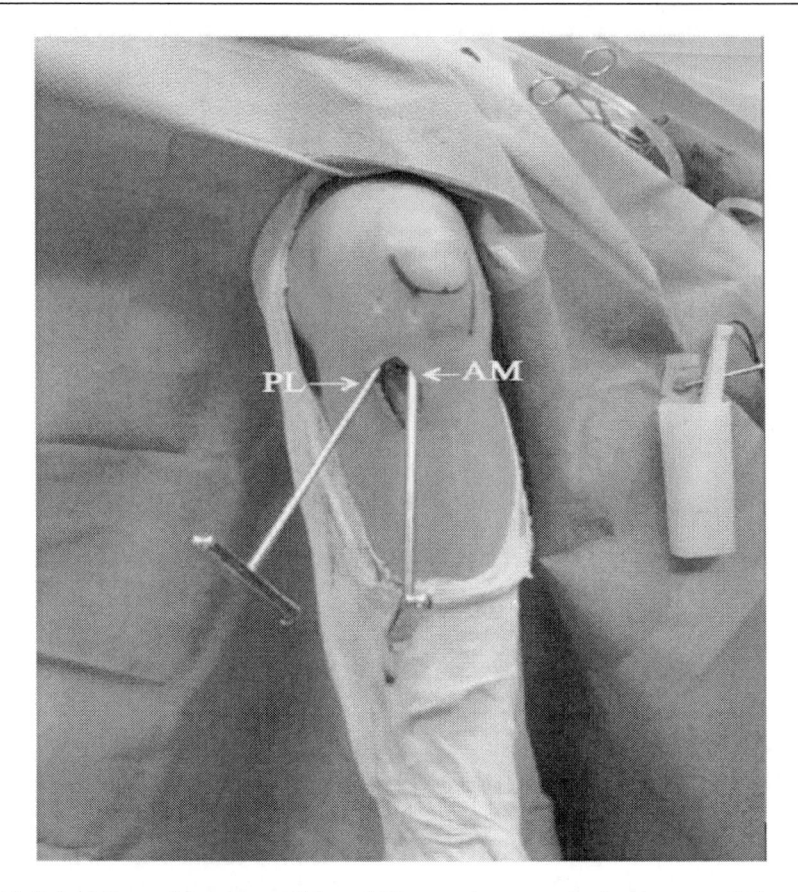

Figure 15. Medial AM tunnel aperture and lateral PL tunnel aperture in the anteromedial aspect of the tibia with a bone bridge larger than 10 mm.

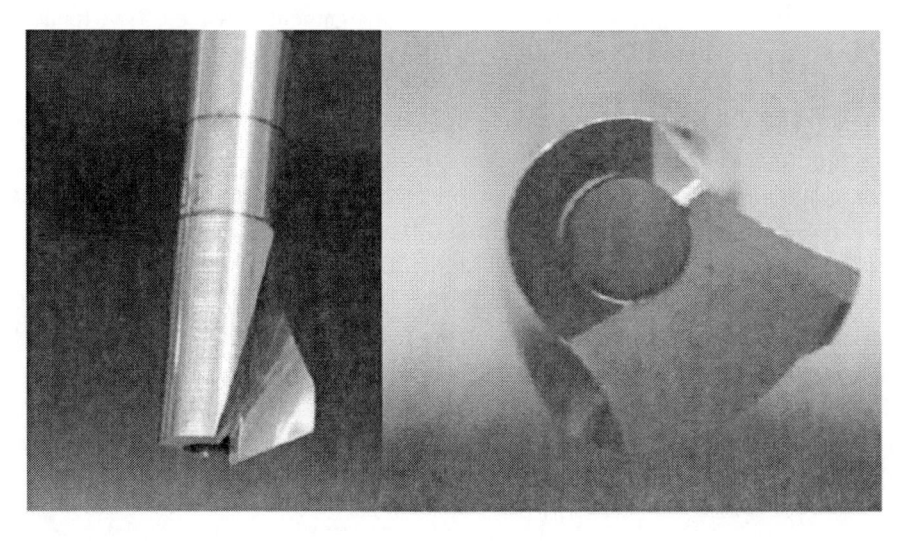

Figure 16. Half moon drill bit.

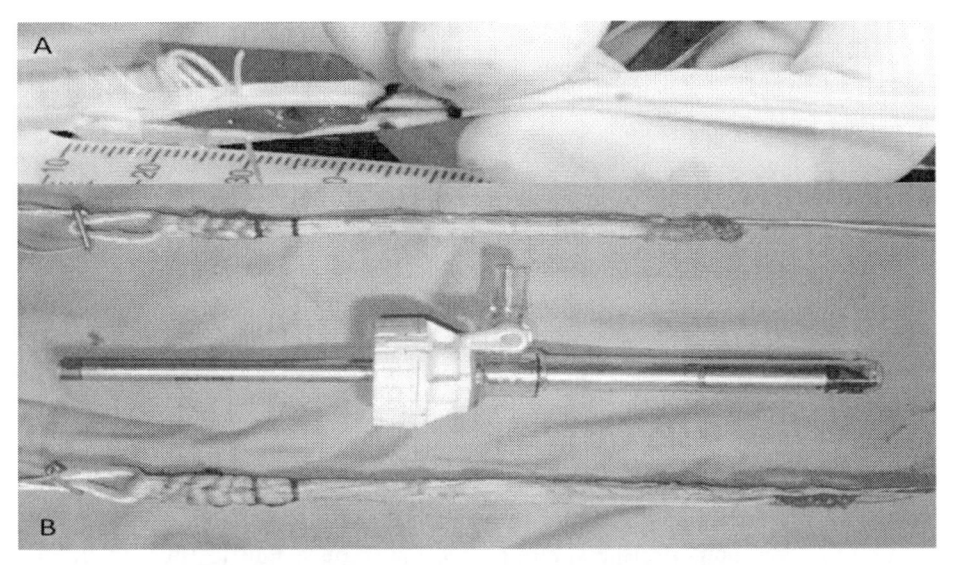

Figure 17. Fibrin clot sutured in the final 2cm ends of the graft. A: Fibrin clost placed between the graft. Notice the detail of the suture. B: Device used to place the fibrin clot between the AM and PL bundle grafts.

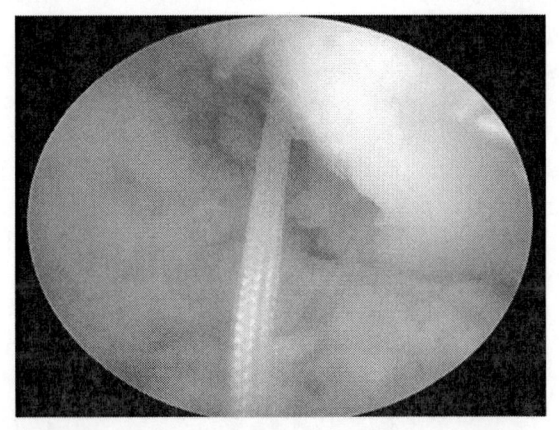

Figure 18. Suture placement to guide PL and AM graft passage.

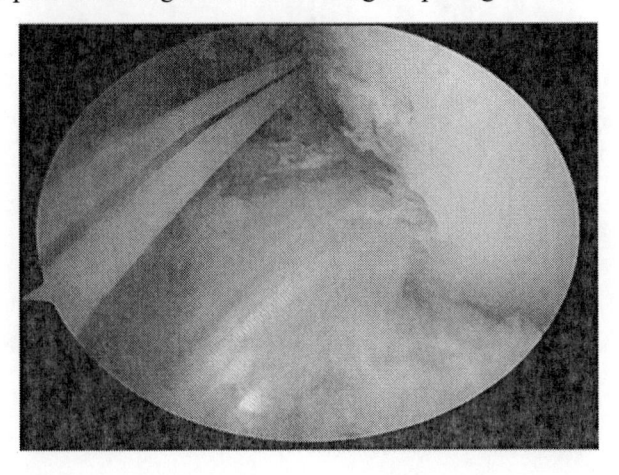

Figure 19. PL graft in place and suture prepared for AM graft passage.

The AM femoral tunnel is typically drilled to a 30-35 mm of length and then the far cortex is breached with a 4.5 mm EndoButton drill. A depth gauge is then used to measure to the far cortex and tunnel length increased accordingly with the 8 mm acorn drill bit by hand depending on length to the far cortex.

During the surgical procedure, the AM and PL grafts are prepared on the back table. Either gracilis and semitendinosus autograft, two tibialis anterior tendon allografts, or two tibialis posterior tendon allografts are typically used. These grafts should be 24-30 cm in length. A fibrin clot is obtained from 60 cc of the patient's venous blood. The clot is placed between the final 2 cm of the graft ends that will be inside the bone tunnels (Figure 17).

The ends of the grafts are sutured with Ultrabraid and Cobraid sutures (Smith and Nephew, Andover, MA) using a whip-stitch, and they are then looped around an EndoButton CL (Smith and Nephew, Andover, MA) to obtain double-stranded grafts. The length of the EndoButton loop is based on the measured femoral tunnel lengths. The tendon grafts are sized to match the diameter of each tunnel.

For the PL bundle graft, a Beath pin with an attached passing suture is placed through the accessory AM portal and with the suture passed out through the PL tibial tunnel using an arthroscopic suture grasper. For the AM bundle graft, a Beath pin with an attached passing suture is placed through the route used for drilling the AM femoral tunnel. A suture grasper is then used to pull the looped suture out through the AM tibial tunnel (Figure 18).

Using the shuttling suture just passed, the PL bundle graft is passed first and the EndoButton flipped on the outer femoral cortex in standard fashion. The AM bundle is then passed in similar fashion (Figure 19).

The grafts are visualized during tensioning to ensure full range of motion and absence of notch or PCL impingement. The knee is then cycled several times. We prefer fixation on the tibial side with bioabsorbable interference screws. The PL bundle is tensioned and fixed with the knee in full extension. A fibrin clot is positioned between the 2 grafts to enhance healing between the two grafts (Figure 20

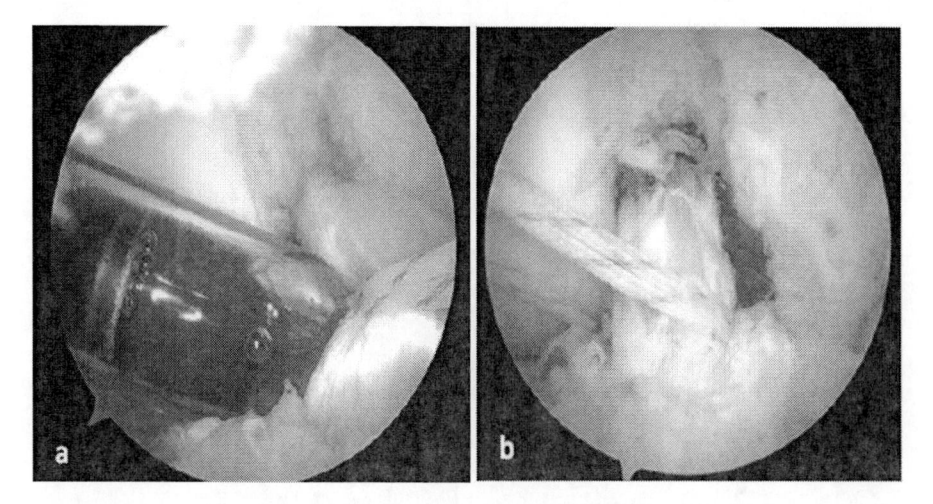

Figure 20. a: Fibrin clot inside the cannula being positioned between the AM and PL grafts. b: Final fibrin clot positioning.

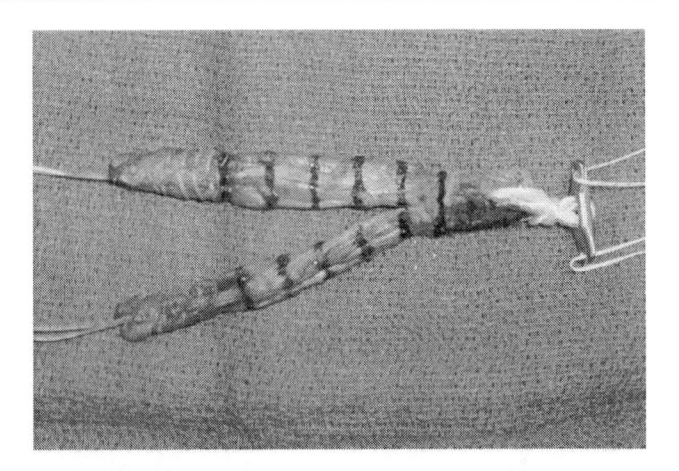

Figure 21. A split quadriceps tendon autograft.

The AM bundle is then tensioned and fixed at 45 degrees of flexion. Final arthroscopic pictures are obtained after all hardware has been placed and a C-arm is used to confirm that the two EndoButtons have been flipped on the lateral femoral cortex.

Surgical Technique (Quadriceps Tendon Autograft with Bone Block)

Double-bundle ACL reconstruction with a quadriceps tendon autograft is similar to the aforementioned procedure but with some key differences. These are seen particularly with respect to graft preparation and femoral tunnel drilling. A graft width of 10 mm is desired for both bone block and tendon width. In addition, the bone block harvested from the proximal portion of the patella should measure at least 20 mm in length and the tendinous portion from the superior aspect of the bone block to the proximal free tendon end should be 60 mm in length for a minimum total graft length of 80 mm. The bone block is fashioned to fit a 10 mm tunnel and placed in the femoral tunnel site. Endobutton-BTB (Smith and Nephew, Andover, NH) fixation is preferred for femoral tunnel fixation. The tendon is then split between the natural plane of the vastus intermedius and rectus femoris 20 mm from the bone block to the free end (Figure 21).

This will create a free tendon end of approximately 7 mm for the AM bundle and a 6 mm free tendon end for the PL bundle. These two limbs are then whip-stitched with heavy suture (E.g. No. 5 Ethibond).

For double-bundle ACL reconstruction with quadriceps tendon autograft, one tunnel is created in the femur to accept the bone block and two tunnels created in the tibia to reproduce the normal tibial insertional anatomy (Figure 22).

Diagnostic arthroscopy and marking of the femoral and tibial insertion sites are preformed as previously described using the same three aforementioned portals. With visualization through the central portal, a thermal device through the accessory AM portal is used to mark the center between the AM and PL footprints. A Steadman awl is then used demarcate the location for tunnel placement and a guidewire is then placed at the marked site (Figure 23).

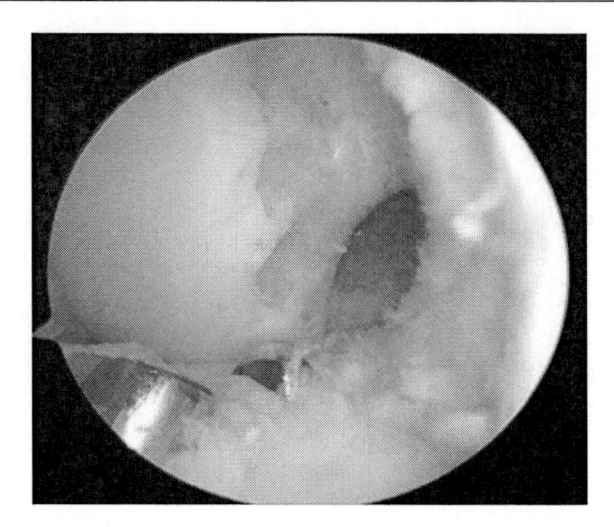

Figure 22. Arthroscopic view showing one femoral tunnel for the quadriceps bone block and two tibial tunnels for the soft tissue of the quadriceps tendon to recreate PL and AM bundles.

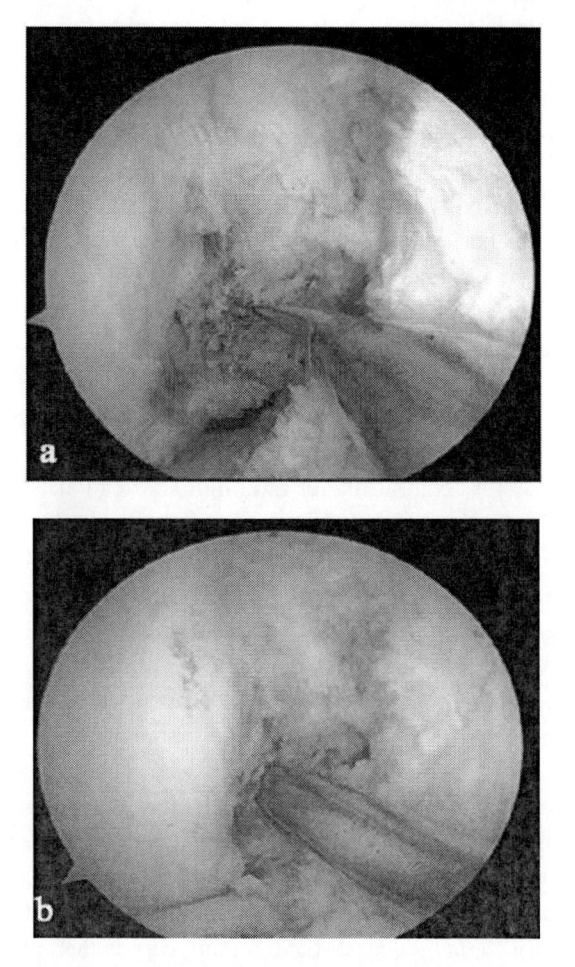

Figure 23. a: Steadman awl. b: Marked position for single femoral tunnel for the double-bundle technique using quadriceps tendon autograft with a bone block .

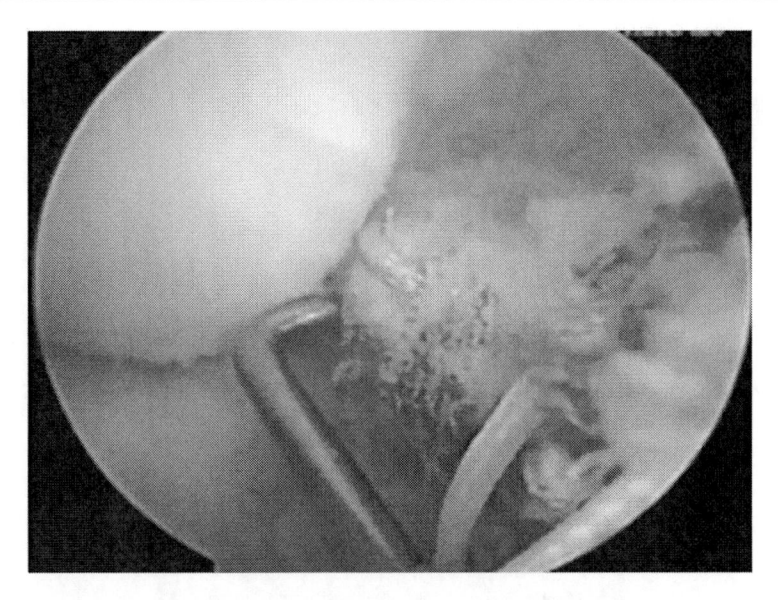

Figure 24. A probe guiding the quadriceps bone block into the femoral tunnel.

The knee is flexed to 120 degrees, and the guidewire is inserted into position. The femoral tunnel is first drilled to a preliminary depth of 25-30 mm with a 5 mm acorn reamer over the guidewire. An Endobutton drill is then used to breach the lateral cortex and the total femoral tunnel length is measured with a depth gauge. The tunnel is dilated by hand to a width of 9 mm with an acorn drill by hand, and then to 10 mm with a dilator. Typically, the tunnel length is 30-35 mm depending on the total distance from the lateral notch to the lateral femoral cortex. Once the femoral tunnel has been created, a 3 cm anteromedial skin incision on the tibia is made for creation and placement of the two tibial tunnels. The technique for this step is as previously described. Once the tibial tunnels are created, a beath pin loaded with a passing suture is introduced through the accessory AM portal into the femoral tunnel and out laterally through the skin. The prepared graft is then brought to the operating field. Prior to graft passage, it is advisable to ensure that the accessory AM portal can accommodate the bone block by placing a 10 mm dilator through the portal and incising and dilating as necessary to ensure that it passes freely. The graft is then passed into the knee joint using the passing sutures from the beath pin. The graft will often need to be guided into the femoral tunnel using a probe or a right-angle clamp (Figure 24).

The Endobutton is then flipped and fluoroscopic images are used to confirm location on the lateral cortex. The PL bundle is brought in first. The draw sutures for the tibial PL bundle are brought into the joint with a hemostat clamp through the accessory AM portal and ice tongs are then used to grasp these sutures into the PL tunnel transtibially. The PL bundle is then brought through the accessory AM portal and down into the PL tunnel (Figure 25a). The AM tibial bundle is brought into the accessory AM and down into the AM tibial tunnel in identical fashion (Figure 25b). As mentioned above, the PL bundle is fixed with the knee in 0 degrees of flexion with a bioabsorbable interference screw and the AM bundle fixed at 45 degrees of flexion with a bioabsorbable interference screw. Final arthroscopic pictures are obtained (figure 25c).

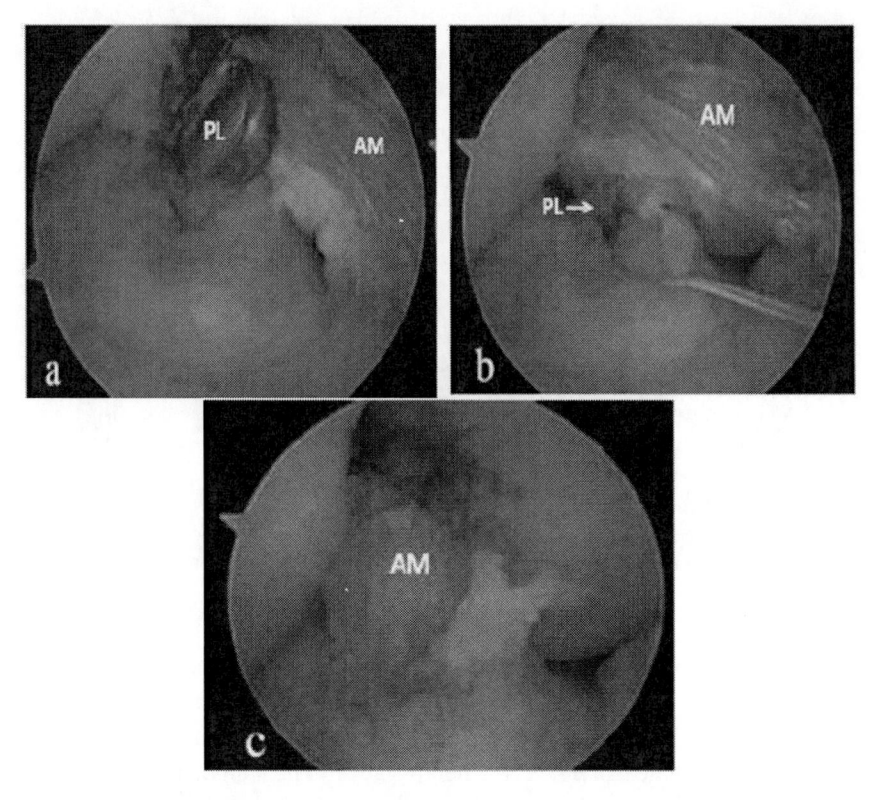

Figure 25. a: Quadriceps PL bundle passage in the tibia. b: suture prepared for quadriceps AM bundle passage. c: Final aspect after tensioning of both bundles.

Post-Op. Recovery

Patients are discharged home on the same day of surgery with pain medication. A cooling-device, such as a Cryocuff (Aircast, Summit, NJ) is placed around the operated knee and the leg is kept elevated.

Rehabilitation

Patients are kept in a hinged knee brace for a total of six weeks. They are locked in full extension for one week and are weight-bearing as tolerated with crutches if no meniscal repair has been performed. Patients are kept touch down weight bearing for four to six weeks if a concomitant meniscal repair has been performed. Continuous passive motion (CPM) is initiated after one week with progression to full flexion if no meniscal repair has been performed, and to a limit of 90 degrees of knee flexion if a meniscal repair has been performed. Heel slides and straight leg raises are initiated immediately. Typically, braces and crutches are weaned at six weeks depending on quadriceps strength. Once quadriceps strength is regained, straight line walking can be initiated at six weeks with progression to straight jogging and riding a stationary bike around three months. Pivoting and cutting is not allowed until at least six months or longer for autografts and seven to eight months for allografts.

Return to sport is typically around nine to twelve months for both autografts and allografts. If the patient desires an earlier return to sport, an MRI is done to evaluate graft maturation and the return to sport decision is based on this imaging and clinical readiness as assessed by the surgeon and physical therapist.

Complications

General complications following double-bundle ACL reconstruction surgery are similar to those seen in single-bundle reconstruction. ACL reconstruction is one of the most commonly performed orthopaedic procedure. Though complications are infrequent, they include hemarthrosis, effusions, neurovascular injury, and wound infection in addition to tibial or femoral fractures and tunnel widening. If a tibial incision is made, the infrapatellar branch of the saphenous nerve can be injured leading to loss of sensation along the anterolateral aspect of the knee.

Anatomic ACL double-bundle reconstruction is a more challenging surgery than traditional single-bundle reconstruction. For this reason, the concept of anatomic ACL reconstruction should be first solidified using a single-bundle technique before attempting the double-bundle approach.

CONCLUSION

ACL reconstruction is one of the most common orthopaedic procedures performed in the United States. Single-bundle reconstruction remains the gold standard for returning athletes to competitive play. Though capable of successfully treating most ACL injuries, non-anatomic single-bundle procedures fail to restore rotational kinematics of the knee and joint stability. The anatomic double-bundle surgical approach resotres the native anatomy and function of both the AM bundle and the PL bundle.

ACL reconstruction should respect individualized aspects of patient anatomy. Hence, individualized anatomic ACL surgery more readily achieves the goal of restoring a patient's native anatomy and knee function following ACL injury. The clinical implications of this restoration of functional anatomy and kinematics on long-term outcomes are current topics of ACL research.

REFERENCES

[1]   Adachi, et al.: Reconstruction of the anterior cruciate ligament: Single- versus double-bundle multistranded hamstring tendons. *J. Bone Joint Surg. Br.* 2004; 86: 515–520.

[2]   Anderson, C. J., Westerhaus, B. D., Pietrini, S. D., Ziegler, C. G., Wijdicks, C. A., Johansen, S., Engebretsen, L., Laprade, R. F. Kinematic impact of anteromedial and posterolateral bundle graft fixation angles on double-bundle anterior cruciate ligament reconstructions. *Am. J. Sports Med.* 2010 Aug.; 38 (8): 1575–83.

[3] Araujo, P. H., Van Eck, C. F., Macalena, J. A., Fu, F. H. Advances in the three-portal technique for anatomic single- or double-bundle ACL reconstruction. *Knee Surg. Sports Traumatol. Arthrosc.* 2011 Feb. 11. [Ahead of Print].

[4] Arnoczky, S. P.: Anatomy of the anterior cruciate ligament. *Clin. Orthop. Relat. Res.* 1983; 172: 19–25.

[5] Bach, J. M., Hull, M. L., Patterson, H. A. Direct measurement of strain in the posterolateral bundle of the anterior cruciate ligament. *J. Biomech.* 1997 March; 30 (3) 281–283.

[6] Belisle, A. L., Bicos, J., Geaney, L., et al. Strain pattern comparison of double- and single-bundle anterior cruciate ligament reconstruction techniques with the native anterior cruciate ligament. *Arthroscopy.* 2007; 23 (11): 1210–1217.

[7] Bellier, G., et al.: Double-stranded hamstring graft for anterior cruciate ligament reconstruction. *Arthroscopy* 2004; 20: 890–894.

[8] Bernstein, J. Early versus delayed reconstruction of the anterior cruciate ligament: A decision analysis approach. *J. Bone Joint Surg. Am.* 2001; 98: e 48 (1-5).

[9] Beynnon, B. D., Johnson, R. J., Abate, J. A., Fleming, B. C., Nichols, C. E. Treatment of anterior cruciate ligament injuries, part I. *Am. J. Sports Med.* 2005; 33 (10): 1579.

[10] Boden, B. P., Dean, G. S., Feagin, J. A. Jr, Garret, W. E. Jr. Mechanisms of anterior cruciate ligament injury. *Orthopedics.* 2000; 23 (6): 573.

[11] Chhabra, A., et al. Anatomic, radiographic, biomechanical, and kinematic evaluation of the anterior cruciate ligament and its two functional bundles. *J. Bone Joint Surg. Am.* 2006; 88: 2–10.

[12] Cuomo, P., Rama, K. R., Bull, A. M., Amis, A. A. (2007) The effects of different tensioning strategies on knee laxity and graft tension after double-bundle anterior cruciate ligament reconstruction. *Am. J. Sports Med.* 35:2083-2090.

[13] Dienst, M., Burks, R. T., Greis, P. E.: Anatomy and biomechanics of the anterior cruciate ligament. Orthop .Clin. North Am. 2002; 33: 605–620.

[14] Ferretti, M, et al. The fetal anterior cruciate ligament: An anatomic and histologic study. *Arthroscopy.* 2007; 23: 278–283.

[15] Fithian, D. C., Paxton, L. W., Goltz, D. H. Fate of the anterior cruciate ligament-injured knee. *Orthop. Clin. North Am.* 2002; 33 (4): 621.

[16] Freedman, K. B., D'Amato, M. J., Nedeff, D. D., et al. Arthroscopic anterior cruciate ligament reconstruction: a meta-analysis comparing patellar tendon and hamstring tendon autografts. *Am. J. Sports Med.* 2003; 31: 2–11.

[17] Frobell, R. B., Roos, E. M., Roos, H. P., Ranstam, J., Lohmander, L. S. A randomized trial of treatment for acute anterior cruciate ligament tears. *N Engl. J. Med.* 2010; 363: 331–342.

[18] Gabriel, M. T. et al. Distribution of in situ forces in the anterior cruciate ligament using a double bundle. *Arthroscopy.* 2000;16: 860–864.

[19] Gabriel, M. T., Wong, E. K., Woo, S. L., et al. Distribution of in situ forces in the anterior cruciate ligament in response to rotator loads. *J. Orthop. Res.* 2004; 22: 85–89.

[20] Gabriel, M. T., Wong, E. K., Woo, S. L., Yagi, M., Debski, R. E. Distribution of in situ forces in the anterior cruciate ligament in response to rotator loads. *J. Orthop. Res. Jan.* 2004; 22 (1): 85-89.

[21] Gardner, E., O'Rahilly, R. The Early development of the knee joint in staged human embryos. *J. Anat.* 1968; 102: 289–299.

[22] Girgis, F. G., Marshall, J. L., Monajem, A: The cruciate ligaments of the knee joint: Anatomical, functional, and experimental analysis. *Clin. Orthop. Relat. Res.* 1975; 106: 216–231.

[23] Hamada, M. et al: Single- versus bi-socket anterior cruciate ligament reconstruction using autogenous multiple-stranded hamstring tendons with endoButton femoral fixation: A prospective study. *Arthroscopy* 2001; 17: 801–807.

[24] Hara, K. et al: Reconstruction of the anterior cruciate ligament using a double bundle. *Arthroscopy* 2000; 16: 860–864.

[25] Hardaker, W. T. Jr, Garrett, W. E. Jr, Bassett, F. H. 3rd. Evaluation of acute traumatic hemarhrosis of the knee joint. *South Med. J.* 1990; 83 (6): 640.

[26] Harner, C. D., Baek, G. H., Vogrin, T. M., Carlin, G. J., Kashiwaguchi, S., Woo, S. L.: Quantitative analysis of human cruciate ligament insertions. *Arthroscopy* 1999; 15: 741–749.

[27] Hurd, W. J., Axe, M. J., Synder-Mackler, L. A 10-year prospective trial of a patient management algorithm and screening examination for highly active individuals with anterior cruciate ligament injury: Part 1, outcomes. *Am. J. Sports Med.* 2008; 36 (1): 40.

[28] Jackson, J. L., O'Malley, P. G. and Kroenke, K. Evaluation of acute knee pain in primary care. *Ann. Intern. Med.* 2003; 139 (7): 575.

[29] Jordan, S. S., DeFrate, L. E., Nha, K. W., Papannagari, R., Gill, T. J., Li, G. The in vivo kinematics of the anteromedial and posterolateral bundles of the anterior cruciate ligament during weightbearing knee flexion. *Am. J. Sports Med.* 2007; 35 (4): 547–554.

[30] Kubo, T. et al.: Anterior cruciate ligament reconstruction using the double-bundle method. *J. Orthop. Surg* .(Hong Kong) 2000; 8: 59 – 63.

[31] Kummer, B., Yamamoto, Y. Funktionelle Anatomie der Kreuzbaender. *Arthroskopie* 1988; 1: 2–10.

[32] Kurosawa, H., Yamakoshi, K., Yasuda, K., Sasaki, T. Simultaneous measurement of changes in length of the cruciate ligaments during knee motion. *Clin. Orthop. Relat. Res.* 1991; 265: 233–240.

[33] Li, G., DeFrate, L. E., Sun, H., Gill, T. J. In vivo elongation of the anterior cruciate ligament and posterior cruciate ligament during knee flexion. *Am. J. Sports Med.* 2004; 32 (6): 1415–1420.

[34] Li, G., Zayontz, S., Most, E., DeFrate, L. E., Suggs, J. F., Rubash, H. E. In situ forces of the anterior and posterior cruciate ligaments in high knee flexion: an in vitro investigation. *J. Orthop. Res.* 2004 March; 22 (2) 293–297.

[35] Mae, T., Shino, K., Matsumoto, N., Nakata, K., Nakamura, N., Iwahashi, T. Force sharing between two grafts in the anatomical two-bundle anterior cruciate ligament reconstruction. *Knee Surg. Sports Traumatol. Arthrosc.* 2006; 14 (6): 505–509.

[36] Mae, T., Shino, K., Matsumoto, N., Natsu-Ume, T., Yoneda, K., Yoshikawa, H., Yoneda, M. (2010) Anatomic double-bundle anterior cruciate ligament reconstruction using hamstring tendons with minimally required initial tension. *Arthroscopy* 26:1289-1295

[37] Maffulli, N., Binfield, P. M., King, J. B., Good, C. J. Acute haemarthrosis of the knee is athletes. A prospective study of 106 cases. *J. Bone Joint Surg. Br.* 1993; 75 (6): 945.

[38] Marcacci, M. et al: Anatomic double-bundle anterior cruciate ligament reconstruction with hamstrings. *Arthoscopy* 2003; 19: 540–546.

[39] Mayr, H. O., Weig, T. G., Plitz, W. Arthrofibrosis following ACL reconstitution – reasons and outcome. *Arch. Orthop. Trauma. Surg.* 2004; 124 (8): 518.

[40] McIntosh, A. L., Dahm, D. L., Stuart, M. J. Anterior cruciate ligament reconstruction in the skeletally immature patient. *Arthroscopy.* 2006; 22 (12): 1325–1330.

[41] Mott, H. W.: Semitendinous anatomic reconstruction for cruciate ligament insufficiency. *Clni. Orthop. Relat. Res.* 1983; 172: 90–92.

[42] Mountcastle, S. B., Posner, M., Kragh, J. F. Jr, Taylor, D. C. Gender differences in anterior cruciate ligament injury vary with activity: epidemiology of anterior cruciate ligament injuries in a young, athletic population. *Am. J. Sports Med.* 2007; 35 (10): 1635.

[43] Muneta, T.: Two-bundle reconstruction of the anterior cruciate ligament using semitendinosus tendon with endobuttons: Operative technique and preliminary results. *Arthroscopy* 1999; 15: 618–624.

[44] Noyes, F. R., Bassett, R. W., Grood, E. S., Butler, D. L. Arthroscopy in acute traumatic hemarthrosis of the knee. Incidence of anterior cruciate tears and other injuries. *J. Bone Joint Surg. Am.* 1980; 62 (5): 687.

[45] O'Rahilly, R. The early prenatal development of the human knee joint. *J. Anat.* 1951; 85: 166–170.

[46] Ockert, B., Haasters, F., Polzer, H., Grote, S., Kessler, M. A., Mutschler, W., and Kanz, K. G. Value of the clinical examination in suspected meniscal injuries. A meta-analysis]. *Unfallchirung.* 2010: 113 (4): 293.

[47] Odensten, M., Gillquist, J. Functional anatomy of the anterior cruciate ligament and a rationale for reconstruction. *J. Bone Joint Surg. Am.* 1984; 67: 257–262.

[48] Palmer, I. On the injuries on the ligaments of the knee joint. A clinical study. *Acta. Chir. Scand.* 2010. 81: 282.

[49] Pearle, A. D., Shannon, F. J., Granchi, C., Wickiewics, T. L., Warren, R. F. Comparison of 3-dimensional obliquity and anisometric characteristics of anterior cruciate ligament graft positions using surgical navigation. *Am. J. Sports Med.* 2008; 36 (8): 1534–1541.

[50] Petersen, W., Tretow, H., Weimann, A., et al. Biomechanical evaluation of two techniques for double-bundle anterior cruciate ligament reconstruction: one tibial tunnel versus two tibial tunnels. *Am. J. Sports Med.* 2007; 35 (2): 228–234.

[51] Radford, W. J., Amis, A. A.: Biomechanics of a double prosthetic ligament in the anterior cruciate deficient knee. *J. Bone Joint Surg. Br.* 1990; 72: 1038–1043.

[52] Robinson, J., Stanford, F. C., Kendoff, D., Stuber, V., Pearle, A. D. Replication of the range of native anterior cruciate ligament fiber length change behavior achieved by different grafts: Measurement using computer assisted navigation. *Am. J. Sports Med.* 2009; 37 (7): 1406–1411.

[53] Sahnghoon, L. *J. Bone Joint Surg. Am.* 2007;89 (Suppl. 3):116-26

[54] Shelbourne, K. D., Gray, T., Wiley, B. V. Results of transphyseal anterior cruciate ligament reconstruction using patellar tendon autograft in tanner stage 3 or 4 adolescents with clearly open growth plates. *Am. J. Sports Med.* 2004; 32 (5): 1218–1222.

[55] Schreiber, V. M., Van Eck, C. F., Fu, F. H. Anatomic Double-bundle ACL Reconstruction. *Sports Med. Arthrosc.* 2010; 18 (1): 27–32.

[56] Smith, B. A., Liesay, G. A., Woo, S. L.: Biology and biomechanics of the anterior cruciate ligament. *Clin. Sports Med.* 1993; 12: 637–670.

[57] Solomon, D. H., Simel, D. L., Bates, D. W., Katz, J. N., and Schaffer, J. L. The rational clinical examination. Does this patient have a torn meniscus or ligament of the knee? Value of the physical exam. *JAMA*. 2001; 286 (13): 1610.

[58] Takeuchi, R. et al.: Double-bundle anatomic anterior cruciate ligament reconstruction using bone-hamstring-bone composite graft. *Arthroscopy* 2002; 18: 550–555.

[59] Van Eck, C. F., Schreiber, V. M., Liu, T. T., and Fu, F. H. 2010. The anatomic approach to primary, revision and augmentation anterior cruciate ligament reconstruction. *KSSTA*. 2010. 18 (9): 1154–1163.

[60] Wu, C., Noorani, S., Vercillo, F., Woo, S. L. Tension patterns of the antero-medial and posterolateral grafts in a double bundle anterior cruciate ligament reconstruction. *J. Orthop. Res*. 2009; 27 (7): 879–884.

[61] Yagi, M. et al.: Biomechanical analysis of an anatomic anterior cruciate ligament reconstruction. Am. J. Sports Med. 2002; 30: 660–666.

[62] Yagi, M., Wong, E. K., Kanamori, A., Deski, R. E., Fu, F. H., Woo, S. L. Biomechanical analysis of an anatomic anterior cruciate ligament reconstruction. *Am. J. Sports Med*. 2002; 30 (5): 660–666.

[63] Yamamoto, Y. et al.: Knee stability and graft function after anterior cruciate ligament reconstruction: A comparison of a lateral and an anatomical femoral tunnel placement. *Am. J. Sports Med*. 2004; 32: 1825–1832.

[64] Yasuda, K. et al: Anatomic reconstruction of the anteriomedial and posterolateral bundles of the anterior cruciate ligament using hamstring tendon grafts. *Arthroscopy* 2004; 20: 1015–1025.

[65] Yasuda, K., Ichiyama, H., Kondo, E., Miyatake, S., Inoue, M., Tanabe, Y. An in vivo biomechanical study on the tension-versus-knee-flexion angle curves of 2 grafts in anatomic double-bundle anterior cruciate ligament reconstruction: Effects of initial tension and internal tibial rotation. *Arthroscopy*. 2008; 24 (3); 276–284.

[66] Yasuda, K., Van Eck, C. F., Hoshino, Y., Fu, F. H., Tashman, S. Anatomic single- and double-bundle anterior cruciate ligament reconstruction, Part 1: Basic Science. *Am. J. Sports Medicine*. DOI: 10.1177/0363546511402659.

[67] Yunes, M., Richmond, J. C., Engels, E. A., et al. Patellar versus hamstring tendons in anterior cruciate ligament reconstruction – a meta-analysis. *Arthroscopy* 2001; 17: 248–257.

[68] Zantop, T., Herbort, M., Raschke, M. J. Fu, F. H., Petersen, W. The role of the anteromedial and posterolateral bundles of the anterior cruciate ligament in anterior tibial translation and internal rotation. *Am. J. Sports Med*. Feb. 2007; 35 (2): 223–227.

[69] Zaricznyj, B.: Reconstruction of the anterior cruciate ligament of the knee using a double tendon graft. *Clin. Orthop. Relat. Res*. 1987; 220: 162–175.

In: The Knee
Editor: Randy Mascarenhas

ISBN: 978-1-61942-268-1
© 2012 Nova Science Publishers, Inc.

Chapter VIII

CURRENT CONCEPTS IN PCL RECONSTRUCTION

Mohamed M. Ahmed, Neil Ghodadra
and Brian Forsythe

University of Illinois at Chicago, Chicago, Illinois, US
Rush University Medical Center, Chicago, Illinois, US
Midwest Orthopedics at Rush, RUMC, Illinois, US

OVERVIEW

Treatment of posterior cruciate ligament injuries may require different approaches ranging from conservative management to surgical reconstruction. With the varying success of surgical treatment, controversy exists as to which approach to use. PCL injuries occur at higher rates than previously believed (PCL injuries comprise 3% of all knee injuries and 37% of trauma cases with acute hemarthrosis[1]), and recent research has provided orthopedic surgeons with a better understanding of treatment algorithms and surgical techniques.

ANATOMY

The posterior cruciate ligament originates from the lateral portion of the medial femoral condyle and inserts one cm below the joint line on the posterior intercondylar tibia. It is shorter than the ACL and has been found to have an average length of 38 mm[47]. Additionally, the PCL has been shown to have a higher tensile strength than the ACL[2]. The primary role of the PCL is to prevent posterior translation of the proximal tibia in relation to the distal femur. Secondary restraints to this posterior translation include the collateral ligaments and the posterolateral corner (PLC). The PCL also acts as a secondary restraint to varus and valgus stress in addition to serving as a restraint to external rotation[12].

The PCL is comprised of two bundles of fibers: the anterolateral bundle (ALB) and the posteromedial bundle (PMB) (Figure 1). These bundles together resist posterior translation of the tibia in both extension and flexion. The PMB has found to be tense in unloaded extension, while the ALB was found to be tense in unloaded flexion[4]. The ALB has been found to be

150% stronger than the PMB, with PMB strength being mainly isometric[2]. The PCL complex also includes the anterior (ligament of Humphrey) and posterior (ligament of Wrisberg) meniscofemoral ligaments, which act as secondary stabilizers against posterior translation of the tibia[34].

The vascular supply to the PCL comes mainly from the middle genicular artery[5] , which branches off the popliteal artery. The PCL is innervated by the popliteal plexus, which is comprised of the posterior articular nerve and the obturator nerve. The posterior articular nerve is a branch of the posterior tibial nerve[6].

Surgeons previously performed PCL reconstruction without using any anatomical landmarks for tunnel placement. The femoral origin of the PCL has been found to be semicircular and concave. Lopes et al found through three-dimensional laser photography that a medial intercondylar ridge existed proximal to the femoral footprint of the PCL in eighteen of twenty human knees[3]. This medial intercondylar ridge serves as the proximal border of the PCL footprint. The ALB footprint was found to have an average area of 118 mm^2 with a standard deviation of 23.95 mm^2, while the PMB footprint was found to have an average area of 90 mm^2 with a standard deviation of 16.13 mm^2. There is also a clear change in slope between the ALB and PMB, termed the medial bifurcate ridge[3]. This ridge separates the two insertion sites of the ALB and the PMB (Figure 2). Consideration of each of these aforementioned landmarks can lead to better anatomical consideration when drilling femoral tunnels in PCL reconstruction.

Mechanism of PCL Injury

A posteriorly directed force to the proximal tibia is the major mechanism for PCL injury[7]. In a study of 587 patients with confirmed PCL insufficiency by Schultz et al, the authors found that 45.3% of injuries were secondary to motor vehicle accidents, 39.9% were due to athletic injury, and 12% resulted from other causes[8]. According to Fowler et al, the most common causative mechanism in isolated PCL injury is forced knee hyperflexion, which results in the PMB remaining intact while the ALB is ruptures[9]. On the other hand, combined PCL injuries result from forced varus or valgus stress on the knee, hyperextension injuries, and knee dislocations. These injuries usually result in tears of multiple ligaments[10].

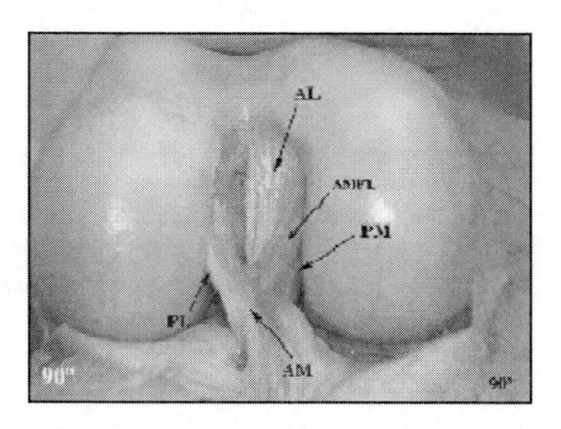

Figure 1. A cadaver knee showing the anterolateral bundle, posteromedial bundle, the anterior meniscofemoral ligament, and the ACL.

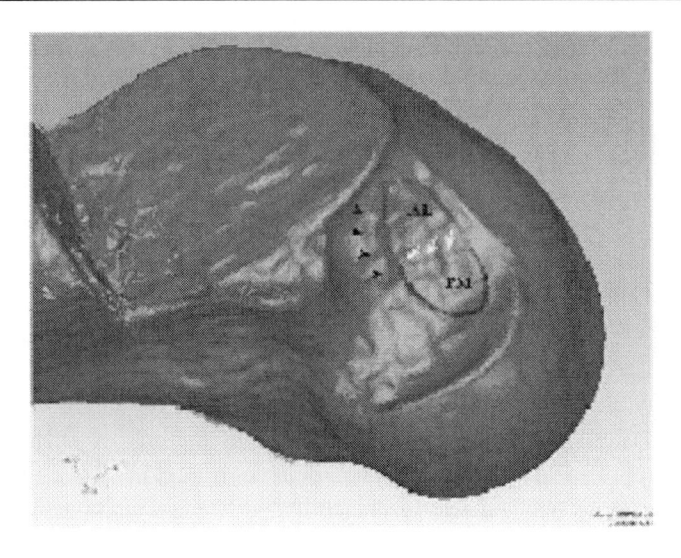

Figure 2. A 3-dimensional image reconstruction showing the femoral footprints of the ALB and PMB. White arrows show the medial bifurcate ridge. Black arrows show the medial intercondylar ridge. The image demonstrates a left knee in flexion from an anterolateral view.

Grading of PCL Injuries

PCL injuries are graded on a scale from I-III[7]

1.   Grade I → 0-5 mm of posterior translation; anterior step off is maintained (partial tear).
2.   Grade II →5-10 mm of posterior translation; medial tibial plateau aligned with medial femoral condyle (partial tear).
3.   Grade III → >10 mm posterior translation; other associated ligamentous injuries (complete tear).

Timing of PCL Injuries

Acute vs. Chronic

1.   Acute → Injury occurred within 3 weeks of diagnosis[7]; usually associated with multi-ligamentous injuries.
2.   Chronic → Injury occurred more than 3 weeks prior to diagnosis; usually associated with grade I or grade II tears.

DIAGNOSIS AND HISTORY

Patients with PCL injuries may present to the clinic with a wide array of symptoms. Patients with chronic PCL insufficiency may present with minimal symptoms, while those with a more acute injury may report severe pain and hemarthrosis[7]. A thorough history must be taken from the patient to accurately assess for PCL injury. Information should be gleaned about the timing and mechanism of injury, as well as symptomatology. There are generally two main venues for PCL injury: high-energy trauma and sporting activity.

Athletic injuries have usually been found to result in isolated PCL tears, while high-energy trauma usually results in multi-ligamentous knee injuries[12]. PCL injury in athletes is most commonly caused by a posteriorly directed force to the proximal tibia with the foot in plantar flexion[12]. High-energy trauma, such as motor vehicle accidents where the dashboard impacts a flexed knee, is a more common cause of PCL injury than athletic injury.

In patients with isolated PCL insufficiency, it has been found that patients rarely report a "pop". Patients may also lack an initial sense of instability[11]. In acute PCL injuries, patients may report pain posteriorly in the knee, along with symptoms of stiffness and swelling. Patients may also report of pain when the knee is in deep flexion[12]. In chronic PCL injuries, patients may report knee pain anteriorly, instability, difficulty walking up and down steps, and pain whilst sprinting and decelerating[13].

PHYSICAL EXAMINATION

Physical examination should begin with assessment of the patient's lower extremity alignment and gait. Patients with a chronic PCL tear or with deficient posterolateral corner (PLC) may present with varus alignment and a varus thrust gait in addition to external rotation. Acute injuries present with effusions, while chronic injuries may or may not.

Posterior Drawer Test

This is the most accurate test for PCL integrity. Rubenstein et al found that the posterior drawer test was the most sensitive test and very specific for diagnosing PCL insufficiency. It was found to be 90% sensitive and 99% specific for PCL injury assessment[23] (Figures 3a. and 3b.).

In a study performed by Sekiya et al, it was hypothesized that a grade III PCL rupture could not be present without associated damage to the PLC. The authors tested ten paired cadaver knees and found that a complete isolated PCL tear resulted in a grade II posterior drawer sign, while a grade III sign was found only with damage to the PLC as well as complete rupture of the PCL[38].

1. Patient must be in the supine position.
2. Hip must be flexed to 45°.
3. Knee must be flexed to 90°.
4. Foot must be in the neutral position.
5. Reduce tibia by pulling anteriorly.
6. Both hands placed behind proximal tibia with a posteriorly directed force applied to the tibia.
7. Position of the medial tibial plateau relative to medial femoral condyle is assessed (Table 1).

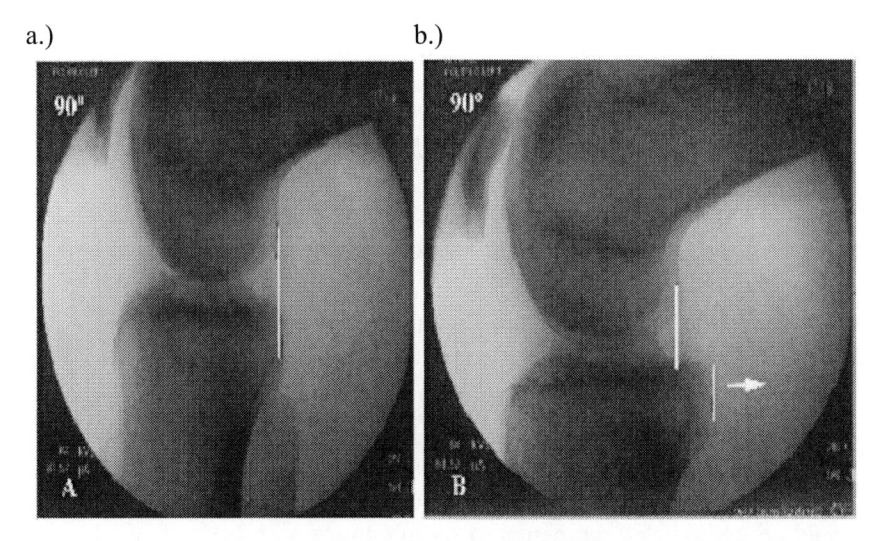

Figure 3. a. Lateral fluoroscopic view of resting knee. b. Lateral fluoroscopic view of knee with an applied posterior drawer force. Notice the translation of the tibia relative to the femur.

Table 1. Posterior drawer grading scale for PCL injury

Displacement of 0 to 5mm → Grade I, II PCL injury, medial tibia plateau anterior to MFC
Displacement of 5mm to 10mm → Grade III PCL injury, medial tibia plateau flush with MFC
Displacement >10mm → Grade III PCL Injury + PLC injury, medial tibia plateau posterior to MFC

Godfrey Test (Posterior Sag Test)

1. Knees and hips are flexed 90°.
2. Legs suspended parallel to examination table.

With a PCL insufficient knee, the examiner will find that the tibia will sag posteriorly relative to the uninjured knee. This is present in both chronic and acute cases.

Quadriceps Active Test

1. Patient must be in the supine position.
2. Knee flexed to 90°.
3. With the foot stabilized, the subject is asked to slide foot down the table.
4. Contraction of quadriceps muscle will cause an anterior shift of tibia in the PCL insufficient knee.

A shift greater than two mm indicates PCL insufficiency[12].

Dial Test

This test determines the integrity of the posterolateral corner (PLC).

1. Patient in supine/prone position.
2. One handle stabilizes the thigh.
3. The other hand applies an external rotation force across the knee through the foot.
4. Assess the external rotation of the tibia tubercle in relation to femur.
5. Test is performed at 30° and 90° flexion.

The injured knee is compared to the intact knee. If there is increased external rotation at 30° and 90° this indicates that there has been injury to the PLC as well as the PCL. However, increased rotation at only 30° of flexion indicates isolated PCL injury[12]. The increase in rotation should generally be 10° or greater to signify injury.

Reverse Pivot Shift Test

This is another test used to assess integrity of the PCL and PLC, in the acute and chronic settings.

1. Patient is supine.
2. Knee is held initially at 90° flexion.
3. Tibia is externally rotated and valgus stress is applied.
4. As the knee is extended the lateral tibial plateau shifts from position of posterior subluxation to a position of reduction as the flexed knee is extended

A positive test results from an anterior shift of the tibia at 20° to 30° of knee flexion when the iliotibial band pulls the proximal tibia forward. The sign disappears when the tibia is internally rotated. The lateral tibia plateau subluxates again as the knee is flexed in the opposite manner.

IMAGING TECHNIQUES

Standard Radiography

Any patient with a significant knee injury should undergo standard radiographs: Anteroposterior (AP), tunnel, 30-degree flexion lateral, and 30-degree anteroposterior axial views should be taken of both knees[7]. With respect to the PCL, potential avulsion fractures at the PCL tibial insertion, as well as other fractures[13] may be evaluated. When dealing with chronic PCL injuries a weight-bearing AP image in neutral and 45° knee flexion should be obtained. Lateral and merchant views should also be taken of the patella. These views help to assess for any degenerative changes in the medial and patellofemoral compartments.

Stress radiography is a useful tool in assessing the amount of posterior tibial translation in adults with PCL injury. In a retrospective study performed by Schulz et al, results from 1041 patients with PCL injuries were analyzed. The results were from stress radiographs using a Telos device (Telos Corp., Greisheim, Germany). Results concluded that posterior tibial translation of 8 mm indicated PCL insufficiency, while translation in excess of 12 mm suggested a multi-ligamentous injury[14] Stress radiography allows for a simple assessment of compartmental knee motion and is an accurate way to measure skeletal displacement while reducing error from soft tissue interposition[13].

Magnetic Resonance Imaging (MRI)

MRI has become the gold standard in diagnosing acute PCL injury. In a large prospective study, it was found that MRI was 99% accurate in diagnosing acute PCL injury as confirmed via arthroscopy[15]. The sensitivity of MRI is less in the setting of chronic PCL insufficiency. This is due to the fact that the PCL has the ability to heal and can regain a normal appearance on MRI within six months of injury[16]. However, a normal appearance of the PCL on MRI does not necessarily imply improvement upon physical examination.

C-Arm Fluoroscopy

Fluoroscopic imaging can be used during PCL reconstruction surgery to help assess pin placement when drilling tunnels (Figures 4, 5a-b).

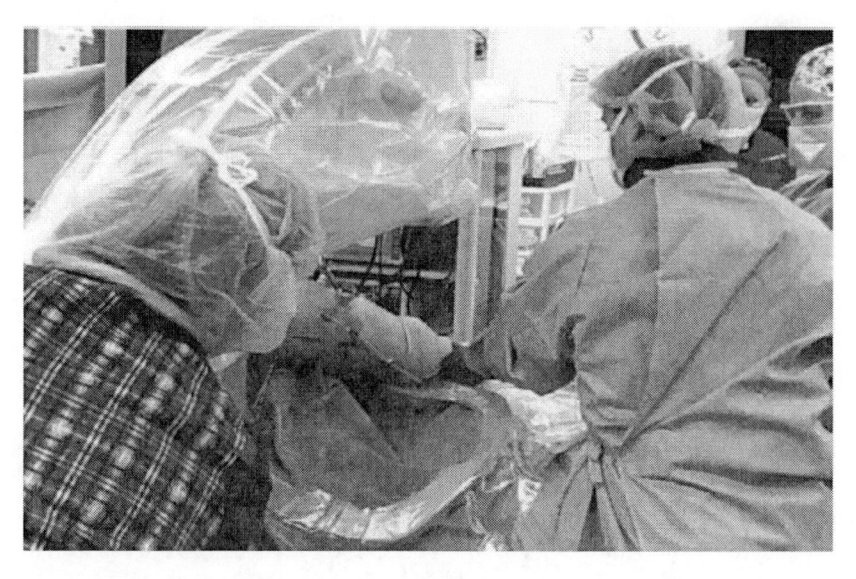

Figure 4. C-Arm fluoroscopic imaging while to assess the pin placement for drilling tunnels during PCL reconstruction.

a)   b)

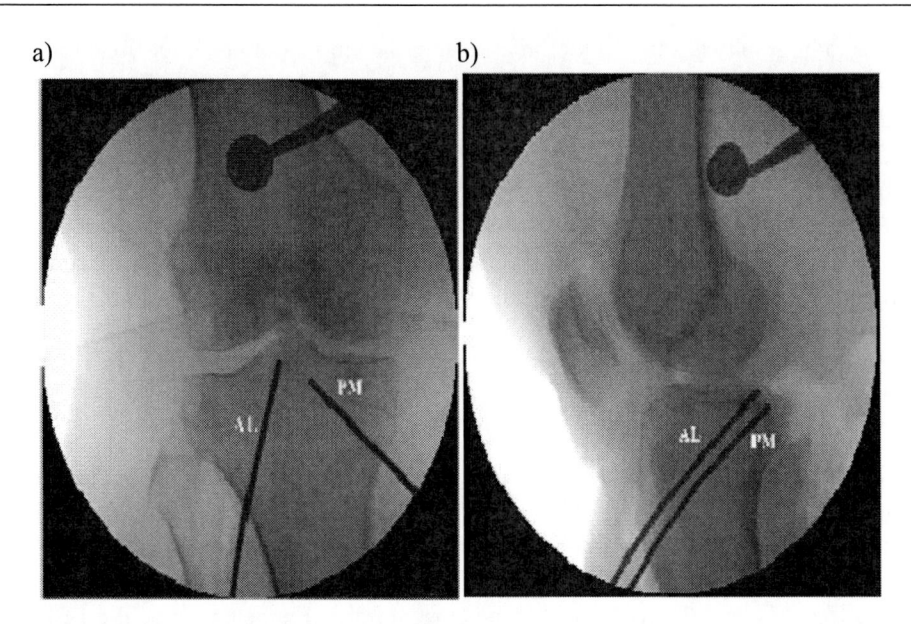

Figure 5. a. Lateral fluoroscopic image of anterolateral and posteromedial tibial pins. b. AP fluoroscopic image of anterolateral and posteromedial tibial pins.

TREATMENT

Isolated PCL tears are treated initially with conservative management, while multi-ligamentous injuries should be approached surgically. In a survey of 78 surgeons of the Herodicus Society conducted by Bach et al, 75% believed that isolated grade II PCL ruptures were best treated with conservative management[22].

In a prospective study by Shelbourne et al, 133 patients with an acute isolated PCL injury were treated with conservative management. After five year follow-up with a subjective survey, it was found that the majority of patients had good results. It was also found that half of patients were able to resume their sport at similar, if not higher levels[17]. In another study performed by Parolie et al, 25 patients with isolated PCL tears from sporting activities were followed. After two years, 80% of patients were satisfied with their level of activity and 68% had returned to previous levels of activity. Conversely, patients with diminished quadriceps strength reported dissatisfaction with their level of activity[18].

Contrary to this promising evidence, other data suggests that patients left with PCL insufficiency are at a higher risk for medial compartment arthritis, meniscal tears, and articular cartilage injury. In another study, 50 patients with isolated PCL insufficiency were treated via conservative management and 20% were found to have meniscal tears or disabling instability[19]. In 40 patients with an average of six years of isolated PCL insufficiency, Keller et al found that 65% had limited activity because of their knee and 43% had difficulty walking[20]. Longer-term studies have suggested that isolated PCL injuries may lead to arthrosis. In a study performed by Dejour et al., it was found that nearly all patients with isolated PCL-deficient knees had degenerative changes after 25 years[21].

This leads to the question of when surgery may be the best option for PCL related injuries. Surgical indications for acute PCL insufficiency include posterior translation of 8

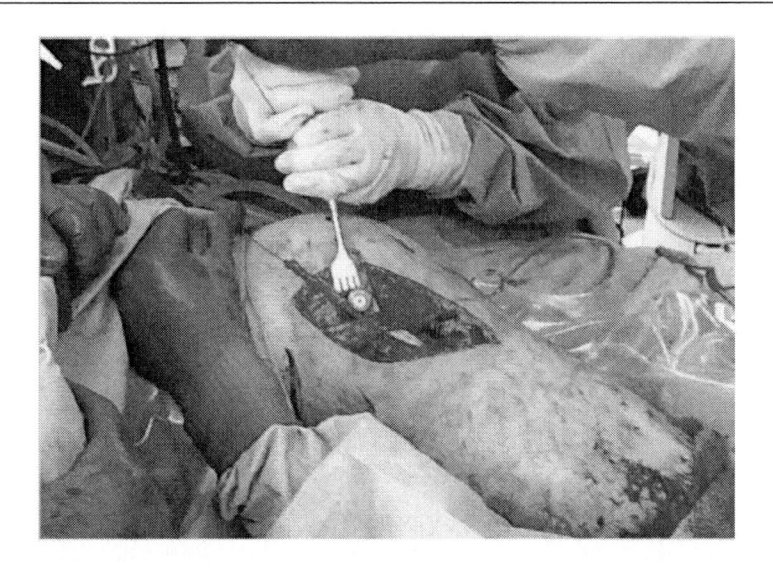

Figure 6.

mm or greater, tibial insertion site avulsions, and multi-ligamentous injuries. In the setting of chronic PCL injury, surgery is required when an isolated PCL tear becomes symptomatic or when there is functional instability present[7]. In the same aforementioned survey performed by Bach et al, it was found that most surgeons operated on isolated grade III injuries, with only 20% of respondents believing that isolated grade III tears do well in long term with conservative management[22].

THE POSTEROLATERAL CORNER (PLC)

It is important to understand the significance of the posterolateral corner (PLC) in ligamentous injuries of the knee. A missed diagnosis of PLC injury may cause failure of ACL and PCL reconstruction. Varying degrees of injury to the lateral collateral ligament (LCL), popliteus, popliteo-fibular ligament, IT band, lateral capsule, and biceps femoris may result in PLC instability and require PLC repair or reconstruction (Figure 6). If the PLC injury is not treated, there is a high risk for recurrent instability and the development of premature degenerative arthritis. In a study performed by Sekiya et al, it was hypothesized that a grade III PCL rupture could not be present without associated damage to the PLC. The authors tested ten paired cadaver knees and found that a complete isolated PCL tear resulted in a grade II posterior drawer sign, while a grade III sign was found only with damage to the PLC as well as complete rupture of the PCL[38].

SURGICAL TECHNIQUES

Due to a degree of persistent posterior knee laxity with the transtibial technique for single-bundle PCL reconstruction, there has been a new focus on finding a technique that better reproduces the biomechanics and anatomy of the intact PCL[24]. There are a variety of considerations that must be assessed before continuing with surgical reconstruction of the

PCL including number of bundles, tibial orientation of graft, graft choice and surgical approach.

Tibial Inlay versus Transtibial Reconstruction

The tibial inlay technique for graft placement has been shown to have many advantages over the transtibial method. In a report by Bergfeld et al, it was found that there was a significant amount of graft thinning with a transtibial approach. This thinning of the graft was attributed to the "killer turn" that the graft must make under cyclic loading[25]. Transtibial PCL reconstruction has also shown increased laxity in cadaveric knees after cyclic loading[26]. With transtibial reconstruction, the graft required an average of 15.6 Newtons more graft tension than with the tibial inlay method. In a test performed by Markolf et al, the effects of cyclic loading on grafts was compared in tibial inlay versus transtibial reconstruction. After 2000 cycles, it was found that all the tibial inlay grafts survived the "killer turn", while 10 out of 31 grafts failed in the transtibial approach[27]. However, the authors did find that the "killer turn" could be avoided in the transtibial approach if a bone block was inserted into the proximal end of the tibial tunnel[30].

In the transtibial technique, it is necessary that the tunnel exit one cm below the joint line, slightly lateral to midline (Figure 7). This location leaves the popliteal artery at great risk for injury. Through the aforementioned studies, it has been determined that there is minimal difference in graft forces and knee laxity following initial fixation between these two methods. It is, however, after cyclic loading that the tibial inlay method appears to be a far superior technique than the transtibial technique. This is because of the thinning, stretching, and increase in knee laxity that is observed in the graft and the knee with the transtibial method.

Another advantage seen with the tibial inlay method is the reproducibility of graft placement. The graft is placed posteriorly on the tibia through a transverse incision in the popliteal skin crease. The inlay trough is found between two bony nodules that border the PCL sulcus[24]. These landmarks allow for reproducibility of anatomic tibial graft placement.

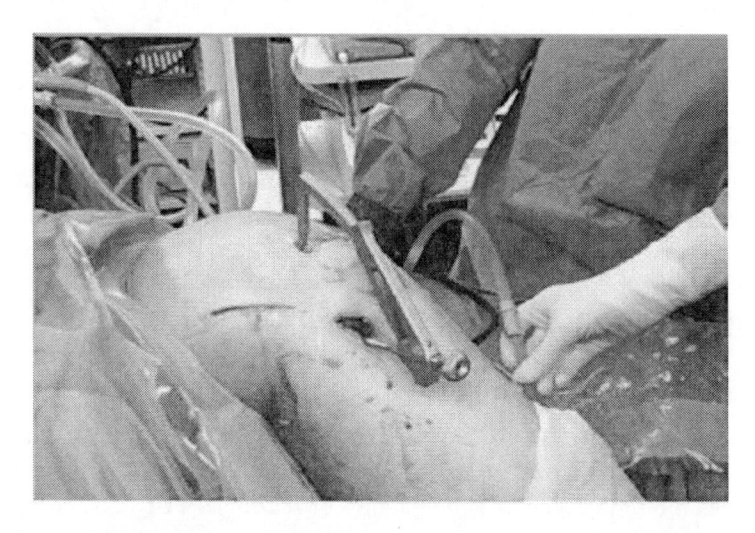

Figure 7.

Table 2. A

Advantages of Transtibial Tunnel	Advantages of Tibial Inlay
Familiar drilling technique because approach is similar to ACL reconstruction Minimally invasive Do not need bone plugs Has been the traditional approach towards PCL reconstruction	Avoids the "killer turn" Better restoration of PCL anatomy Thinning and stretching avoided Reproducible graft placement

Table 2. B

Disadvantages of Transtibial Tunnel	Disadvantages of Tibial Inlay
Neurovascular risk due to blind drilling "Killer Turn" for graft passage.	Usually done through posterior approach, which leads to the possibility of greater neurovascular risk Patient positioning

Arthroscopic versus Open Surgical Approach

Most arthroscopic procedures in PCL reconstruction are performed with a transtibial technique. As mentioned previously, this transtibial method subjects the graft to thinning as it passes the "killer turn" and can lead to subsequent graft laxity The open inlay technique adds a few complexities to PCL reconstruction. Patient positioning is the greatest difficulty seen with the open inlay technique. This is difficult in patients that are large or suffering from multiple trauma[24]. In open tibial inlay procedures, the patient must be in a lateral decubitus position or moved intra-operatively from prone to supine due to the posterior approach that is required for surgery[28]. The biggest disadvantage to the posterior approach required in open tibial inlay reconstruction of the PCL is the risk for vascular injury. Another disadvantage of the posterior approach are the incisions in the posterior capsule, popliteus muscle belly, and oblique popliteal ligament that are required. According to Park et al, if these structures are compromised there will be increased laxity and a subsequent increase in posterior translation of the tibia[48].

Mariani et al developed a fully arthroscopic inlay reconstruction technique, which in essence combines all the advantages of an inlay procedure, while avoiding the disadvantages of a posterior approach[31]. Their technique avoids the "killer turn" associated with a transtibial approach, while also avoiding injury to the neurovascular bundle. The technique describes a transeptal approach, which grants safe access to the posterior compartment while also providing exceptional visualization of the PCL tibial attachment. This technique provides several other advantages. It allows for direct visualization throughout the entirety of the procedure and there is less disruption of the surrounding soft tissue and bone. It is important to note that this technique is very technically challenging and that it requires great experience

Table 3. A

Advantages of arthroscopic surgery	Advantages of open knee surgery
More familiar technique with transtibial tunnel Avoid disrupting surrounding soft tissue and bone Less invasive Avoid open posterior approach when done with tibial inlay	More familiar technique when doing tibial inlay Can use screw fixation

Table 3. B

Disadvantages of arthroscopic surgery	Disadvantages of open knee surgery
Not a well studied approach when doing tibial inlay Requires exceptional surgical skill and experience when used with tibial inlay Requires further refinement in instruments for tibial inlay[24]	Patient positioning is difficult Must make incision in posterior capsule, the popliteus muscle belly, and the oblique popliteal ligament Neurovascular risk with posterior approach

and surgical skill. The authors of this study now use this technique for primary PCL reconstruction and have thus far had favorable results in a limited series.

In a study done by Zehms et al, ten paired cadaver knees were compared following PCL reconstruction with an arthroscopic inlay procedure versus a standard open double-bundle PCL tibial inlay procedure. It was found that both the arthroscopic and open approach restored knee stability and that there was no difference in posterior displacement of the knee following both procedures[32]. It has been theorized that one down side to the arthroscopic approach to tibial inlay procedures is the use of a suture fixation. The use of suture fixation has generally been regarded as inferior to the screw fixation used in open inlay procedures. However, in a cadaveric study performed by Campbell et al, it was found that initial and early fixation with an arthroscopic approach was similar to that of an open inlay approach.

Single-Bundle versus Double-Bundle Grafts

The PCL is composed of two bundles that are distinct: the anterolateral bundle (ALB) and the posteromedial bundle (PMB). The historical use of a single-bundle or double-bundle technique has largely been predicated upon injury pattern. In acute multi-ligamentous PCL injuries, the single-bundle technique has generally been used (Figure 8b). The single graft is placed to imitate the biomechanics and anatomy of the ALB because it has been found that the ALB is stronger and comprises the bulk of the posterior cruciate ligament. The ALB has been found to have 150% the strength of the PMB, with the PMB mainly being isometric. The single-bundle technique is also used in acute and chronic PCL tears when the meniscofemoral ligaments and the PMB are still intact[33]. In knees where the ALB, PMB and the meniscofemoral ligaments are ruptured, the double bundle technique is generally used (Figure 8a). According to Chhabra et al, these cases are usually chronic in nature and present with severe posterior knee laxity[33].

In the survey of surgeons done by Bach et al, it was found that the majority of surgeons that did more than ten PCL reconstructions annually performed the double-bundle technique[22]. The double-bundle technique is theorized to lead to better replication of the biomechanics and anatomy of the PCL and thus better improve stabilization against posterior translation of the proximal tibia. Harner et al found that the double-bundle technique most closely restored normal kinematics of the knee[46] in a laboratory study. However, there have also been studies that demonstrate weaknesses in the argument for reconstructing both the ALB and PMB. In a biomechanical study performed by Markolf et al, it was found that performing a double-bundle PCL reconstruction using a tibial inlay method improved laxity when compared to the single-bundle technique. However, this was at the expense of an increase in graft forces and subsequent lengthening of the graft that possibly negated any advantages seen with reduction in laxity[27]. Thus McAllister et al concluded that the single most important component in PCL reconstruction was reconstruction of the ALB, with PMB reconstruction viewed strictly as an adjunct[24].

In a prospective study conducted by Wang et al, the single-bundle and double-bundle techniques were compared in 35 patients after a 2-year follow-up. In the single-bundle patients, Lysholm and Tegner scores were 88 and 4.5 respectively. In the double-bundle patients, Lysholm and Tegner scores were 89 and 5.2. Average posterior drawer tests revealed 1.16 mm of posterior trnaslation in single-bundle patients and 1.13 mm in double bundle patients. The authors of this study concluded that both techniques produced similar clinical results and high levels of patient satisfaction[35].

In closing, Harner et al recommend the double-bundle technique in cases of isolated PCL injury. In cases that are multi-ligamentous and require reconstruction of the ACL and the PCL, single-bundle reconstruction is recommended secondary to the risk of tunnel widening and coalescence of the tibial tunnels[29].

a)   b)

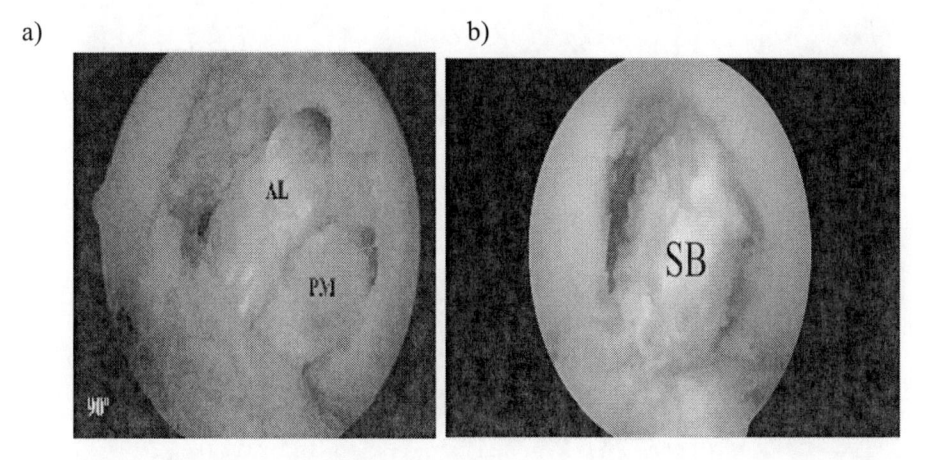

Figure 8. a. Double-bundle reconstruction of the anterolateral and posteromedial bundles of the PCL. b. Single-bundle reconstruction of the PCL.

GRAFT CHOICE

Graft choices are usually made to best mirror the large cross-sectional area of the PCL. There are many options for graft use in PCL in reconstruction. Bone-patellar tendon-bone or hamstring grafts have been suggested for use in single-bundle reconstruction, but other graft choices are larger in cross-sectional area and seem to be the preferred choice of most surgeons. These include Achilles tendon-bone, quadriceps tendon-bone, and tibialis anterior and posterior tendon grafts. In the survey conducted by Bach et al, biomechanical graft strength was listed as the most important factor when choosing a graft[22].

In the argument regarding use of autograft or allograft tissue, the trend in PCL reconstruction seems to lean towards using allograft because of the need for a larger and biomechanically stronger graft. However, graft strength needs to be balanced against consideration of risk of disease transmission and longer incorporation time seen with the use of allograft tissue. With this longer incorporation time, there also appears to be a tendency for the graft to stretch with time[36]. The two diseases that are of greatest concern with respect to disease transmission are HIV and hepatitis and although the chances of contracting these two diseases from allograft use are minimal, the risk still exists and should be discussed with the patient before surgery[37].

The advantages of using allograft are the lack of graft harvest site morbidity, shorter surgical time, smaller incision requirements and reduced quadriceps and hamstring weakness. On the other hand, advantages of autograft use include lack of risk of disease transmission and faster graft incorporation time. The survey performed by Bach et al revealed that most surgeons use an Achilles tendon allograft for both acute and chronic PCL reconstruction (Figures 9a and 9b). In the chronic cases, the second most popular graft choice was patellar tendon autograft[22].

a)   b)

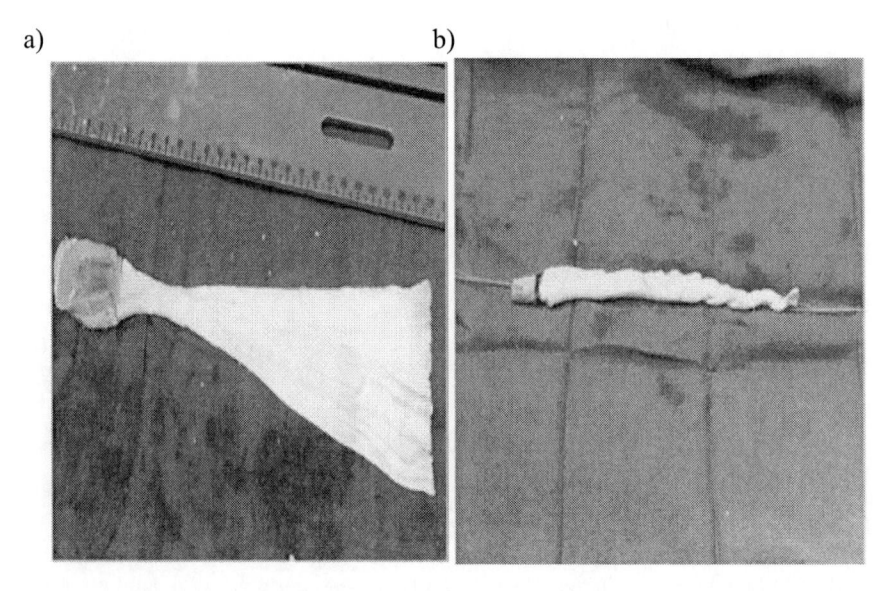

Figure 9. a. Achilles tendon allograft before preparation. b. Achilles tendon allograft after preparation.

Table 4. A

Advantages of allograft	Advantages of autograft
No harvest site morbidity	No risk of disease transmission
Shorter surgical time	Faster graft incorporation time
Less hamstring and quadriceps weakness	
Smaller incisions	

Table 4. B

Disadvantages of allograft	Disadvantages of autograft
Risk of disease transmission (i.e. HIV, hepatitis)	Longer surgical time
Longer incorporation time	Donor site morbidity
Risk of stretching of graft	More incisions
	Increased hamstring and quadriceps weakness

CONSERVATIVE MANAGEMENT

Low-grade (I/II) PCL injuries are treated conservatively. Isolated grade III PCL injuries without injury to the posterolateral corner are initially treated conservatively. Reconstruction is only considered (in isolated grade III injuries) after the patient has failed a minimum of 3 months of conservative management, for symptoms of instability. Combined injuries to the PCL (usually grade III) and posterolateral corner are treated operatively.

Physical therapy focused on quadriceps strengthening is utilized while unopposed hamstring contraction is avoided. The goal of conservative management is to strengthen the muscles around the knee. Closed-chain kinetic exercises and open-chain kinetic quadriceps exercises were found by Lutz et al to be the best approach to conservative management, as these exercises reduced forces on the patellofemoral and tibiofemoral compartments while strengthening the musculature around the knee[39]. As mentioned previously, it should be noted that patients may be at increased risk for medial and patellofemroal compartment chondrosis, meniscal tears, and articular cartilage injury with conservative management of PCL injury.

POST-OPERATIVE REHABILITATION

In the first month of post-operative rehabilitation, the patient is placed in a hinged knee brace. The primary focus of the rehabilitation program is to allow for healing of soft-tissue and bony structures. Early, protected range of motion of the affected knee should be encouraged to minimize the effects of immobilization[29]. After one week, the brace is unlocked and the patient begins closed-kinetic chain mini squat exercises, straight leg raises, and open-kinetic chain quadriceps exercises under the guidance of a physical therapist or trainer. From six to eight weeks after surgery, the patient can discontinue use of the brace if adequate quadriceps strength has been achieved. Activity is still restricted to $90°$ knee flexion at this stage. Between 9 and 36 weeks after surgery, the patient can begin using a treadmill, swimming, and pool jogging. The breaststroke should be avoided when swimming. According to Harner et al, the patient should undergo either a sport-specific training regimen, work hardening program, or job restructuring at 36 weeks after surgery in an effort to return the patient back to work or their previous level of sporting activity[29].

COMPLICATIONS

Due to the anatomy of the PCL and its location, the neurovascular risk when performing surgery is increased. The popliteal artery lies 29.1 mm from the center of the PCL and 9.1 mm from the proximal PCL fovea[41]. This anatomy becomes particularly important when drilling transtibial tunnels, as it has been found that the average distance between the tibial tunnel and the popliteal artery was approximately 7.4 mm[42]. Injury to the popliteal artery or tibial nerve could result in loss of the limb and may even be fatal in some cases. Another complication to be considered following PCL reconstruction is the possibility of osteonecrosis. This usually occurs due to an interruption in the extraosseous blood supply to the medial femoral condyle secondary to femoral tunnel placement[43]. Additionally, there is the possibility for a fracture to occur in the femur or tibia if the tibial or femoral tunnels are too large[44].

Stiffness can result in the loss of flexion following PCL reconstruction. This can be caused by arthrofibrosis, improper tunnel placement, poor graft tensioning or a lack of proper post-operative rehabilitation[45]. While these are all causes for stiffness and loss of knee flexion, they can also result in loosening and residual posterior laxity in the PCL-reconstructed knee. As mentioned previously, the biggest factor when encountering residual post-operative posterior laxity is usually a missed diagnosis of a PLC injury. This persistent posterior laxity may also lead to anterior knee pain[44]. Anterior knee pain can also be caused by bone-patellar tendon-bone graft harvest [44]. An additional but rare complication to be considered is heterotopic ossification secondary to femoral tunnel reaming.

Table 5.

Complications in PCL Surgery
Neurovascular Injury
Disease transmission with allograft
Stiffness (reduced flexion)
Loosening (increased posterior laxity)
Anterior Knee Pain
Heterotopic Ossification
Osteonecrosis
Fracture

CONCLUSION

The lack of concensus of knowledge found in PCL treatment stems from the relative infrequency of PCL injuries. With this low incidence of PCL injury, there is generally a greater level of inexperience with most surgeons performing less than ten PCL reconstructions a year. Nevertheless, an increasing level of importance placed on PCL research has led to a better understanding of the PCL and the development of better surgical techniques for treating patients with PCL injury.

Though a consensus for treatment of PCL injuries still seems far away, there does appear to be a trend in that direction for PCL reconstruction. In cases of grade I and II tears, conservative management is almost always successful. Grade III tears can be managed conservatively, however when they coincide with an injury to the PLC surgical intervention is usually necessary.

Currently the transtibial technique is the most popular method employed, in part because of its familiarity and similarity to ACL reconstruction. A single-bundle reconstruction is generally chosen in the setting of multi-ligamentous knee injury to avoid tunnel coalescence, while a double-bundle graft is recommended in isolated PCL ruptures due to restoration of the anatomy and biomechanics of the native PCL. The graft of choice for most surgeons seems to be Achilles tendon allograft secondary to its larger cross-sectional area and greater biomechanical strength.

While the aforementioned recommendations are based on survey data, available biomechanical and lab data suggests that the best approach to surgical treatment of PCL injuries may be a double-bundle arthroscopic tibial inlay technique. This approach avoids many of the complications seen with the transtibial method, namely the "killer turn". It also avoids the risks involved with the posterior surgical approach seen in the open tibial inlay procedure, as well as patient positioning issues. This procedure also has been shown to have comparable biomechanical outcomes to transtibial and open inlay methods. Nevertheless, incorporation of this method into mainstream practice has been limited, as it requires great experience and surgical skill.

In conclusion, a concrete recommendation as to which technique or graft to choose cannot be given based upon the current level of evidence of the available literature. Orthopaedic surgeons should assess each PCL injury as a unique case and analyze their findings to determine the best approach for treatment. This should include history and physical examination findings, imaging results and arthroscopic diagnosis. When surgical reconstruction is indicated, the Orthopedist should utilize the technique he or she is most familiar and comfortable with.

REFERENCES

[1]   Fanelli, G. C., Edson, C. J. Posterior cruciate ligament injuries in trauma patients: part II. *Arthroscopy* 1995;11:526–52.

[2]   Miller, M. D. *Review of Orthopaedics*. 4th ed. Philadelphia: Elsevier; 2004.

[3] Lopes, O. V. Jr, Ferretti, M., Shen, W., Ekdahl, M., Smolinski, P., Fu, F. H. Topography of the femoral attachment of the posterior cruciate ligament. *J. Bone Joint Surg. Am.* 2008;90: 249–255.

[4] Fox, R. J., Harner, C. D., Sakane, M., Carlin, G. J., Woo, S. L. Determination of the in situ forces in the human posterior cruciate ligament using robotic technology. A cadaveric study. *Am. J. Sports Med.* 1998;26:395–401.

[5] Edwards, A., Bull, A. M., Amis, A. A. The attachments of the fiber bundles of the posterior cruciate ligament: an anatomic study. *Arthroscopy* 2007;23:284–290

[6] Kennedy, J. C., Alexander, I. J., Hayes, K. C. Nerve supply of the human knee and its functional importance. *Am. J. Sports Med.* 1982;10:329–335.

[7] Fanelli, G. C., Beck, J. D., Edson, C. J. Current concepts review: the posterior cruciate ligament. *J. Knee Surg.* 2010;23:61–72.

[8] Schulz, M. S., Russe, K., Weiler, A., Eichhorn, H. J., Strobel, M. J. Epidemiology of posterior cruciate ligament injuries. *Arch. Orthop. Trauma Surg.* 2003;123:186–191.

[9] Fowler, P. J., Messieh, S. S. Isolated posterior cruciate ligament injuries in athletes. *Am. J. Sports Med.* 1987;15:553–557.

[10] Fanelli, G. C. Posterior cruciate ligament injuries in trauma patients. *Arthroscopy* 1993;9:291–294.

[11] DeLee, J. C., Drez, D. Jr., Miller, M. D. Orthopaedic Sports Medicine: Principles and Practice. 2nd ed. Philadelphia: *Saunders;* 2003.

[12] McAllister, D. R., Petrigliano, F. A. Diagnosis and treatment of posterior cruciate ligament injuries. *Curr. Sports Med. Rep.* 2007;6:293–299.

[13] Margheritini, F., Mariani, P. P. Diagnostic evaluation of posterior cruciate ligament injuries. *Knee Surg. Sports Traumatol. Arthrosc.* 2003;11:282–288.

[14] Schulz, M. S., Steenlage, E. S., Russe, K., Strobel, M. J. Distribu- tion of posterior tibial displacement in knees with posterior cruciate ligament tears. *J. Bone Joint Surg. Am.,* 2007;89:332–338.

[15] Gross, M. L., Grover, J. S., Bassett, L. W., Seeger, L. L., Finerman, G. A. Magnetic resonance imaging of the posterior cruciate ligament. Clinical use to improve diagnostic accuracy. *Am. J. Sports Med.* 1992;20:732–737.

[16] Servant, C. T., Ramos, J. P., Thomas, N. P.: The accuracy of mag- netic resonance imaging in diagnosing chronic posterior cruciate ligament injury. *Knee* 2004, 11:265–270.

[17] Shelbourne, K. D., Davis, T. J., Patel, D. V. The natural history of acute, isolated, nonoperatively treated posterior cruciate ligament injuries. A prospective study. *Am. J. Sports Med.* 1999;27:276–283.

[18] Parolie, J. M., Bergfeld, J. A. Long-term results of nonoperative treatment of isolated posterior cruciate ligament injuries in the athlete. *Am. J. Sports Med.* 1986;14:35–38.

[19] Boynton, M. D., Tietjens, B. R. Long-term follow-up of the untreated isolated posterior cruciate ligament-deficient knee. *Am. J. Sports Med.* 1996;24:306–310.

[20] Keller, P. M., Shelbourne, K. D., McCarroll, J. R., Rettig, A. C. Nonoperatively treated isolated posterior cruciate ligament injuries. *Am. J. Sports Med.* 1993;21:132–136.

[21] Dejour, H., Walch, G., Peyrot, J., et al. The natural history of rupture of the posterior cruciate ligament. Fr. *J. Orthop. Surg.* 1988;2:112–120.

[22] Dennis, M. G., Fox, J. A., Alford, J. W., Hayden, J. K., Bach, B. R. Posterior cruciate ligament reconstruction: current trends *J. Knee Surg.* 2010;17:133–139.

[23] Rubinstein, R. A. Jr, Shelbourne, K. D., McCarroll, J. R., VanMeter, C. D., Rettig, A. C. The accuracy of the clinical examination in the setting of posterior cruciate ligament injuries. *Am. J. Sports Med.* 1994;22:550–557.

[24] McAllister, D. R., Miller, M. D., Sekiya, J. K., Wojtys, E. M. Posterior cruciate ligament biomechanics and options for surgical treatment. Instr. *Course Lect.* 2009;58:377-388.

[25] Bergfeld, J. A., McAllister, D. R., Parker, R. D., et al: A biomechanical comparison of posterior cruciate ligament reconstruction techniques. *Am. J. Sports Med.* 2001; 29: 129-136.

[26] McAllister, D. R., Markolf, K. L., Oakes, D. A, et al: A biomechanical comparison of tibial inlay and tibial tunnel postererior cruciate ligament reconstruction techniques: Graft pretension and knee laxity. *Am. J. Sports Med.* 2002;30:312-317.

[27] Markolf, K. L., Zemanovic, J. R., McAllister, D. R.: Cyclic loading of posterior cruciate ligament replacements fixed with tibial tunnel and tibial inlay methods. *J. Bone Joint Surg. Am.* 2002; 84:518-524.

[28] Miller, M. D., Kline, A. J., Gonzales, J., et al.: Vascular risk associated with posterior approach for posterior cruciate ligament reconstruction using the tibial inlay technique. *J. Knee Surg.* 2002;15:137-140.

[29] Forsythe, B., Harner, C., Martins, C. A., Shen, W., Lopes, O. V., Fu, F. H. Topography of the femoral attachment of the posterior cruciate ligament. surgical technique. *J. Bone Joint Surg. Am.* 2009;91:89-100.

[30] Markolf, K. D. M. Zoric, B. McAllister, D.., Effects of bone block position and orientation within the tibial tunnel for posterior cruciate ligament graft reconstructions: a cyclic loading study of bone-patellar tendon-bone allografts. *Am. J. Sports Med.*, 2003;31: 673-679.

[31] Mariani, P. P., Margheritini, F. Full arthroscopic inlay reconstruction of posterior cruciate ligament. Knee Surg. Sports Traumatol. *Arthrosc.* 2006;14:1038-1044.

[32] Zehms, Whiddon, Miller, Quinby, Montgomery, Campbell, Sekiya. Comparison of a double bundle arthroscopic inlay and open inlay PCL reconstruction using clinically relevant tools. *Arthroscopy* 2008;4:472-480.

[33] Chhabra, A., Kline, A. J., Harner, C. D. Single-bundle versus double-bundle posterior cruciate ligament reconstruction: scientific rationale and surgical technique. *Instr. Course Lect.* 2006;55:497-507.

[34] Gupte, C. M., Bull, A. M., Thomas, R. D., Amis, A. A. The meniscofemoral ligaments: secondary restraints to the posterior drawer. Analysis of anteroposterior and rotary laxity in the intact and posterior-cruciate-deficient knee. *J. Bone Joint. Surg. Br.* 2003;85:765–773.

[35] Wang, C. J., Chen, H. S., Huang, T. W. Outcome of arthroscopic single bundle reconstruction for complete posterior cruciate ligament tear. *Injury* 2003;34:747–751.

[36] Sabrina, M. Strickland, M., John, D. MacGillivray, M. D., Russell, F. Warren, M. D. Anterior cruciate ligament reconstruction with allograft tendons. *Orthopedic clinics of North America.* 2003;34:41-47.

[37] Miller, S. L., Gladstone, J. N. Graft selection in anterior cruciate ligament reconstruction. *The Orthopedic clinics of North America* 2002;33:675-683.

[38] Sekiya, J. K., Whiddon, D. R., Zehms, C. T., Miller, M. D. A clinically relevant assessment of posterior cruciate ligament and posterolateral corner injuries. *J. Bone Joint Surg. Am.* 2008;90:1621-1627.

[39] Lutz, G. E., Palmitier, R. A., An, K. N., Chao, E. Y. S. Comparison of tibiofemoral joint forces during open-kinetic-chain and closed-kinetic-chain exercises. *J. Bone Joint Surg. Am.* 1993; 75:732–739.

[40] Fanelli, G. C., Monahan, T. Complications in posterior cruciate ligament and posterolateral corner surgery. *Oper. Tech. Sports Med.* 2001;9:96–99.

[41] Cosgarea, A. J., Kramer, D. E., Bahk, M. S., et al. Proximity of the popliteal artery to the PCL during simulated knee arthroscopy: implications for establishing the posterior trans-septal portal. *J. Knee Surg.* 2006;19:181–185.

[42] Matava, M. J., Sethi, N. S., Totty, W. G. Proximity of the posterior cruciate ligament insertion to the popliteal artery as a function of the knee flexion angle: implications for posterior cruciate ligament reconstruction. *Arthroscopy.* 2000;16:796–804.

[43] Reddy, A. S., Frederick, R. W. Evaluation of the intraosseous and extraosseous blood supply to the distal femoral condyles. *Am. J. Sports Med.* 1998;26:415–419.

[44] Zawodny, S. R., Miller, M. D. Complications of posterior cruciate ligament surgery. *Sports Med. Arthrosc. Rev.* 2010;18:269-274.

[45] Irrgang, J. J., Harner, C. D. Loss of motion following knee ligament reconstruction. *Sports Med.* 1995;19:150–159.

[46] Harner, C. D., Janaushek, M. A., Kanamori, A., et al. Biomechanical analysis of a double-bundle posterior cruciate ligament reconstruction. *Am. J. Sports Med.* 2000;28:144–151.

[47] Girgis, F. G., Marshall, J. L., Monajem, A. The cruciate ligaments of the knee joint. Anatomical, functional and experimental analysis. *Clin. Orthop. Relat. Res.* 1975;106:216–231.

[48] Park, S. E., Stamos, B. D., DeFrate, L. E., Gill, T. J. ,. Li, G. The effect of posterior knee capsulotomy on posterior tibial translation during posterior cruciate ligament tibial inlay reconstruction. *Am. J. Sports Med.* 2004; 32:1514–1519.

In: The Knee
Editor: Randy Mascarenhas

ISBN: 978-1-61942-268-1
© 2012 Nova Science Publishers, Inc.

Chapter IX

MENISCAL TEARS: ANATOMY, DIAGNOSIS, AND TREATMENT

K. Chan and O. R. Ayeni

McMaster University, Section of Orthopaedic Surgery,
Hamilton, Ontario, Canada

INTRODUCTION

Meniscal injuries are common and can lead to significant morbidity. Historically, these injuries were managed with a total meniscectomy. However, knowledge of the anatomy and function of the meniscus has advanced considerably since the days when it was thought to be the functionless vestiges of a leg muscle[1]. On the contrary, the meniscus is now known to be an integral component of the complex biomechanics of the knee. This is reflected in the various interventions and techniques employed to preserve the meniscus, and arthroscopic treatment of meniscal tears has become one of the most common procedures in the United States[2]. It is the goal of this chapter to review our understanding of the meniscus and the associated treatment of meniscal injuries.

ANATOMY

From a gross anatomical perspective, the menisci are C-shaped or semi-circular fibrocartilaginous structures that are located between the femoral condyles and the tibial plateau. When viewed in cross-section, the menisci are wedge-shaped structures with a thick convex surface peripherally that is attached to the joint capsule. This surface tapers centrally to a thin free edge. The anterior and posterior horns of each meniscus are attached to the tibial surface via insertional ligaments. The superior surface of each meniscus is concave to conform to the shape of the femoral condyles, whereas the inferior surface is flat on the tibial plateau.

The medial and lateral menisci are uniquely shaped. The medial meniscus has a more semi-circular shape, with the posterior horn wider than the anterior horn. The anterior horn attaches approximately 6 to 8 mm anterior to the anterior cruciate ligament (ACL) at the intercondylar fossa, whereas the posterior horn inserts just anterior to the posterior cruciate ligament (PCL)[3]. In contrast, the lateral meniscus is more circular in shape and demonstrates a more uniform width along its course. It covers proportionally more of the tibial plateau than the medial meniscus. The anterior horn of the lateral meniscus inserts anterior to the lateral tibial spine, while the posterior horn attaches just anterior to the insertion of the posterior horn of the medial meniscus[3]. In contrast to the medial meniscus, there is a loose attachment of the lateral meniscus to the joint capsule peripherally, which is interrupted by the popliteus tendon as it passes posterolaterally. This allows for increased movement of the lateral meniscus during normal knee range of motion[2].

The lateral meniscus may possess attachments to the femur via meniscofemoral ligaments. The two ligaments that connect the posterior horn of the lateral meniscus to the intercondylar area of the femur are the posterior meniscofemoral ligament (of Wrisberg) and the anterior meniscofemoral ligament (of Humphrey). These ligaments are named for their anatomic position relative to the PCL. There is considerable variation in the reported incidence of the meniscofemoral ligaments[4]. Objective evidence of their function in the knee is also lacking[4]. However, it is speculated that they may play a role in moving the lateral meniscus during knee motions to increase tibiofemoral congruency and decrease contact pressures[4].

MENISCAL MICROANATOMY

The fibrocartilaginous meniscus is composed of 75% water[5]. Of its dry weight, 75% is mainly type I collagen[5]. The collagen fibrils are organized into three distinct zones[6]. The most superficial tibial and femoral surfaces contain a meshwork of thin collagen fibrils with no preferred orientation. Beneath this, there is a lamella-like layer of collagen that is arranged in a radial direction near the periphery, while the rest of the layer demonstrates a more random orientation. The central portion represents the main region of each meniscus and features predominantly collagen bundles that are organized circumferentially. This reflects the functional role of the meniscus in load-bearing.

From a clinical standpoint, meniscal blood supply has significant implications in evaluating the repairability of tears. At birth, the entire meniscus is well vascularized[2]. However, as it matures with age, the meniscal blood supply changes dramatically. The work of Arnoczky and Warren[7] has provided a clear understanding of the vascularity of the adult meniscus. According to them, the lateral, medial, and middle genicular arteries provide blood supply to each meniscus. These vessels form a peri-meniscal capillary plexus in the capsular and synovial tissues, which supply the peripheral 10-25% of the lateral meniscus and 10-30% of the medial meniscus. In addition, the anterior and posterior horns of each meniscus is well vascularized by a covering of synovial tissue. The posterolateral aspect of the lateral meniscus does not contain penetrating vessels around the popliteal tendon.

The characteristics of meniscal blood supply have led to terminology that describes zones of vascularity. Particularly, the "red zone" refers to the most peripheral regions of the meniscus that possess a good vascular bed. The most central avascular portion is called the "white zone" and the middle portion is the "red-white zone". As alluded to previously, these zones have profound effects on the potential for healing following meniscal injuries and repair.

The meniscal neuroanatomy is not as well described as the vascularity. There appears to be nerve fibres in the peripheral one-third of each meniscus, which may contribute to nociception[8]. In addition, the anterior and posterior horns of the menisci are populated by mechanoreceptors that likely play a role in proprioception[2, 9, 10]

MENISCAL FUNCTIONS

The meniscus has several important biomechanical functions in the knee joint. Firstly, it acts as a load-bearing structure. The meniscus has been shown in in-vitro studies to carry at least 50-70% of the load[11]. During knee flexion, this can increase to 85%[11]. Similarly, the meniscus can act as a shock absorber to protect the underlying articular cartilage. The ability of the meniscus to transmit and dissipate forces is derived from its anatomic shape, which increases the contact areas at the knee joint and decreases the force across the central portion of each compartment[5]. In addition, the circumferentially oriented collagen in each meniscus can effectively convert and dissipate vertical forces into horizontal "hoop stresses"[5].

The meniscus also functions to improve joint stability by creating a socket[2]. The anatomic shape of each meniscus increases the congruency between the rounded femoral condyles and the flat tibial plateau. In addition, it limits excess motion in all directions. Finally, the meniscus can help lubricate the knee joint. Although the exact mechanism for this is unclear, it may be related to fluid exudation across the meniscus, similar to articular cartilage[10].

EPIDEMIOLOGY

Meniscal tears are common with an estimated incidence of 60 to 70 per 100,000[2]. In fact, arthroscopic knee surgery to address meniscal pathology has become one of the most common surgical procedures[12]. Meniscal tears occur more frequently in males than females[2]. Young, athletic patients are more likely to sustain acute traumatic tears, whereas degenerative tears tend to occur in patients who are older than 40 years of age[2].

CLINICAL FEATURES

The diagnosis of a meniscal tear can usually be made from a combination of careful history, physical examination, and selected diagnostic tests. Traumatic tears are frequently associated with twisting or hyper-flexion injuries. Patients may complain of acute pain, swelling, and mechanical symptoms such as locking or catching. A locked knee or loss of motion with a mechanical block to extension can be associated with a displaced bucket handle tear. In contrast, patients with degenerative meniscal tears may present with a chronic history of mild joint swelling, pain, or mechanical symptoms.[2]

The physical examination of a patient with a suspected meniscal injury should follow basic principles, including the examination of the joint above and below the knee. A focused exam of the knee may begin with inspection of the joint to assess for swelling or quadriceps atrophy. Evaluating the range of motion is important to determine if there is any locking or mechanical block to joint motion. In addition, several provocative manoeuvres have been described to identify torn menisci. The most widely used one is the McMurray test (Figure 1). A positive exam for the medial meniscus is demonstrated by a palpable click during external rotation of the tibia and passive flexion to extension of the knee. Similarly, the lateral meniscus can be tested by internally rotating the tibia and passively moving from flexion to extension. The literature supports an approximate sensitivity of 26% and specificity of 94% for the McMurray test[13]. Palpating for joint line tenderness may be of diagnostic value as well. Ergen[14] found that the sensitivity and specificity of joint line tenderness in identifying tears were 92% and 97%, respectively; for the lateral meniscus, and 86% and 67%, respectively, for the medial meniscus.

Karachalios et al[15] also described a new provocative manoeuver for the early detection of meniscal tears called the Thessaly test, which involves dynamic reproduction of load transmission through the knee. The patient is instructed to stand on the affected knee and rotate internally and externally three times at 5° and 20° of flexion. A positive test occurs when the patient experiences medial or lateral joint-line discomfort, locking, or catching. In their original article, Karachalios et al[15] reported an accuracy rate with knee flexion at 20° of 94% for medial meniscus tears and 96% for the lateral meniscus.

However, other authors have found much lower accuracy rates for the Thessaly test. Konan et al[16] showed rates of only 61% for the medial meniscus and 80% for the lateral meniscus. In their study, the authors found that joint line tenderness had a much higher diagnostic accuracy (81% for the medial meniscus and 90% for the lateral meniscus)[16]. Despite these findings, Konan et al[16] supported the notion that a combination of standard tests is the most helpful in diagnosing meniscal tears, which is echoed by other authors[2, 17].

a)   b)

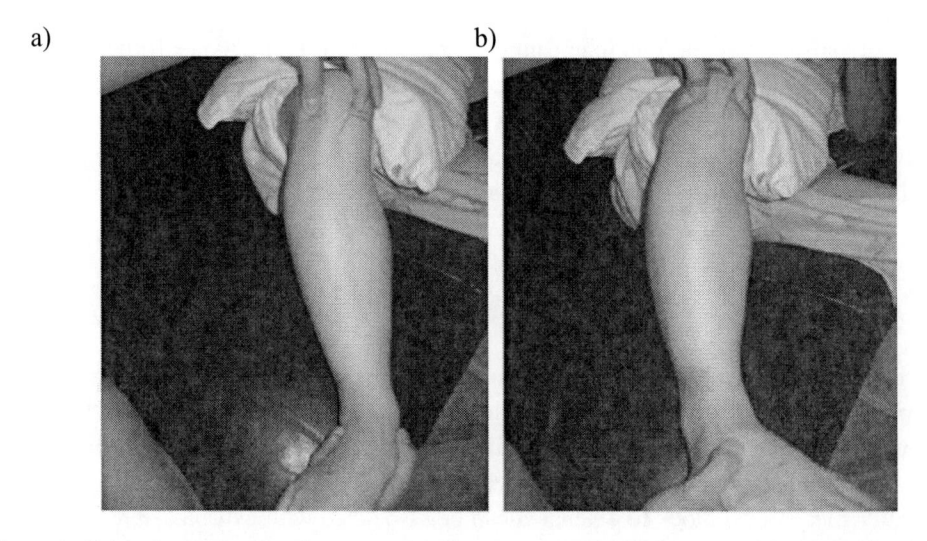

Figure 1. Physical examination demonstrating the McMurray's test. (A) A positive exam for the medial meniscus is demonstrated by a palpable click during external rotation of the tibia and passive flexion to extension of the knee. (B) Similarly, the lateral meniscus can be tested by internally rotating the tibia and passively moving from flexion to extension.

Imaging studies that can be used include plain radiographs, arthrography, and magnetic resonance imaging (MRI). Although plain radiographs cannot be used to diagnose meniscal tears, they are still useful in defining bony pathologies such as degenerative joint changes. This may serve as an adjunct to the history and physical examination to sort through the differential diagnosis of a patient with knee pain.[2] Arthrography is now infrequently used due to the advent of MRI, which is considered to have an accuracy of detecting meniscal tears of 89% to 98%[18]. As a result, most patients with a suspected meniscal injury require an MRI for evaluation (Figures 2-4).

It is worth remembering that asymptomatic meniscal tears are not uncommon findings on MRI and can be managed non-operatively[19]. In a study by Boden et al[20], the authors found that 16% of asymptomatic individuals had a meniscal tear on MRI. The prevalence increased with age from 13% in those under age 45 to 36% in individuals older than 45[20]. This highlights the importance of correlating radiological findings with relevant clinical features to formulate an appropriate treatment plan.

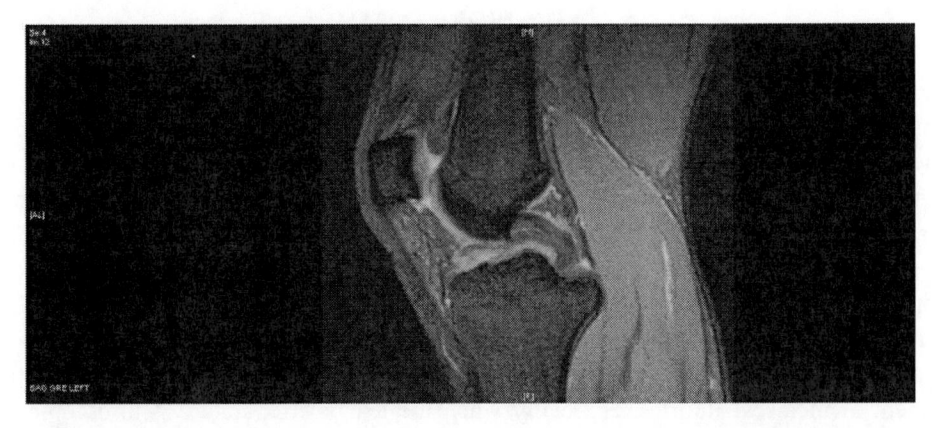

Figure 2. MRI of the left knee demonstrating a "double PCL" sign, which is suggestive of a displaced bucket-handle meniscal tear.

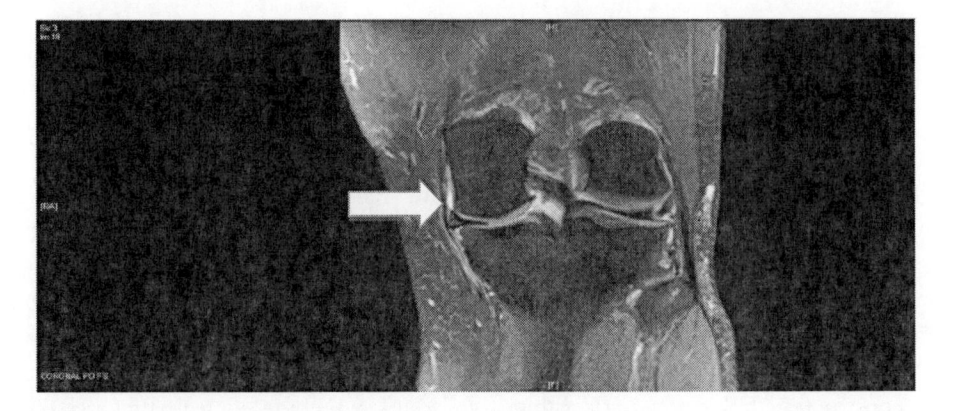

Figure 3. MRI showing a degenerative medial meniscal tear (white arrow).

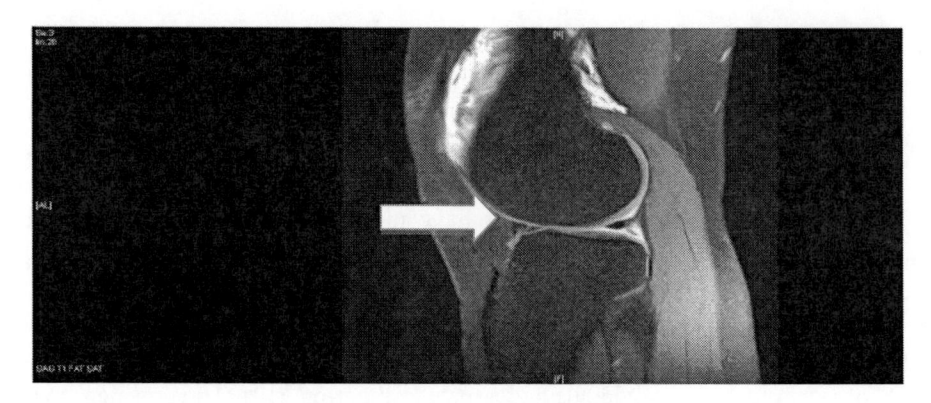

Figure 4. A sagittal T2-weighted MRI of the knee demonstrating a tear of the anterior horn of the lateral meniscus (white arrow).

MENISCECTOMY

Historically, meniscal injuries were managed surgically with a total meniscectomy, even for minor pathology. However, our understanding of the importance of the meniscus has led to the development of various meniscus-preserving techniques. Fairbanks[21] was one of the first to document the negative changes that occurred following a total meniscectomy. He described changes in the knee that were consistent with early degenerative arthritis including joint space narrowing, ridge formation, and flattening of the femoral condyles. In his article, he reported that "meniscectomy is not wholly innocuous"[21].

Total meniscectomy is infrequently performed today for the aforementioned reasons. However, partial arthroscopic meniscectomy remains an important surgical option for the treatment of meniscal injuries, especially when the tear is irreparable. Arthroscopic partial meniscectomy should be pursued only after two important questions have been addressed[12]: (1) is surgery indicated? and (2) if so, can a repair be done? The general indications for surgical intervention include a symptomatic meniscal tear that has failed non-operative treatment[12].

In deciding whether a meniscal repair is possible, various factors need to be considered. These include vascular zones, tear type, tear chronicity, presence or absence of secondary tears, and associated ACL rupture[12] (See Figure 5). The ideal tear to repair is a vertical longitudinal tear within the peripheral 3 mm with a concomitant ACL reconstruction[12]. The most commonly accepted general indications for repair are[2, 12]: (1) complete vertical longitudinal tears > 1 cm long; (2) tears with rim widths of 3 or 4 mm; (3) unstable tears; (4) no degenerative tears (ie. meniscal tissue to be repaired remains of good quality); and (5) concurrent ligament stabilization procedure or in a patient with a stable knee. An unstable tear is defined as one in which the meniscal fragment can be subluxed into the joint by more than 3 mm[12]. Tears in the peripheral 4 or 5 mm can be considered for repair if there is a concurrent ACL reconstruction[12]. Short tears (less than 1 cm long) or incomplete tears that are stable can be left alone[12].

a)   b)

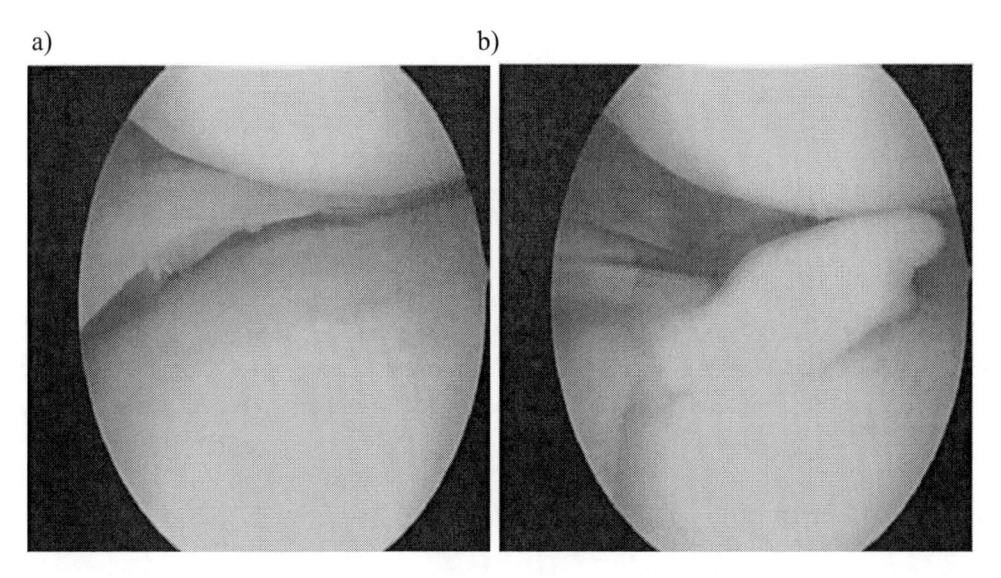

Figure 5. Intraoperative arthroscopic images of the medial meniscus, (A) demonstrating a tear in the white zone. (B) The tear is probed and noted to be unstable. This tear was subsequently managed with a partial meniscectomy.

If partial meniscectomy is warranted, the general guidelines for arthroscopic resection include removal of meniscal fragments if they can be pulled past the inner margins of the meniscus towards the centre of the joint; while the remaining rim should be contoured or smoothed to prevent further tearing[12, 22]. An arthroscopic probe should be used liberally to test the mobility and texture of the remaining meniscus[22].

Results of partial meniscectomy have largely been positive in the short-term with a quoted success rate of 95%[12]. However, longer-term studies may question whether the favorable outcomes are sustained. For example, Schimmer et al[23] found a 91.7% rate of excellent or good results at 4 years of follow-up, which decreased to 78.1% at 12 years. They also found that associated articular cartilage damage at the time of meniscectomy had the greatest effect on long-term outcomes[23]. A systematic review by Petty and Lubowitz[24] of studies with a minimum of eight years follow-up after partial meniscectomy found that all included studies had a statistically significant incidence of radiographic evidence of osteoarthritis. Interestingly, though, they noted that these changes did not correlate with clinical symptoms of osteoarthritis or clinical outcomes[24]. Burks et al[25] also studied clinical and radiological outcomes after partial meniscectomy with a mean follow-up of 14.7 years. They reported an 88% rate of excellent or good outcomes[25]. In addition, the authors found that patients did worse if they had ACL deficiency at the time of partial meniscectomy[25].

Overall, it would appear that arthroscopic partial meniscectomy can yield favorable outcomes and should remain a mainstay for the treatment of meniscal tears, especially when repair cannot be accomplished.

MENISCAL REPAIR

Dr. Thomas Annandale has been credited as the first to perform a meniscal repair in 1883 using an open technique[12]. The advancement of arthroscopic technology has allowed today's orthopaedic surgeons to preserve meniscal tissue without the inherent risks of open surgery. Arthroscopic meniscal repair techniques include inside-out, outside-in, and all-inside procedures.

When a repair is performed, the meniscal bed should be prepared regardless of the technique used[12, 22]. This involves abrasion of the tear site and perimeniscal synovium using a small powered shaver or rasp to promote bleeding and healing[12]. Better healing rates have also been achieved using nonabsorbable sutures oriented vertically rather than horizontally[12].

Inside-Out Technique

The inside-out technique was popularized by Dr. Henning in the 1980's. It is a well-established procedure that can be used for most meniscal tears. Compared to the increasingly popular all-inside technique, the inside-out method offers the advantage of being able to repair complex tears more easily[26]. This is because all-inside devices often utilize a blunt and thicker needle, which requires greater pressure to pass through the meniscus and can cause displacement of meniscal fragments during reduction attempts[26]. In addition, the sharp thin needles used in the inside-out technique provide the opportunity to adjust and correct the reduction of meniscal tears since they can be partially passed and if necessary, backed out to make another attempt[26]. The disadvantages of the inside-out technique include the potential for neurovascular injury and the need for accessory incisions.

The inside-out procedure can be further subdivided into single- or double-barrel passage techniques[12]. The latter was developed by Clancy and Graf. It offers the advantage of a faster procedure at the potential expense of being a less secure repair, since it may not be possible to individually direct each throw of the suture for better reduction of tear fragments[12].

In general, the inside-out technique uses sutures with long flexible needles on each end. The needle is then passed through the meniscal fragments after being positioned with arthroscopically directed cannulas. It is retrieved using an accessory medial or lateral incision as it exits the joint capsule. The second needle is advanced in a similar fashion after the guide is positioned on the other side of the tear. Finally, the suture can be tied over the joint capsule.

The literature has generally supported the use of the inside-out technique[26]. Horibe et al[27] repaired 278 torn menisci using this method and reported only 9 patients with tibiofemoral symptoms at the time of second-look arthroscopy (mean interval of 8 months). Of those evaluated by repeat arthroscopy, they found that 73% of the repaired menisci had healed completely[27]. Rubman et al[28] evaluated 198 torn menisci and reported that 80% were asymptomatic at follow-up after arthroscopic inside-out repair. Of the 91 repairs evaluated arthroscopically after a mean of 18 months postoperatively, 23 (25%) were classified as healed, 35 (38%) as partially healed, and 33 (36%) as failed[28].

Outside-In Technique

The outside-in technique was developed by Warren[29] as a way to decrease the risk of peroneal nerve injury during arthroscopic repair of the lateral meniscus using the inside-out method. This procedure is particularly useful for repairs of the anterior and middle thirds of the meniscus[22, 30]. For tears of the posterior meniscus, the outside-in technique may be difficult in terms of allowing placement of sutures perpendicular to the meniscal surface. As a result, the inside-out or all-inside methods may be more appropriate in posterior meniscal tears[30]. The outside-in technique also obviates the need for rigid cannulas, which reduces the risk of articular cartilage damage during cannula insertion[30]. In addition, this technique avoids the need for larger accessory incision as with the inside-out technique[30].

The outside-in procedure requires the use of an 18-gauge spinal needle, sutures, and an arthroscopic grasper. Under arthroscopic guidance, the spinal needle is passed percutaneously through the joint capsule and across the meniscal tear. The needle should come through the inner segment of the meniscus on either the femoral or tibial surface. Curved needles may facilitate passage through posterior meniscal tears and avoid the need for a posterior starting point and the risk of neurovascular injury[30]. A second needle is then inserted in a similar fashion across the meniscal tear to achieve proper suture orientation. A number-0 polydioxanone suture is then advanced through the needles and pulled out from an anterior knee portal. A knot is then tied to the suture and pulled back into the joint against the superior or inferior surface of the meniscus to repair the tear. Tying one set of sutures prior to the insertion of the next is recommended in order to avoid tangling the sutures inside the joint[30]. The placement of adjacent suture sets should alternate between the tibial and femoral surfaces to evenly align the meniscal repair edges[30]. Each set of sutures should be spaced approximately 3 or 4 mm apart[30]. Finally, the adjacent free ends of the sutures are tied over the joint capsule through a small incision.

Morgan et al[31] were one of the first authors to use objective examination with second-look arthroscopy to evaluate meniscal healing after repair with the outside-in technique[30]. In their study with 74 repaired menisci, the overall rate of healing was 84%[31]. The authors also reported that visual evidence of healing was seen by approximately 4 months[31]. Mariani et al[32] studied the same repair technique in a series of 22 patients in conjunction with ACL reconstruction. They reported good clinical results in 77.3% of patients after a mean follow-up of 28 months[32]. In a more recent long-term study with mean follow-up of 11.7 years, the authors showed good clinical outcomes in 36 of 41 patients[33]. In this series, several clinical outcomes were evaluated and included the International Knee Documentation Committee (IKDC) form, the modified Lysholm score, the SF-36 (short form 36) score, a visual analogue scale (VAS) for patients satisfaction, and another VAS for patients pain perception[33]. These results suggest that the clinical success of the outside-in technique may be maintained in the long-term.

All-Inside Technique

The all-inside technique has become a popular method of meniscal repair. It is performed entirely under arthroscopic visualization and is typically used for unstable vertical longitudinal tears of the posterior meniscus[22]. This technique has evolved dramatically with the advancement of arthroscopic technology. Miller and Hart[34] described the various generations of all-inside meniscal repair techniques, and this serves as a useful paradigm.

First-generation all-inside meniscal repair techniques utilize suture hooks that are similar to those used in rotator cuff surgery[34]. This necessitates a 70° arthroscope placed through a posterolateral or posteromedial working portal. Second-generation techniques are exemplified in the T-Fix (Smith and Nephew), which involves passing sutures that are attached to small peripheral bars through spinal needles[34]. A series of sutures are placed using the T-Fix and adjacent sutures are tied to repair the meniscus. Kocabey et al[35] has studied the clinical outcomes after using the T-Fix. In a series of 52 patients with a mean follow-up of 10.3 months, the authors showed excellent results in 96% of patients using clinical examination findings as outcomes[35].

The third-generation of all-inside techniques includes various bioabsorbable, sutureless devices that are deployed through cannulas or specialized guns[34]. The most common one is the Meniscal Arrow (Bionx Implants), which has a barbed design and is made of poly-L-lactic acid (see Figure 6). Many surgeons use these devices in combination with inside-out sutures in a hybrid technique[34]. The sutures are used for most of the repairs, while the all-inside devices are employed for the difficult-to-reach posterior tears.

a)   b)

c)   d)

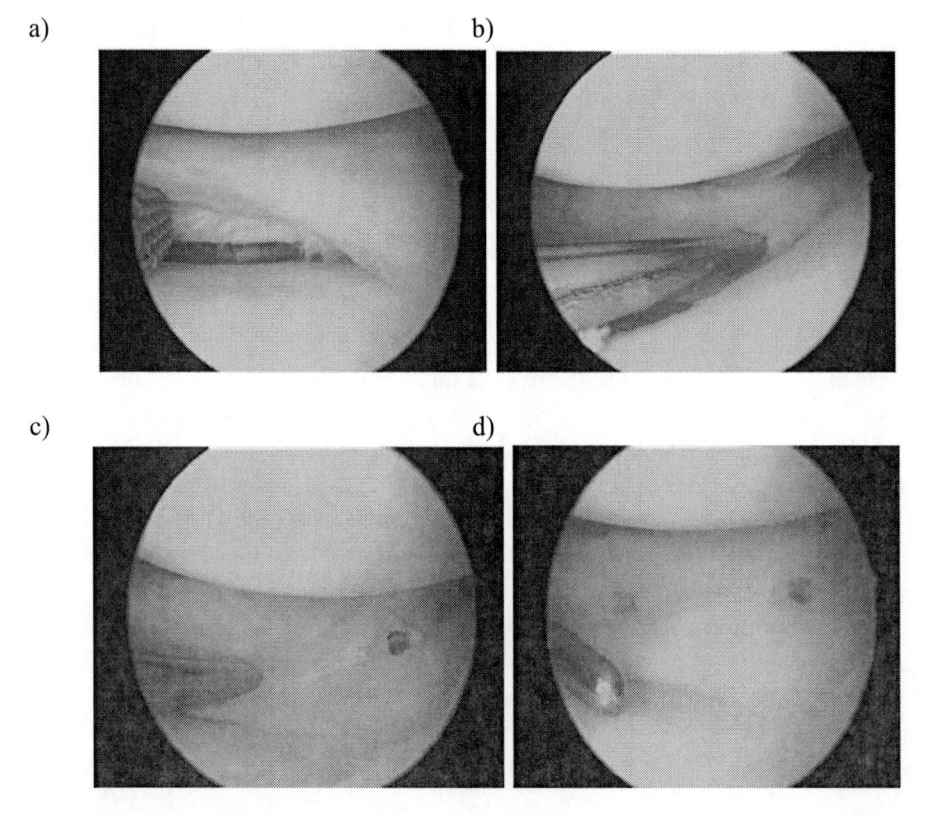

Figure 6. Intraoperative arthroscopic images demonstrating (A) a peripheral vertical longitudinal tear that was (B) amenable to repair. (C) A meniscal arrow was used to repair the tear. (D) Final arthroscopic image of the reduced and repaired meniscal tear.

Ellerman et al[36] prospectively studied 113 consecutive patients after all-inside meniscal repair with a bioabsorbable arrow. At a mean follow-up of 33 months, a 20% failure rate was identified[36]. The authors concluded that the clinical results were similar to traditional suture techniques[36]. A meniscal arrow may be preferred due to its simplicity, efficiency, and the avoidance of accessory incisions[36]. In contrast, Kurzweil et al[37] followed 60 consecutive patients with a mean follow-up of 54 months and reported a 28% failure rate. As a result, the authors in this series questioned the effectiveness of bioabsorbable arrows in meniscal repair[37].

Finally, fourth generation all-inside repair devices allow tensioning of the repair against an anchor and are designed with lower profiles to limit iatrogenic injury to surrounding structures such as the articular cartilage[34]. Examples of devices that fit into this category include the FasT-Fix (Smith and Nephew) and the RapidLoc (Mitek). The ability to tension repairs is attractive because the proper amount of tensioning allows better reduction of meniscal fragments. One study using the FasT-Fix showed good clinical outcomes in 90.2% of patients followed for a mean of 18 months[38]. In this series, the authors' criteria for clinical success included the absence of joint-line tenderness, locking, swelling, and a negative McMurray test[38]. In addition, Tegner scores, Lysholm knee scores, and KT-1000 arthrometry were used to assess clinical outcomes[38].

Given the variety of all-inside repair techniques, Lozano et al[39] conducted a systematic review of the literature from January 1966 to July 2006 to examine the effectiveness of the various devices. Interestingly, the authors found no substantial differences in the failure rates among these devices. However, 77% of the included studies were case series. Due to the paucity of randomized controlled trials, the authors could not make definite conclusions about the different all-inside repair devices.

In addition, there have been several studies comparing all-inside and inside-out repair techniques. One prospective, randomized controlled trial has recently compared these procedures[40]. After a mean follow-up of 28 months, the authors found no statistically significant difference in the retear rate between the two techniques[40]. Choi et al[41] also compared these two techniques in a prospective cohort study and found no difference in meniscal healing rates following repair performed via either technique during concomitant ACL reconstruction at a mean follow-up of 35.7 months. Another prospective cohort study by Spindler et al[42] found equivalent failure rates using the inside-out or the all-inside techniques after a median follow-up of 68 months for the former and 27 months for the latter. Based on these results, it would appear that similar clinical outcomes can be achieved using either repair technique.

Contemporary Meniscal Repairs

The continual advancement of meniscal repair techniques and the appreciation for the menisci as integral components of normal knee function has encouraged orthopaedic surgeons to push the boundaries of current repair indications. The classic teaching has been that only peripheral vertical longitudinal tears are amendable to meniscal repair[43]. Radially oriented tears that extend to the periphery have historically been treated with partial meniscectomy[43]. As alluded to previously, though, partial meniscectomies are associated with an increased incidence of early knee degeneration. In addition, an interesting in-vitro study by Bedi et al[43] showed that large radial tears of the meniscus are not functionally equivalent to meniscectomies. In their study, the authors used a dynamic cadaver model to demonstrate that even radial tears extending to 90% of the medial meniscal rim width did not significantly increase the mean or peak contact pressures over the medial tibial plateau, but instead caused a posterocentral shift in the location of the peak contact pressure. However, a partial meniscectomy led to an increase in the mean and peak contact pressures, as well as a further posterior shift in the location of the peak contact pressures when compared to the 90% torn and repaired menisci. These results highlight the importance of preserving and repairing torn menisci. More recently, studies have shown that radially oriented tears can be repaired if the meniscal bed is adequately prepared, fragments are tightly sutured, and adjuncts such as exogenous fibrin clots are added to promote healing[43, 44, 45].

CONCLUSION

Our understanding of the human meniscus has advanced considerably with time. It is now recognized that the meniscus plays a critical role in the biomechanics of the knee. When indicated, meniscal repair should be done to preserve this important structure using the various techniques described. With the constant advances in technology, there are a number of techniques and tools available for repair. Although no technique has been established as a gold standard, future randomized trials will delineate the best techniques and outcomes.

REFERENCES

[1] Sutton, J. B. Ligaments: Their nature and morphology, Ed 2. London, H.K. Lewis and Co., 1897.

[2] Greis, P. E., Bardana, D. D., Holmstrom, M. C., and Burks, R. T. Meniscal injury: I. Basic science and evaluation. *J. Am. Acad. Orthop. Surg*. 2002; 10: 168-176.

[3] Johnson, D. L., Swenson, T. M., Livesay, M. S., Aizawa, H., Fu, F. H., and Harner, C. D. Insertion-site anatomy of the human meniscus: Gross, arthroscopic, and topographical anatomy as a basis for meniscal transplantation. *Arthroscopy*. 1995; 11: 386-394.

[4] Gupte, C. M., Bull, A. M. J., Thomas, R. D., and Amis, A. A. A review of the function and biomechanics of the meniscofemoral ligaments. *Arthroscopy*. 2003; 19(2): 161-171.

[5] Wojtys, E. M. and Chan, D. B. Meniscus structure and function. AAOS *Instructional Course Lectures*. 2005; 54: 323-330.

[6] Petersen, W. and Tillmann, B. Collagenous fibril texture of the human knee joint menisci. *Anat. Embryol*. 1998; 197: 317-324.

[7] Arnoczky, S. P. and Warren, R. F. Microvasculature of the human meniscus. *Am. J. Sports Med*. 1982; 10: 90-95.

[8] Mine, T., Kimura, M., Sakka, A., and Kawai, S. Innervation of nociceptors in the menisci of the knee joint: an immunohistochemical study. *Arch. Orthop. Trauma. Surg*. 2000; 120: 201-204.

[9]   Assimakopoulos, A. P., Katonis, P. G., Agapitos, M. V., and Exarchou, E. I. The innervation of the human meniscus. *Clin. Orthop. Relat. Res*. 1992; 275: 232-236.

[10]   Rodkey, W. G. Basic biology of the meniscus and response to injury. AAOS *Instructional Course Lectures*. 2000. 49; 189-193.

[11]   Ahmed, A. M. and Burke, D. L. In-vitro measurement of static pressure distribution in synovial joints. Part I: Tibial surface of the knee. *J. Biomech. Eng*. 1983; 105: 216-225.

[12]   McGinty, J. B. *Operative arthroscopy*, ed 3. Philadelphia, PA. Lippincott-Raven, 2003, pp 218-231.

[13]   Stratford, P. W. and Binkley, J. A review of the McMurray test: Definition, interpretation, and clinical usefulness. *J. Orthop. Sports Phys. Ther*. 1995; 22(3): 116-120.

[14]   Eren, O. T. The accuracy of joint line tenderness by physical examination in the diagnosis of meniscal tears. *Arthroscopy*. 2003; 19(8): 850-854.

[15]   Karachalios, T., Hantes, M., Zibis, A. H., Zachos, V., Karantanas, A. H., and Malizos, K. N. Diagnostic accuracy of a new clinical test (the Thessaly test) for early detection of meniscal tears. *J. Bone Joint Surg*. 2005; 87-A(5): 955-962.

[16]   Konan, S., Rayan, F. and Haddad, F. S. Do physical diagnostic tests accurately detect meniscal tears? Knee Surg. Sports Traumatol. *Arthrosc*. 2009; 17: 806-811.

[17]   Solomon, D. H., Simel, D. L., Bates, D. W., Katz, J. N., and Schaffer, J. L. The rational clinical examination. Does this patient have a torn meniscus or ligament of the knee? Value of the physical examination. *JAMA*. 2001; 286(13): 1610-1620.

[18]   Gray, S. D., Kaplan, P. A. and Dussault, R. G. Imaging of the knee. Current status. *Orthop. Clin. North Am*. 1997; 28(4): 643-658.

[19]   Fabricant, P. D. and Jokl, P. Surgical outcomes after arthroscopic partial meniscectomy. *J. Am. Acad. Orthop. Surg*. 2007;15:647-653.

[20]   Boden, S. D., Davis, D. O., Dina, T. S., Stoller, D. W., Brown, S. D., Vailas, J. C., and Labropoulous P. A. A prospective and blinded investigation of magnetic resonance imaging of the knee. Abnormal findings in asymptomatic subjects. *Clin. Orthop. Relat. Res*. 1992; 282: 177-185.

[21]   Fairbanks, T. J. Knee joint changes after meniscectomy. *J. Bone Joint Surg*. 1948; 30: 664-670.

[22]   Greis, P. E., Holmstrom, M. C., Bardana, D. D., and Burks, R. T. Meniscal injury: II. Management. *J. Am. Acad. Orthop. Surg*. 2002; 10: 177-187.

[23]   Schimmer, R. C., Brülhart, K. B., Duff, C., and Glinz, W. Arthroscopic partial meniscectomy: a 12-year follow-up and two-step evaluation of the long-term course. *Arthroscopy*. 1998; 14(2): 136-142.

[24]   Petty, C. A., Lubowitz, J. H. Does arthroscopic partial meniscectomy result in knee osteoarthritis? A systematic review with a minimum of 8 years' follow-up. *Arthroscopy*. 2011; 27(3): 419-424.

[25]   Burks, R. T., Metcalf, M. H. and Metcalf, R. W. Fifteen-year follow-up of arthroscopic partial meniscectomy. *Arthroscopy*. 1997; 13: 673-679.

[26]   Lindenfeld, T. Inside-out meniscal repair. *Instr. Course Lect*. 2005; 54: 331-336.

[27] Horibe, S., Shino, K., Nakata, K., Maeda, A., Nakamura, N., and Matsumoto, N. Second-look arthroscopy after meniscal repair. Review of 132 menisci repaired by an arthroscopic inside-out technique. *J. Bone Joint Surg. Br.* 1995; 77(2): 245-249.

[28] Rubman, M. H., Noyes, F. R. and Barber-Westin, S. D. Arthroscopic repair of meniscal tears that extend into the avascular zone. A review of 198 single and complex tears. *Am. J. Sports Med.* 1998; 26(1): 87-95.

[29] Warren, R. F. Arthroscopic meniscus repair. Arthroscopy. 1985; 1: 170-172.

[30] Rodeo, S. A. Arthroscopic meniscal repair with use of the outside-in technique. *Instr. Course Lect.* 2000; 49: 195-206.

[31] Morgan, C. D., Wojtys, E. M., Casscells, C. D., and Casscells, S. W. Arthroscopic meniscal repair evaluated by second-look arthroscopy. *Am. J. Sports Med.* 1991; 19(6): 632-637.

[32] Mariani, P. P., Santori, N., Adriani, E., and Mastantuono, M. Accelerated rehabilitation after arthroscopic meniscal repair: A clinical and magnetic resonance imaging evaluation. *Arthroscopy.* 1996; 12(6): 680-686.

[33] Abdelkafy, A., Aigner, N., Zada, M., Elghoul, Y., Abdelsadek, H., and Landsiedl, F. Two to nineteen years follow-up of arthroscopic meniscal repair using the outside-in technique: A retrospective study. *Arch. Orthop. Trauma Surg.* 2007; 127(4): 245-252.

[34] Miller, M. D. and Hart, J. A. All-inside meniscal repair. *Instr. Course Lectures.* 2005; 54: 337-340.

[35] Kocabey, Y., Nyland, J., Isbell, W. M., and Caborn, D. N. Patient outcomes following T-Fix meniscal repair and a modifiable, progressive rehabilitation program, a retrospective study. *Arch. Orthop. Trauma Surg.* 2004; 124(9): 592-596.

[36] Ellermann, A., Siebold, R., Buelow, J. U., and Sobau, C. Clinical evaluation of meniscus repair with a bioabsorbable arrow: A 2- to 3-year follow-up study. *Knee Surg. Sports Traumatol. Arthrosc.* 2002; 10(5): 289-293.

[37] Kurzweil, P. R., Tifford, C. D. and Ignacio, E. M. Unsatisfactory clinical results of meniscal repair using the meniscus arrow. *Arthroscopy.* 2005; 21(8): 905.

[38] Kotsovolos, E. S., Hantes, M. E., Mastrokalos, D. S., Lorbach, O., and Paessler, H. H. Results of all-inside meniscal repair with the FasT-Fix meniscal repair system. *Arthroscopy.* 2006; 22(1): 3-9.

[39] Lozano, J., Ma, C. B. and Cannon, W. D. All-inside meniscus repair. *Clin. Orthop. Relat. Res.* 2007; 455: 134-141.

[40] Bryant, D., Dill, J., Litchfield, R., Amendola, A., Giffin, R., Fowler, P., and Kirkley, A. Effectiveness of bioabsorbable arrows compared with inside-out suturing for vertical, reparable meniscal lesions: a randomized clinical trial. *Am. J. Sports Med.* 2007; 35(6): 889-896.

[41] Choi, N. H., Kim, T. H. and Victoroff, B. N. Comparison of arthroscopic medial meniscal suture repair techniques: inside-out versus all-inside repair. *Am. J. Sports Med.* 2009; 37(11): 2144-2150.

[42] Spindler, K. P., McCarty, E. C., Warren, T. A., Devin, C., and Connor, J. T. Prospective comparison of arthroscopic medial meniscal repair technique: Inside-out suture versus entirely arthroscopic arrows. *Am. J. Sports Med.* 2003; 31(6): 929-934.

[43] Bedi, A., Kelly, N. H., Baad, M., Fox, A. J., Brophy, R. H., Warren, R. F., and Maher, S. A. Dynamic contact mechanics of the medial meniscus as a function of radial tear, repair, and partial meniscectomy. *J. Bone Joint Surg. Am.* 2010; 92(6): 1398-1408.

[44] Haklar, U., Kocaoglu, B., Nalbantoglu, U., Tuzuner, T., and Guven, O. Arthroscopic repair of radial lateral meniscus [corrected] tear by double horizontal sutures with inside-outside technique. *Knee.* 2008; 15(5): 355-359.

[45] Van Trommel, M. F., Simonian, P. T., Potter, H. G., and Wickiewicz, T. L. Arthroscopic meniscal repair with fibrin clot of complete radial tears of the lateral meniscus in the avascular zone. *Arthroscopy.* 1998; 14(4): 360-365.

In: The Knee
Editor: Randy Mascarenhas

ISBN: 978-1-61942-268-1
© 2012 Nova Science Publishers, Inc.

Chapter X

PATELLOFEMORAL INSTABILITY: EVALUATION AND MANAGEMENT

M. Kleiner, S. Safier and E. J. Kropf

Temple Univesity Department of Orthopaedic Surgery,
Philadelphia, PA, US

INTRODUCTION

Patellar dislocation represents a common injury with a variety of causal factors. The incidence of patellofemoral instability is estimated to be approximately 5.8 per 100,000 with an increased incidence in adolescents of approximately twenty-nine per 100,000(1,2). It has been suggested that the recurrence rates after nonoperative treatment of an acute patellar dislocation range from 15-44% (2). However, once a second dislocation occurs, the rate of future instability events increases to nearly 50% (1). The extent of disability that occurs after an acute dislocation event should not be underestimated. Many patients experiencing patellar instability are young, active individuals that injure themselves during sporting activity. It has been shown that these individuals have definite limitations to return to their previous activity levels with a significant decrease in return to strenuous athletic activities even after six months of recovery (3). Because of the relatively low rate of re-dislocation after a primary event, a trial of conservative management with focus on regaining range of motion and strength should certainly be attempted. Once a second dislocation event occurs, more emphasis should be placed on causality and the possible benefit that can be gleaned from surgical treatment.

Patellofemoral instability is multifactorial in origin. The stability of the patellofemoral articulation relies on the interplay between several anatomical factors. These include limb alignment and rotation, overall congruence of the patella within the femoral trochlear groove, and multiple soft tissue constraints including the medial patellofemoral ligament, the vastus medialis insertion and the medial and lateral retinaculum. In order to effectively treat patellofemoral instability, a thorough understanding of the pathogenesis of patellofemoral instability and the relationship of these anatomical factors to potential derangements should be well understood.

ANATOMY

The stability of the patellofemoral joint is largely influenced by the congruence between the articular surface of the patella and the femoral trochlear groove. The lateral facet of the trochlea is highest anteriorly and decreases its height distally and posteriorly, leading to increased stability in extension and early flexion (4). In higher degrees of flexion, higher degrees of stability are conferred by the component vectors of the quadriceps and patellar tendons. In addition, greater forces are transmitted to the patellar articular surface in these higher degrees of flexion.

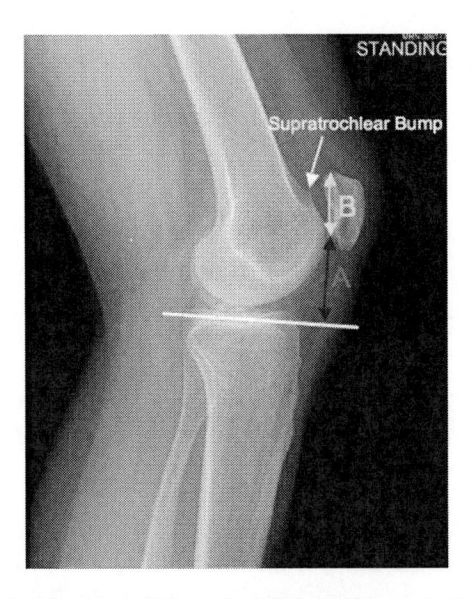

Figure 1. 30° flexion weight-bearing lateral view of a left knee demonstrating clear patella alta and a supratrochlear bump. The Blackburn-Peele index is depicted (A/B).

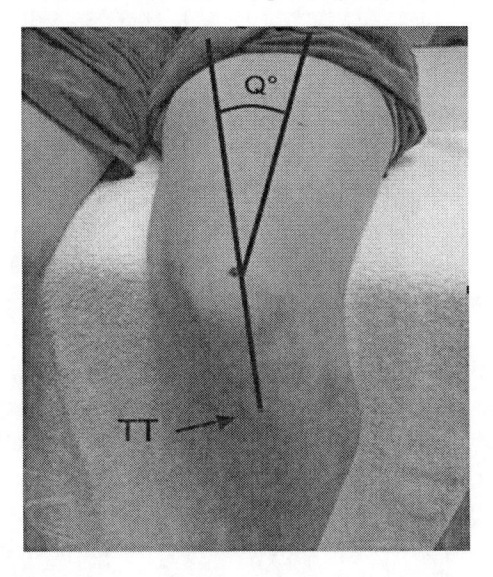

Figure 2. The seated Q angle is measured at the intersection of a line drawn from ASIS to center of patella and a line from the center of the patella to the tibial tubercle (TT).

Patella alta (Figure 1) has also been implicated in increased patellofemoral instability because the patella does not engage with the trochlea until higher degrees of flexion.

It has been noted that dislocation events occur without elicitation by trauma more frequently in patients with patella alta than in patients without patella alta (5).

The quadriceps angle, or Q angle, is formed by the intersection of a line drawn from the ASIS to the center of the patella and a line drawn from the center of the patella to the tibial tuberosity. The Q angle can be evaluated in the standing or seated position (Figure 2).

This angle increases during full extension due to the external rotation ("screw-home") mechanism of the tibia. In a knee with inherent instability, this can result in a greater propensity for patellar dislocation as the knee moves into higher degrees of flexion.

The medial patellofemoral ligament (MPFL) is an important stabilizing structure on the medial aspect of the knee. It provides 50-60% of lateral restraint in early degrees of flexion, particularly around 20 degrees (6). In addition, it has been found that when the MPFL is sectioned, as much as 50% of the resistance to lateral patellar translation is lost. Furthermore, when the MPFL is repaired, it can restore appropriate balance to the patella (7).

The vastus medialis obliquus (VMO) and vastus lateralis obliquus (VLO) also play an important role in the stability and tracking of the patella. An imbalance between the VMO and VLO can lead to patellar instability, largely because their combined vectors summate to a force that is parallel to the long axis of the femur. Furthermore, it has been shown that the vastus medialis is particularly prone to weakness with injury to the quadriceps mechanism, leading to relative overpull of the lateral stabilizers and potential lateral instability.

PHYSICAL EXAMINATION

Evaluation of suspected patellofemoral instability should begin with a thorough history and physical. The patient will often report painful episodes of the knee "giving out" or "popping out." These episodes may or may not coincide with traumatic events or athletic activities. An acute dislocation may be followed by immediate swelling and pain within the knee, which is attributable to the tense hemarthrosis that develops from tearing of the capsule. While the majority of patellar dislocations will self-reduce, occasionally the patella will be palpable lateral to the lateral femoral condyle and will require manual reduction with or without some form of sedation. A thorough examination during the acute phase of the injury will be extremely difficult due to the pain and discomfort experienced by the patient. However, by visual inspection only, the presence or absence of a significant knee effusion can be noted. Tenderness along the medial patellofemoral ligament and lateral femoral condyle should also be inspected for on exam and documented. Other provocative tests may be intolerable to the patient in the acute setting.

In cases of chronic instability, there are a few key clues that should lead to a diagnosis of patellofemoral instability. Again, the Q angle should be measured as a quick means of assessing amount of lateral pull experienced by the patella. The normal Q angle values are approximately 15 degrees in women and 10 degrees in men.

Another sign of lateral patellar maltracking is the so-called J sign. The patella engages the trochlea in approximately 30 to 40 degrees of flexion. An observed abrupt lateral shift of the patella as the patient extends the knee from 90 degrees of flexion represents a positive J sign. A positive J sign is most indicative of patella alta, as the lateral translation that is seen is caused by the patella exiting the groove near terminal extension. The manual translation test (Figure 3) can also be used to assess for patellar instability.

The principle of this test is that the examiner should not be able to translate the patella more than half of its width in either direction. The ability to do so corresponds to instability. Alternatively, one can divide the patella into quadrants. More than two quadrants of lateral translation is considered a positive test for lateral instability. Finally, a patient with patellar instability may have a positive apprehension test, in which the patient senses a feeling of imminent dislocation with an applied lateral force with the knee in approximately 30 degrees of flexion (8). A dynamic or "moving patellar apprehension test" has been described and may yield higher sensitivity and specificity when properly performed in the office setting (9).

IMAGING

As with all knee injuries, radiographs and advanced imaging studies are a key part of the evaluation of a patient with suspected patellofemoral instability. Routine radiographs should include posteroanterior weight bearing films at full extension and 30°, a 30° flexion weight-bearing lateral, and Merchant ("sunrise") views. The flexion lateral view (Figure 1) will provide the best assessment of patella alta. The Blackburn-Peele index, which evaluates the ratio between perpendicular distance from the lower articular margin of the patella to the tibial plateau (A) and the length of articular surface of patella (B), has shown the greatest inter-observer reliability for assessment of patella alta (10,11). On a true lateral radiograph, trochlear hypoplasia is seen by the "crossing sign" when the shallowest point of the trochlea crosses the anterior aspect of the femoral condyles. A supratrochlear spur will be present in some cases and the "double contour" sign is seen in cases of medial femoral condyle hypoplasia (12).

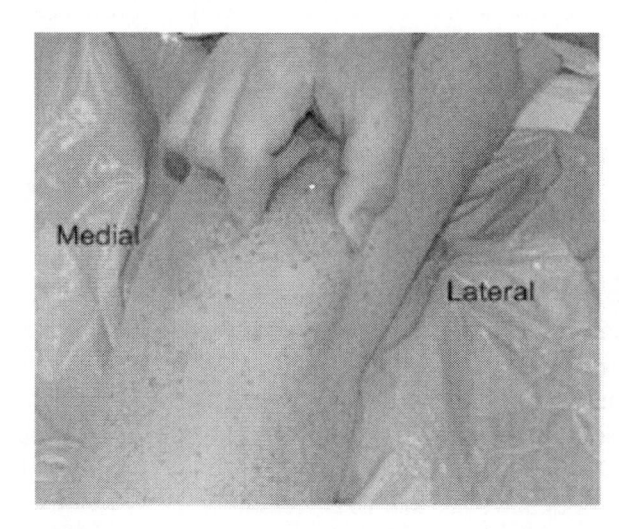

Figure 3. The manual translation test is performed at full extension and with the knee in 30° of flexion. The degree of translation is assessed in both medial and lateral directions and reported in quadrants of the patella. A side-to-side comparison is always performed.

Axial or Merchant views (Figure 4) are extremely helpful for assessment of patellar tilt, subluxation, and trochlear dysplasia.

The congruence angle measures the fit between the intercondylar surface and the patellar articular surface, and typically measures 6 to 11 degrees medially (13). Another measurement that can be made from Merchant views is the sulcus angle, which is formed by joining the highest points of the lateral and medial femoral condyles with the lowest point of the intercondylar sulcus. This should be approximately 138 degrees +/- 6 degrees, with measurements greater than 145 degrees indicating significant trochlear dysplasia (14,15).

In all cases of suspected chondral injury, advanced imaging with magnetic resonance imaging (MRI) should be performed (Figure 5).

We typically will perform MRI in all potential operative cases to evaluate the integrity of the medial patellofemoral ligament (Figure 6). MRI has been shown to be 85% sensitive and 70% specific for detection of injuries to the medial patellofemoral ligament, which is most often avulsed off its medial femoral epicondylar origin (16,17).

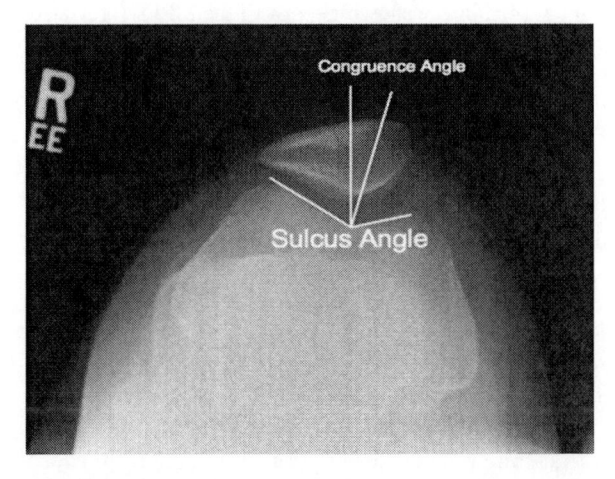

Figure 4. Axial view of the right patella. The sulcus angle can be measured to determine trochlear depth. The congruence angle is a measure of subluxation, not patellar tilt.

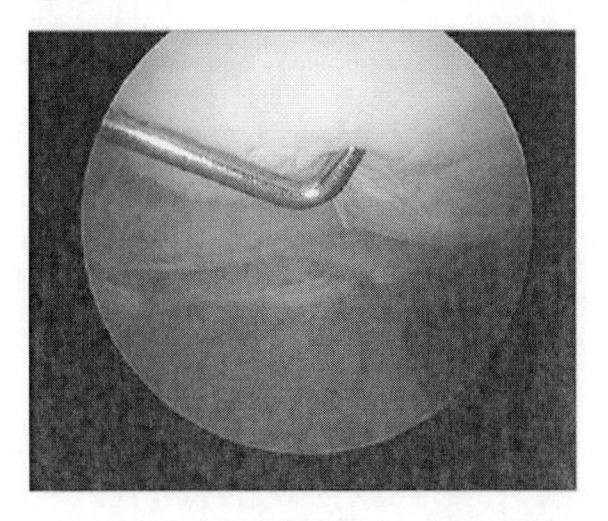

Figure 5. Arthroscopic image of a left knee depicting medial patellar facet injury following acute first time patellar dislocation.

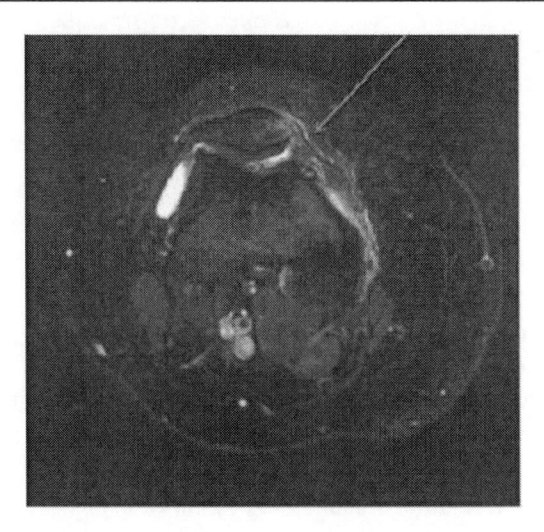

Figure 6. Axial T2-weighted MRI image showing a tear of the MPFL (blue arrow) from its patellar insertion with increased signal intensity representing edema.

The tibial tubercle- trochlear groove (TT-TG) distance can be calculated with cross sectional imaging at these two levels. Historically, this measurement has been performed with selective computed tomography scanning, but with simple processing of appropriate MRI images, this calculation can be accurately determined with MRI. A TT-TG distance that exceeds 20 mm predicts a high rate of patellar instability (12).

Non-Operative Management

Although there is some debate in the literature regarding the appropriate treatment regimen following a first-time patellar dislocation, it is generally accepted that most patients should be managed with an initial period of non-operative treatment and rehabilitation (18). Initial goals of therapy include reduction in swelling and effusion, muscle (specifically vastus medialis) recruitment and strengthening, and a gradual return of full range of motion. No studies have shown reduction in re-dislocation rates with initial immobilization, but such treatment likely allows some time for the medial structures to scar down. Stiffness may develop and the patient should be monitored closely to avoid such complication.

To date, two prospective trials have shown no difference in long-term rates of re-dislocation or subluxation when comparing results of early medial repair versus nonoperative management of patellar dislocation (19, 20). The presence of a displaced osteochondral fragment on radiographs or MR imaging represents an absolute indication for immediate operative fixation or removal of the fragment. In this setting, many authors advocate early retinacular and/or MPFL repair or reconstruction. If no osteochondral fragment is present, the injury can be managed with an initial period of immobilization followed by aggressive knee rehabilitation (21).

Prophylactic knee braces designed to limit lateral patellar dislocation are readily available and widely utilized, but their efficacy is largely unclear (22). While initial rehabilitative efforts should be maximized, certain circumstances, anatomic concerns or patient factors may tip the scales towards operative management. Among these factors to be considered include the presence of an osteochondral lesion, substantial disruption of the medial stabilizers, a laterally subluxated patella with a contralateral normally aligned limb, and patients who remain symptomatic following appropriate rehabilitation(23). Once a patient experiences a second dislocation, the subsequent risk of patellar dislocation increases significantly. At this point, surgical options should be considered for most healthy, active patients who wish to return to their prior level of function and sport. In a recent meta-analysis, Smith et al found that the operative treatment of patellar dislocation led to a higher risk of patellofemoral arthritis and a lower risk of redislocation than nonoperative treatment (24). The clinical significance of these results probably varies based on individual patient factors and expectations, and should be tailored to individual patient needs.

SURGICAL MANAGEMENT

The decision to proceed with surgical treatment of patellofemoral instability must be made with specific attention to the underlying cause of the disorder. The cause will most often be identified based on the history and physical examination along with appropriate imaging studies. It should be determined pre-operatively whether the disability results from a purely traumatic event in an otherwise anatomically normal knee versus a low-energy mechanism in a patient with significant anatomic predisposition to patellar instability. For example, a significant patellar tilt seen on Merchant views without a history of trauma may respond to a lateral release whereas patellar subluxation associated with malalignment may respond better to a distal realignment procedure.

Over 100 different procedures have been described to address patellofemoral instability. For ease of discussion, procedures can be divided into proximal and distal procedures. Commonly performed proximal realignment procedures include: 1) lateral retinacular release; 2) medial "reefing" or imbrication; and 3) MPFL reconstruction. Distal realignment typically refers to some version of a tibial tubercle realignment osteotomy (Elmsie Trillat, Maquet or Fulkerson anteriomedialization osteotomy).

Lateral Retinacular Release

The use of an isolated lateral release (Figure 7) for the treatment of lateral patellar instability is controversial and not without potential complications despite the seemingly straightforward nature of the procedure.

Poor outcomes after lateral release can be related to hemarthrosis, reflex sympathetic dystrophy, and medial subluxation. An isolated lateral release should be reserved for patients with true lateral patellar compression syndrome, which is characterized by an appropriate history and significant patellar tilt without subluxation, trochlear dysplasia or any other anatomic anomalies noted on roentenographic examination or CT Scan (25). Studies have shown that isolated lateral release for patellar instability yields poor results in long-term follow-up (26).

There is a role for lateral release in combination with medial patellofemoral ligament repair or reconstruction, especially when the tibial tubercle-to-trochlear groove distance is

a)   b)

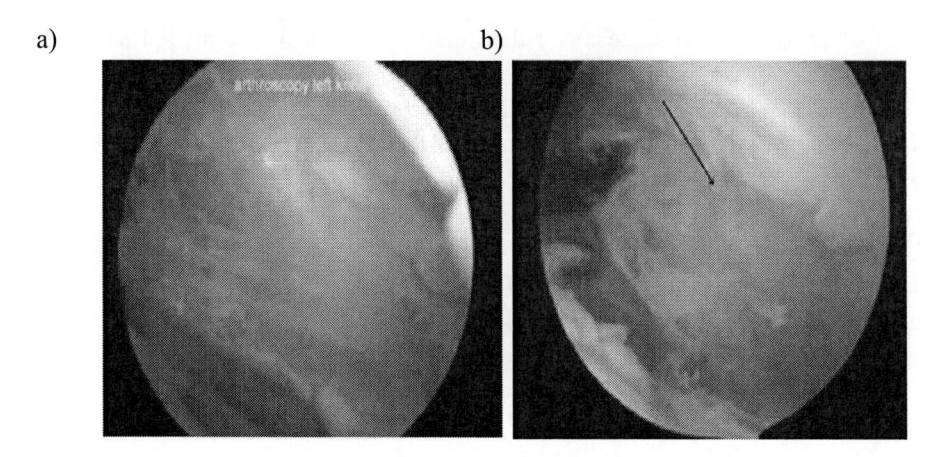

Figure 7. Arthroscopic view of lateral knee capsule a. before and b. after lateral release. The black arrow indicates the site of surgical dissection.

less than 20 mm (27). In such cases, lateral release is necessary to properly balance to the proximal soft tissue sleeve following medial imbrication. Aggressive lateral release has been associated with medial patellar instability, which can be a devastating post-operative complication.

Medial Patellofemoral Ligament Repair and Reconstruction

Following traumatic patellar dislocation, some degree of injury to the MPFL nearly always occurs. Therefore medial patellofemoral ligament repair or reconstruction may be warranted (28). The morphology of medial patellofemoral ligament tears has been shown to be similar between the adult and pediatric population. Accordingly, recurrent pediatric patellar dislocations can be managed similarly to those of their adult counterparts by repair or reconstructive procedures (29). In the pediatric population, MPFL reconstruction may be the only viable surgical option when open physeal growth plates contraindicate distal tubercle osteotomy.

There is some long-term data suggesting that the good surgical results often quoted in the pediatric population may be misleading. Patient satisfaction does not always reflect the low post-operative rate of dislocation that gets reported (30). The presence of trochlear dysplasia should also be noted and managed accordingly. Isolated trochlear dysplasia without evidence of concomitant patella alta or tibial tubercle-trochlear groove distance can be managed with trochleoplasty.(15).

Advocates of direct MPFL repair often cite good success rates as well as less likelihood of overload of the patellofemoral joint due to overtensioning of the graft used for reconstruction (31). According to one study, non-anatomic MPFL repair leads to a greater chance of redislocation, but when done correctly, the success rate is high (32). Another randomized controlled trial of 80 patients cautions that MPFL repair to the adductor tubercle does not decrease the risk of dislocation or even subjective functional outcome scores with the exception of specific subjective patella stability scores when compared with non-operative treatment (33).

Late reconstruction of the medial patellofemoral ligament is another viable surgical treatment option for chronic patellar instability. A recent review of the literature indicates that MPFL reconstruction performed with semitendinosus autografts is likely to improve a patient's ability to get back to their normal activities of daily living without significant limitation. However there is some caution regarding its efficacy in terms of full return to sporting activities (34). One study with five years of mean follow-up showed that reconstruction with free semitendinosus autograft prevents instability, joint deterioration and painful episodes (35). While the semitendinosus tendon appears to be the most commonly used autograft, some surgeons have also used gracillis tendon with positive results (36). Patellar tendon autograft and tibialis anterior allograft reconstructions have also been described.

While there are many methods described for reconstruction of the medial patellofemoral ligament, the overall consensus is that reconstruction results in excellent functional outcomes (37). In one study with patients without any predisposing factors for dislocation, reconstruction using hamstring autograft through transverse patellar tunnels was shown to be a reliable treatment option based on patient outcomes after a mean of just over three years (38). The dual tunnel technique, utilizing two tunnels at the medial border of the patella and one at the adductor tubercle of the femur, has produced good results without significant complications such as patellar fracture or re-dislocation (39). There is some debate over reconstruction by static or dynamic means, with some evidence that subjective outcomes in patients treated with dynamic reconstruction are better than patients treated with rigid reconstructive techniques (40).

While reconstruction carries with it some inherent risk of patellar fracture, medial subluxation, and redislocation, the results appear to be favorable for the management of recurrent dislocations without significant anatomic abnormalities. Another potential pitfall of reconstruction of the MPFL is over-narrowing of the patellofemoral joint space, though this can be guarded against by avoiding over-tensioning of the graft.

Tibial Tubercle Osteotomy

When significant anatomic predisposition to instability exists, osteotomy procedures should be considered. There are numerous procedures available for the treatment of patellofemoral instability due to osseous abnormalities, with each one carrying its own unique profile of risks and benefits. The choice of which procedure to use is based on the underlying reason for the instability, which is determined based on history, physical exam findings, and appropriate imaging studies.

There have been several versions of distal realignment/tibial tubercle osteotomy described, with each having varying degrees of success. The tibial tubercle can be transferred either directly medially (Elmsie-Trillat procedure) or anteromedially as described by Fulkerson. The goal of anteromedialization of the tibial tubercle is to treat instability and pain due to distal or lateral patellar articular damage by unloading the distal cartilage and lateral facet (41). Commonly, distal realignment procedures are combined with other proximal realignment procedures in order to correct recurrent patellar dislocation (42).

a)   b)

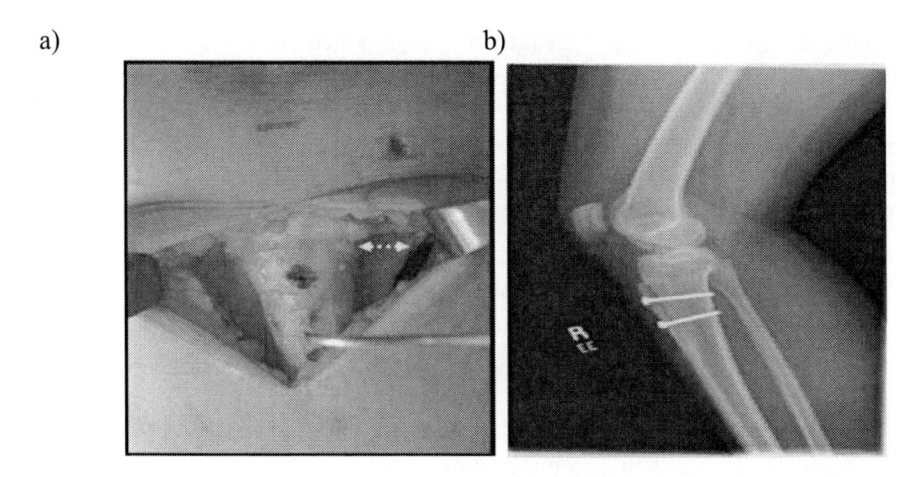

Figure 8. a. Intraoperative view of tibial tubercle osteotomy. Note the degree of medialization depicted by the dashed line.b. Postoperative image of the same patient showing appropriately placed hardware.

Elmsie-Trillat Procedure (Medialization Osteotomy)

Medial transfer of the tibial tubercle (Figure 8) along with lateral release (Elmsie-Trillat procedure) has been used with some success for the treatment of patellar instability and can be performed with or without a medial capsulorraphy (43).

It has been lauded for its ability to improve the patellar congruence angle and maintain it over time (44). A long-term follow-up study of the Elmsie-Trillat procedure by Nakagawa suggested that the procedure yielded intermediate results, with better Fulkerson scores seen at the time of first follow-up than at final follow-up. The authors recommended that the procedure be performed before the onset of degenerative changes in the patellofemoral joint. In addition, they suggested that there was a greater chance of re-dislocation and poor scores when more time had elapsed between the first dislocation and time of fixation (45). It has been suggested that medial tibial tubercle transfer is better for patients with patellar maltracking and anterior knee pain than for patients with isolated patellar instability (46). It has also been noted that symptoms of patients undergoing the Elmsie-Trillat procedure often deteriorate over the long term and most often come from worsening of patellofemoral joint pain rather than recurrent instability (45).

Fulkerson (Anteromedialization/AMZ) Osteotomy

The Fulkerson osteotomy was developed to address the overload of the patellofemoral joint that occurs with isolated medial tibial tubercle transfer. When the patient is appropriately selected, knee pain secondary to malalignment and a degenerative patellar articular surface can be effectively treated by anteromedialization that allows the individual to resume normal activities with substantially diminished pain (47).

By moving the tubercle anteriorly, the joint is offloaded such that less force is driven across the articular surface and the lateral facet offloaded at lower flexion angles with equalization of pressure between the medial and lateral facets at higher flexion angles (48).

The femoral trochlea also experiences significantly less force after anteromedialization of the patella, particularly in the lateral and central areas (49). As opposed to the Elmsie-Trillat procedure, it has been observed that patients who have isolated instability pre-operatively do better than patients with pain or those with pain and instability. The same study noted good results with long-term follow-up and better outcomes associated with male sex, healthy patellar articular cartilage, and pre-operative symptoms of instability (48). Better results are seen with lower Outerbridge scores, but the procedure has been shown to produce satisfactory results even in elderly patients (50).

Other than re-dislocation, the most disastrous complication resulting from anteromedialization of the tibial tubercle is probably fracture distal to the screws placed for fixation. Several authors have reported fracture of the tibia after Fulkerson osteotomy, a potentially devastating event for the patient (51,52). In order to help prevent tibial fracture, patients should be restricted to partial weight bearing for six to eight weeks after the surgery. Other aspects of rehabilitation should probably be tailored to the individual patient's expectations and goals with range of motion, strength, proprioception, and return to sports of particular importance (53). All osteotomy procedures should be approached with a serious assessment of the patient's metabolic bone condition. Diabetics and smokers represent relative contraindications because of a high risk of non-union following osteotomy.

Trochleoplasty

In the case of a shallow femoral trochlea, patients can be treated with isolated soft tissue procedures or with groove-deepening trochleoplasty. Medial patellofemoral ligament reconstruction is recommended for patellofemoral instability when patella alta or increased tibial tubercle-trochlear groove distance are not present. Trochleoplasty should be reserved for severe trochlear dysplasia that is recalcitrant to other stabilization techniques (15). Performing a trochloplasty carries the risk of articular damage, arthrofibrosis, and poor subjective outcomes. The procedure should thus be used with caution.

CONCLUSION

Patellofemoral instability is a complex problem with a variety of causes. The underlying cause of the instability, whether traumatic or due to limb malalignment or both, should be determined to help guide treatment. Initial treatment for traumatic instability should focus on rehabilitation and strengthening of the quadriceps, particularly the vastus medialis obliquus. Recurrent traumatic instability should likely be managed with repair or reconstruction of the medial patellofemoral ligament for best results. The presence of limb malalignment or osseous abnormalities often requires a more sophisticated procedure to treat the instability, with a combination of proximal and distal realignment procedures often being necessary.

REFERENCES

[1] Fithian, D. C., Paxton, E. W., Stone, M. L., Silva, P., Davis, D.K., Elias, D. A., et al. Epidemiology and natural history of acute patellar dislocation. *Am. J. Sports Med.* 2004 Jul.-Aug.;32(5):1114-21.

[2] Hawkins, R. J., Bell, R. H., Anisette, G. Acute patellar dislocations. the natural history. *Am. J. Sports Med.* 1986 Mar.-Apr.;14(2):117-20.

[3] Atkin, D. M., Fithian, D. C., Marangi, K. S., Stone, M. L., Dobson, B. E., Mendelsohn, C. Characteristics of patients with primary acute lateral patellar dislocation and their recovery within the first 6 months of injury. *Am. J. Sports Med.* 2000 Jul.-Aug.;28(4):472-9.

[4] Colvin, A. C., West, R. V. Patellar instability. *J. Bone Joint Surg. Am.* 2008 Dec.;90(12):2751-62.

[5] Geenen, E., Molenaers, G., Martens, M. Patella alta in patellofemoral instability. *Acta. Orthop. Belg.* 1989;55(3):387-93.

[6] Desio, S. M., Burks, R.T., Bachus, K. N. Soft tissue restraints to lateral patellar translation in the human knee. *Am. J. Sports Med.* 1998 Jan.-Feb.;26(1):59-65.

[7] Hautamaa, P. V., Fithian, D. C., Kaufman, K. R., Daniel, D. M., Pohlmeyer, A. M. Medial soft tissue restraints in lateral patellar instability and repair. *Clin. Orthop. Relat. Res.* 1998 Apr.;(349):174-82. (349):174-82.

[8] Lubowitz, J. H., Bernardini, B. J., Reid, J. B.,3rd. Current concepts review: Comprehensive physical examination for instability of the knee. *Am. J. Sports Med.* 2008 Mar.;36(3):577-94.

[9] Ahmad, C. S., McCarthy, M., Gomez, J. A., Shubin Stein, B. E. The moving patellar apprehension test for lateral patellar instability. *Am. J. Sports Med.* 2009 April; 37(4)791-796.

[10] Seil, R., Muller, B., Georg, T., Kohn, D., Rupp, S. Reliability and interobserver variability in radiological patellar height ratios. *Knee Surg. Sports Traumatol. Arthrosc.* 2000;8:231-6.

[11] Berg, E. E., Mason, S. L., Lucas, M. J. Patellar height ratios. A comparison of four measurement methods. *Am. J. Sports Med.* 1996;24:218-21.

[12] Dejour, H., Walch, G., Nove-Josserand, L., Guier, C. Factors of patellar instability: an anatomic radiographic study. *Knee Surg. Sports Traumatol. Arthrosc.* 1994;2:19-26.

[13] Merchant, A. C., Mercer, R. L., Jacobsen, R. H., Cool, C. R. Roentgenographic analysis of patellofemoral congruence. *J. Bone Joint Surg. Am.* 1974 Oct.;56(7):1391-6.

[14] Dejou,H., Walch, G., Nove-Josserand, L., Guier, C. Factors of patellar instability: An anatomic radiographic study. *Knee Surg. Sports Traumatol. Arthrosc.* 1994;2(1):19-26.

[15] Bollier, M., Fulkerson, J. P. The role of trochlear dysplasia in patellofemoral instability. *J. Am. Acad. Orthop. Surg.* 2011 Jan.;19(1):8-16.

[16] Sanders, T. G., Morrison, W. B., Singleton, B. A., Miller, M. D., Cornum, K. G. Medial patellofemoral ligament injury following acute transient dislocation of the patella: MR findings with surgical correlation in 14 patients. *J. Comput. Assist. Tomogr.* 2001 Nov.-Dec.;25(6):957-62.

[17] Nomura, E., Horiuchi, Y., Inoue, M. Correlation of MR imaging findings and open exploration of medial patellofemoral ligament injuries in acute patellar dislocations. *Knee*. 2002 May;9(2):139-43.

[18] Wilk, K. E., Davies, G. J., Mangine, R. E., Malone, T. R. Patellofemoral disorders: A classification system and clinical guidelines for nonoperative rehabilitation. *J. Orthop. Sports Phys. Ther*. 1998 Nov.;28(5):307-22.

[19] Nikku, R., Nietosvaara, Y., Kallio, P. E., Aalto, K., Michelsson, J. E. Operative versus closed treatment of primary dislocation of the patella. similar 2-year results in 125 randomized patients. *Acta. Orthop, Scand*. 1997 Oct.;68(5):419-23.

[20] Nikku, R., Nietosvaara, Y., Aalto, K., Kallio, P. E. Operative treatment of primary patellar dislocation does not improve medium-term outcome: A 7-year follow-up report and risk analysis of 127 randomized patients. *Acta. Orthop*. 2005 Oct.;76(5):699-704.

[21] Mehta, V. M., Inoue ,M,. Nomura, E., Fithian, D. C. An algorithm guiding the evaluation and treatment of acute primary patellar dislocations. *Sports Med. Arthrosc*. 2007 Jun.;15(2):78-81.

[22] Cherf, J., Paulos, L. E. Bracing for patellar instability. *Clin. Sports Med*. 1990 Oct.;9(4):813-21.

[23] Stefancin, J. J., Parker, R. D. First-time traumatic patellar dislocation: A systematic review. *Clin. Orthop. Relat. Res*. 2007 Feb.;455:93-101.

[24] Smith, T. O., Song, F., Donell, S. T., Hing, C. B. Operative versus non-operative management of patellar dislocation. A meta-analysis. *Knee Surg. Sports Traumatol. Arthrosc*. 2011 Jan. 14.

[25] Clifton, R., Ng, C. Y., Nutton, R. W. What is the role of lateral retinacular release? *J. Bone Joint Surg. Br*. 2010 Jan.;92(1):1-6.

[26] Verdonk, P., Bonte, F., Verdonk, R. Lateral retinacular release]. *Orthopade*. 2008 Sep.;37(9):884-9.

[27] Tom, A., Fulkerson, J. P. Restoration of native medial patellofemoral ligament support after patella dislocation. *Sports Med. Arthrosc*. 2007 Jun.;15(2):68-71.

[28] Boden, B. P., Pearsall, A. W., Garrett, W. E.,Jr, Feagin, J. A.,Jr. Patellofemoral instability: Evaluation and management. *J. Am. Acad. Orthop. Surg*. 1997 Jan.;5(1):47-57.

[29] Balcarek, P., Walde, T. A., Frosch, S., Schuttrumpf, J. P., Wachowski, M. M., Sturmer, K. M., et al. Patellar dislocations in children, adolescents and adults: A comparative MRI study of medial patellofemoral ligament injury patterns and trochlear groove anatomy. *Eur. J. Radiol*. 2010 Jul. 15.

[30] Luhmann, S. J., O'Donnell, J. C., Fuhrhop, S. Outcomes after patellar realignment surgery for recurrent patellar instability dislocations: A minimum 3-year follow-up study of children and adolescents. *J. Pediatr. Orthop*. 2011 Jan.-Feb.;31(1):65-71.

[31] Fabbriciani, C., Panni, A. S., Delcogliano, A. Role of arthroscopic lateral release in the treatment of patellofemoral disorders. *Arthroscopy*. 1992;8(4):531-6.

[32] Camp, C. L., Krych, A. J., Dahm, D. L., Levy, B. A., Stuart, M. J. Medial patellofemoral ligament repair for recurrent patellar dislocation. *Am. J. Sports Med*. 2010 Nov.;38(11):2248-54.

[33] Christiansen, S. E., Jakobsen, B. W., Lund, B., Lind, M. Isolated repair of the medial patellofemoral ligament in primary dislocation of the patella: A prospective randomized study. *Arthroscopy*. 2008 Aug.;24(8):881-7.

[34] Fisher, B., Nyland, J., Brand, E., Curtin, B. Medial patellofemoral ligament reconstruction for recurrent patellar dislocation: A systematic review including rehabilitation and return-to-sports efficacy. *Arthroscopy.* 2010 Oct.;26(10):1384-94.

[35] Ellera Gomes, J. L., Stigler Marczyk, L. R., Cesar de Cesar, P., Jungblut, C. F. Medial patellofemoral ligament reconstruction with semitendinosus autograft for chronic patellar instability: A follow-up study. *Arthroscopy.* 2004 Feb.;20(2):147-51.

[36] Goorens, C. K., Robijn, H., Hendrickx, B., Delport, H., De Mulder, K., Hens, J. Reconstruction of the medial patellofemoral ligament for patellar instability using an autologous gracilis tendon graft. *Acta. Orthop. Belg.* 2010 Jun.;76(3):398-402.

[37] Buckens, C. F., Saris, D. B. Reconstruction of the medial patellofemoral ligament for treatment of patellofemoral instability: A systematic review. *Am. J. Sports Med.* 2010 Jan.;38(1):181-8.

[38] Ronga, M., Oliva, F., Longo, U. G., Testa, V., Capasso, G., Maffulli, N. Isolated medial patellofemoral ligament reconstruction for recurrent patellar dislocation. *Am. J. Sports Med.* 2009 Sep.;37(9):1735-42.

[39] Toritsuka, Y., Amano, H., Mae, T., Uchida, R., Hamada, M., Ohzono, K., et al. Dual tunnel medial patellofemoral ligament reconstruction for patients with patellar dislocation using a semitendinosus tendon autograft. *Knee.* 2010 May 29.

[40] Gomes, J. E. Comparison between a static and a dynamic technique for medial patellofemoral ligament reconstruction. *Arthroscopy.* 2008 Apr.;24(4):430-5.

[41] Fulkerson, J. P. Diagnosis and treatment of patients with patellofemoral pain. *Am. J. Sports Med.* 2002 May-Jun.;30(3):447-56.

[42] Wootton, J. R., Cross, M. J., Wood, D. G. Patellofemoral malalignment: A report of 68 cases treated by proximal and distal patellofemoral reconstruction. *Injury.* 1990 May;21(3):169-73.

[43] Tomatsu, T., Imai, N., Hanada, T., Nakamura, Y. Simplification of the elmslie-trillat procedure for patellofemoral malalignment. is medial capsulorraphy necessary? *Int. Orthop.* 1996;20(4):211-5.

[44] Shelbourne, K. D., Porter, D. A., Rozzi, W. Use of a modified elmslie-trillat procedure to improve abnormal patellar congruence angle. *Am. J. Sports Med.* 1994 May-Jun.;22(3):318-23.

[45] Nakagawa, K., Wada, Y., Minamide, M., Tsuchiya, A., Moriya, H. Deterioration of long-term clinical results after the elmslie-trillat procedure for dislocation of the patella. *J. Bone Joint Surg. Br.* 2002 Aug.;84(6):861-4.

[46] Diks, M. J., Wymenga, A. B., Anderson, P. G. Patients with lateral tracking patella have better pain relief following CT-guided tuberosity transfer than patients with unstable patella. *Knee Surg. Sports Traumatol. Arthrosc.* 2003 Nov.;11(6):384-8.

[47] Fulkerson, J. P., Becker, G. J., Meaney, J. A., Miranda, M., Folcik, M. A. Anteromedial tibial tubercle transfer without bone graft. *Am. J. Sports Med.* 1990 Sep.-Oct.;18(5):490,6; discussion 496-7.

[48] Pritsch, T., Haim, A., Arbel, R., Snir, N., Shasha, N., Dekel, S. Tailored tibial tubercle transfer for patellofemoral malalignment: Analysis of clinical outcomes. *Knee Surg. Sports Traumatol. Arthrosc.* 2007 Aug.15(8):994-1002.

[49] Kuroda, R., Kambic, H., Valdevit, A., Andrish, J. T. Articular cartilage contact pressure after tibial tuberosity transfer. A cadaveric study. *Am. J. Sports Med.* 2001 Jul.-Aug.;29(4):403-9.

[50] Carofino, B. C., Fulkerson, J. P. Anteromedialization of the tibial tubercle for patellofemoral arthritis in patients > 50 years. *J. Knee Surg.* 2008 Apr.;21(2):101-5.

[51] Fulkerson, J. P. Fracture of the proximal tibia after fulkerson anteromedial tibial tubercle transfer. A report of four cases. *Am. J. Sports Med.* 1999 Mar.-Apr.;27(2):265.

[52] Eager, M. R., Bader, D. A., Kelly, J. D.,4th, Moyer, R. A. Delayed fracture of the tibia following anteromedialization osteotomy of the tibial tubercle: A report of 5 cases. *Am. J. Sports Med.* 2004 Jun.;32(4):1041-8.

[53] Salari, N., Horsmon, G. A., Cosgarea, A. J. Rehabilitation after anteromedialization of the tibial tuberosity. *Clin. Sports Med.* 2010 Apr.;29(2):303,11, ix.

In: The Knee
Editor: Randy Mascarenhas

ISBN: 978-1-61942-268-1
© 2012 Nova Science Publishers, Inc.

Chapter XI

Treatment of Combined Knee Pathology: Malalignment, Instability and Cartilage Loss

Rachel M. Frank, Brian Forsythe and Neil Ghodadra

Rush University Medical Center, Department of Orthopaedics,
Chicago, Illinois, US
OAK Orthopaedics, Frankfort, Illinois, US

Introduction

Patients presenting with knee pain may have multiple concurrent etiologies. With advancements in surgical techniques, implant designs, and imaging modalities, the ability to successfully perform complex procedures in even the most challenging patient is improving. However patients with multiple coexisting knee pathologies remain a difficult patient group, especially with regard to determining which (if any) of the lesions is the cause of symptoms. Cartilage lesions may be simply incidental in nature, and the decision to treat is based upon their confirmed contribution to patients' symptomatology.

The combination of tibial-femoral malalignment, ligament instability, and chondral/meniscal damage presents multiple challenges.[1] Corrective procedures for each of these problems performed in isolation have historically produced adequate results, however combined procedures to treat varied pathologies may augment repairs and in fact prove essential for the success of any single procedure.[1] For a patient with severe cartilage damage, uni-compartmental knee arthroplasty or total knee arthroplasty has clearly and consistently demonstrated good to excellent outcomes with regard to pain relief and restoration of function. However, arthroplasty is not ideal for the young and active moderate to high-demand patient[1] due to the potential for component loosening and wear. Thus, consideration of patient expectations in this difficult patient population is one of the key components to a successful outcome.

Many surgical options are available for the patient with multiple knee pathologies and are often used in combination. Specifically, varus malalignment can be addressed with a high tibial osteotomy (HTO) that unloads the diseased medial compartment, while valgus malalignment can be treated with a distal femoral osteotomy (DFO) that unloads the diseased lateral compartment. Ligamentous pathology can be addressed with direct repair or reconstruction. Articular cartilage pathology can be treated with a variety of procedures including debridement, microfracture, autologous chondrocyte implantation, and osteochondral autograft/allograft. Finally, meniscal deficiencies can be treated with direct repair or allograft transplantation.

The young, athletic patient with uni-compartmental knee osteoarthritis warrants an in-depth discussion, as such patients are notoriously difficult to treat. Non-operative solutions are often temporizing at best, while operative solutions often require significant future activity modifications or provide incomplete relief of symptoms. Historically, high tibial osteotomy has been performed to correct the angular deformity associated with rickets, polio, and post-traumatic deformities.[2, 3] Today, HTO is most commonly used to treat isolated medial compartment knee osteoarthritis. More recently, HTO has been used as a concomitant malalignment corrective procedure in patients undergoing cartilage and/or meniscus surgery in an attempt to off-load the compartment in which cartilage surgery is performed.

Good-to-excellent results with HTO have been reported in the literature, but there are several potential drawbacks. First, the procedure is not ideal if there is more than one affected compartment. Although it may effectively offload the most diseased compartment, it may also place increased stress in other compartments (ie, lateral, patello-femoral). Second, reported results of HTO progressively worsen over time, whereas medium to long-term arthroplasty results are excellent.[4] Furthermore, some literature suggests that patients with total knee replacements do not do as well as those with high tibial osteotomies, but these findings may be historical based on post-operative rehabilitation concerns.[5]

Recently, there has been a renewed interest in HTO because of the growing number of chronologically and physiologically young patients with medial compartment disease. Arthroplasty is certainly not the ideal option as running and impact activities are not recommended following arthroplasty, but such activities are permitted following HTO. In fact, pending other concomitant knee pathologies and corrective surgeries, there are no major activity restrictions following HTO. Further, with HTO, newer techniques and instrumentation such as locking plates with variable screw angles have improved fixation and early post-operative results and patient satisfaction. HTO has also been instrumental in treating patients who previously had contraindications for meniscal and/or chondral reconstructive procedures secondary to tibiofemoral malalignment.[1]

For all of these procedures, whether performed in isolation or concurrently, proper patient selection and determining which lesion(s) is responsible for generating symptoms are crucial. As mentioned above, treating incidental lesions must be avoided.

Pathophysiology

In a knee with multiple pathologies (meniscus, instability, articular cartilage, malalignment), each entity must be considered individually with respect to its influence on the overall health of the knee. Menisectomy is a commonly performed procedure in sports medicine. It is minimally invasive and can produce satisfactory outcomes in a majority of patients, especially those desiring a quick return to activity. However, the procedure is not without risks when it comes to the long-term health of the knee. Subtotal menisectomy decreases joint contact area[6] and increases peak stress.[6] Following subtotal or total menisectomy, there is a fourteen-times increased relative risk of developing unicompartmental arthritis.[7-9] Furthermore, the literature has demonstrated worse outcomes associated with[10, 11] young age, chondral damage found at time of menisectomy, ligamentous instability,[12-14] and/or tibio-femoral malalignment. Additionally, meniscal repair as well as meniscal transplantation have worse outcomes when performed with untreated concomitant instability, malalignment, and/or articular cartilage disease[1, 15-18]

Articular cartilage injury leads to an increase in degenerative joint disease, especially when bipolar ("kissing lesions"). Full-thickness chondral injuries can be extremely problematic, causing knee swelling, night/rest pain, and severe activity-related pain. Injuries causing instability (including cruciate and collateral ligament tears) also contribute to degenerative changes of the knee,[19] although recent studies have questioned the supposed causative association between such injuries and the development of osteoarthritis.

Knee malalignment causes excessive loading of articular cartilage, which can lead to degenerative joint disease. Varus malalignment[20] leads to medial tibial cartilage volume and thickness losses, as well as increases in tibial and femoral denuded bone. The osteotomy procedure alters the biomechanical axis by shifting load away from the damaged compartment. The pathophysiologic principle of this procedure is to correct the weight-bearing axis if possible to avoid rapid and irreversible progression of uni-compartmental degenerative joint disease.[21-23] Accordingly, in the patient with isolated medial compartment disease typically associated with varus tibio-femoral malalignment, a valgus producing HTO can unload the medial compartment, possibly delaying the onset of medial compartment osteoarthritis.

Patient Presentation

Patients with such complex, combined knee pathologies will typically complain of unilateral knee pain. Often, their symptoms are chronic in nature, as it takes time for any one of these isolated injuries to have an additive affect on another. This goes to the core of the complexity of treating patients with multiple knee pathologies. Diagnosing and treating any injury occurring in isolation is usually rather straightforward, however multiple concurrent injuries tend to expedite the development of degenerative disease. As such, these patients may also present following at least one, if not more, previous (and unsuccessful) surgical interventions. Only occasionally do these types of patients present acutely following a traumatic event. Other common components of the patient presentation are outlined in Table 1.

Table 1. Common patient presentations

Symptom	Common in:
Intermittent pain ("comes and goes")	Articular cartilage injury, malalignment
Swelling, rest pain	Articular cartilage injury, malalignment
Mechanical symptoms (clicking, locking)	Meniscus injury
Joint line pain and tenderness to palpation	Meniscus, articular cartilage, ligament injury
Sensation of instability	Ligament injury, meniscus injury
Multi-ligament injury	Ligamentous injury

The history of the patient with combined knee pathologies will not be as straight-forward as that of the typical sports-medicine patient who presents with a defined traumatic twisting, pivoting, or instability event. As such, it is vital for the clinician to be suspicious for a knee with combined pathology.

Physical Examination

For any patient with combined knee pathology, a standard physical examination of both knees should be performed to compare strength, sensation, and stability of the injured knee with that of the contralateral knee. Patients with a unilateral joint effusion are likely to have cartilage pathology, although this physical examination finding is not specific. Patients with tenderness to palpation posterior to the midline of joint line are more likely to have meniscal pathology, while those with tenderness anterior to the midline of joint line may have patellofemoral or chondral pathology. Nevertheless, with combined pathology, symptoms can be difficult to differentiate. Most patients will have preserved strength and range-of-motion, unless their degenerative disease has progressed far enough to cause weakness and/or stiffness. Certain provocative tests may aid in the diagnosis of ligamentous pathology. In particular, the pivot shift, Lachman and anterior drawer tests can identify ACL injury, while the posterior drawer test can show PCL pathology and varus/valgus stress tests will identify collateral ligament damage. Anteromedial rotatory instability should be assessed with the knee in 90 degrees of flexion with the patient supine. Posterolateral rotatory instability should be assessed with the patient prone while applying external rotation to both knees in 30 and 90 degrees of flexion for side-to-side comparison.

Leg length and gait should be assessed in every patient as well, as these findings may have significant implications on surgical planning. The presence of clinical genu valgum or varum should also be assessed.

Imaging

Imaging for patients with combined knee pathologies can include radiographs, magnetic resonance imaging (MRI), and/or computed tomography (CT). A standard radiographic series can evaluate joint space, articular surfaces, and knee alignment. Standard weight-bearing anterior-posterior (AP) views are taken in extension, while posterior-anterior (PA) views are taken in 45 degrees of flexion. Other helpful views include flexion lateral and merchant views. The weight-bearing long-leg alignment films are extremely important in ruling out mechanical axis problems as a cause of patient symptoms.

MRI is useful for examining soft tissue integrity. Specific sequences can be used to identify articular cartilage, menisci, ligamentous structures, and other intra-articular structures and pathology (Figure 1). Bone marrow edema seen on MRI can be indicative of uni-compartmental overload. CT scans can be helpful as adjunctive imaging modalities, especially in the patient with prior surgery (ie, bone tunnels in previous ACL reconstruction). Other imaging modalities, including bone scans, may provide information regarding degenerative activity in the condyles/plateaus/patella.

TREATMENT OPTIONS

A variety of both non-operative and surgical techniques exist for patients with combined knee pathologies. Non-operative approaches include activity modification, rest, physical therapy, non-steroidal anti-inflammatories (NSAIDs), corticosteroid injections, hyaluronic acid injections, and more recently, platelet rich plasma therapy. While often effective at symptomatic relief, these modalities typically only provide temporary relief. Surgical management for these patients is not as straightforward as that for any of these pathologies in isolation, and particular attention must be given to surgical indications. To reiterate, treatment should be aimed at lesions which are truly responsible for a given patient's symptoms, and not those which are simply incidental in nature. This is especially important during diagnostic arthroscopy procedures, when a previously unknown cartilage injury may be detected, but may simply be an incidental finding that is not responsible for any symptoms.

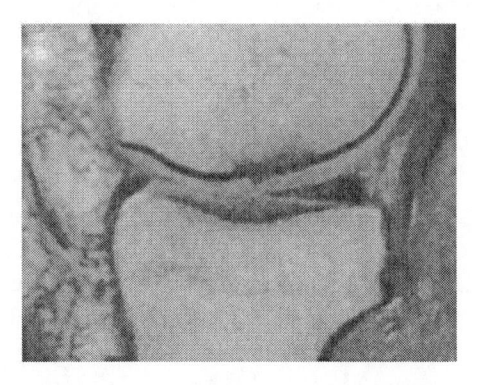

Figure 1. MRI of symptomatic cartilage leasion of femoral condyle with reactive edema in adjacent marrow.

Combined procedures will only be effective in patients with appropriate indications for surgery. Patients who are young and active are ideal for these procedures, while older less active patients may benefit more from arthroplasty. Furthermore, only patients who demonstrate an ability to tolerate and comply with rehabilitation protocols should be considered for surgery. Relative contraindications for such procedures include generalized osteoarthritis, an inability to comply with rehabilitation, unrealistic patient expectations, and obesity. Understanding patient expectations is crucial, as the patient must understand that their knee will still not be a normal knee and that activity restrictions following several of these procedures may exist.

Surgical approaches for patients with combined knee pathologies depend on the specific pathologies. Treatments may be performed in one operative setting or may be staged. The various surgical options include osteotomy (for malalignment), ligamentous repair or reconstruction (for ligament instability), articular cartilage debridement, microfracture, autologous chondrocyte implantation and osteochondral autograft/allograft transplantation (for articular cartilage disease), and meniscus debridement, repair, or transplantation (for meniscus pathology).

Malalignment

As mentioned above, high tibial osteotomy (HTO) procedures treat varus malalignment by decreasing the biomechanical load in the medial compartment of the knee. Similarly, distal femoral osteotomy procedures (DFO) treat valgus malalignment by decreasing the biomechanical load in the lateral compartment (Figure 2). Long-leg radiographs are needed in these cases to determine the required degree of correction. There are several specific indications when considering HTO in the varus malaligned knee. HTO can be helpful in treating medial compartment degenerative joint disease in traumatic, subacute, or chronic cases. HTO can also be used to treat osteochondritis dissecans refractory to non-operative therapy, as the treatment allows for unloading of the damaged medial femoral condyle. In patients with osteonecrosis/avascular necrosis, which more commonly occurs in the older patient population, arthroplasty is a more common treatment option. However, in this particular patient population, HTO may decrease pain, postpone the need for arthroplasty, and lead to regression of underlying necrosis when performed with concomitant drilling and/or bone grafting.[24] HTO can also be used in the treatment of chronic posterolateral instability, as primary stabilizing procedures may fail if there is varus malalignment leading to excessive tension on the reconstruction.[25-27] Concomitant HTO with cartilage restoration procedures has been increasing in popularity, as malalignment is a contraindication to performing such procedures in isolation. Specifically, outcomes are worse in patients with tibiofemoral malalignment undergoing chondral/meniscal reconstruction, and biomechanical and clinical studies have shown the benefits of restoring alignment prior to or concomitant with chondral/meniscal restorative procedures.[28-33] The issue of correcting alignment following failed ACL reconstruction has also received a recent increase in attention. With such patients, one must consider malalignment and thus medial compartment overload as a factor leading to failure of the initial ACL reconstruction. In these patients, correcting the weight-bearing axis with HTO prior to or during the ACL revision may be appropriate. However, it is important that the treating surgeon be experienced with these cases so as to not to disrupt the sagittal plane alignment and cause increased strain on the revision graft.

Relative contraindications to HTO include multi-compartmental degenerative disease. Even mild lateral compartment disease at the time of HTO can be detrimental to the success of the procedure. Similarly, patellofemoral compartment disease is a relative contraindication and if the HTO is the procedure of choice, it may be possible to concomitantly perform a Maquet (anterior) or Fulkerson (anteromedial) tibial tubercle osteotomy to treat the patellofemoral disease. Other relative contraindications to HTO include lateral meniscus deficiency, inflammatory arthritis (as this leads to tricompartmental degenerative joint disease), and patients unwilling to comply with the prescribed rehabilitation following HTO.

Ligamentous Instability

With regard to the patient with combined cartilage and ligament injury, ligamentous repair/reconstruction is an appropriate and often necessary surgical option. ACL and collateral ligament reconstruction are good surgical options in the appropriately indicated patient. Important considerations in the pre-operative planning for revision ACL reconstruction include planning of tunnel placement and consideration of treatment of other damaged structures. With primary and revision posterior cruciate ligament (PCL) injuries, the surgeon should be aware of the integrity of the posterolateral corner (PLC). Finally, medial collateral ligament (MCL) injuries are rarely treated operatively, but are important to consider in patients with long-term instability.

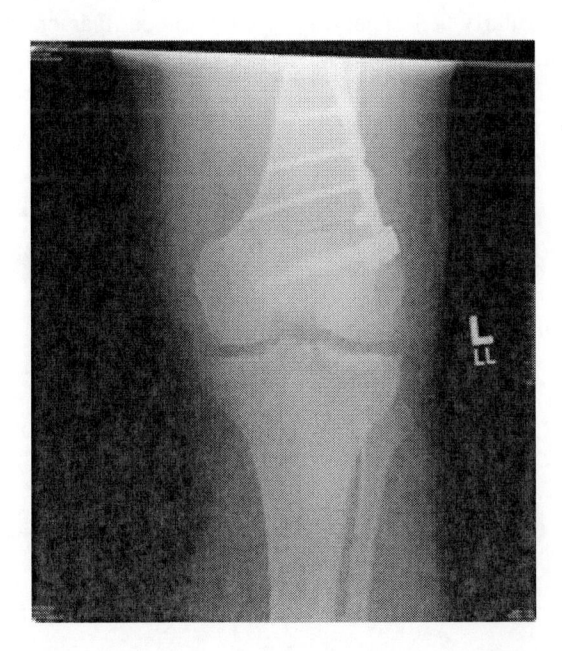

Figure 2. Radiograph illustrating post-operative findings consistent with DFO.

Articular Cartilage Disease

There are several surgical techniques for articular cartilage disease. The single most important consideration includes determining which lesions are symptomatic and which are simply incidental in nature. Operative treatment typically starts with debridement, which is considered a first-line arthroscopic approach that producing palliative results. Microfracture is a reparative procedure that is best for small (<2 cm^2) unipolar lesions. This marrow stimulating technique is highly dependent on appropriate technical execution and has over two decades of successful outcomes reported in the literature (Figure 3).[34, 35] The key to the success of this procedure is the creation of vertical walls to contain mesenchymal stem cell clot that attempts to fill in the full-thickness chondral defect with fibrocartilage. Similar in theory to microfracture are autologous chondrocyte implantation (ACI) and matrix-induced autologous chondrocyte implantation (MACI). Unlike the single-staged microfracture procedure, ACI/MACI is a reparative two-stage procedure best used for large condylar lesions (>4 cm^2) or patellar lesions without significant bony involvement (Figure 4). This technique utilizes the patient's own articular cartilage cells to fill in full-thickness cartilage defects with hyaline/fibrocartilage secured down with a periosteal flap and can be particularly useful in the patellofemoral joint. For medium-sized articular cartilage lesions, (2-4cm^2) reconstructive procedures such as osteochondral autograft transfer (OATS) and osteochondral allograft transplantation are useful. The OATS procedure is typically used on medium-sized lesions that can be treated with one or two donor site plugs taken from the non-weight-bearing region of the ipsilateral knee and transferred to the damaged area. With osteochondral allograft transplantation, donor plugs are utilized instead of those from the patient's own knee. This can be particularly beneficial during a combined ligament or meniscus procedure, as autograft transfer may add further insult to the knee. This technique is best for medium-sized lesions (greater than 1-2 cm) or those that are uncontained or associated with significant bony loss in addition to the chondral disease (Figure 5).

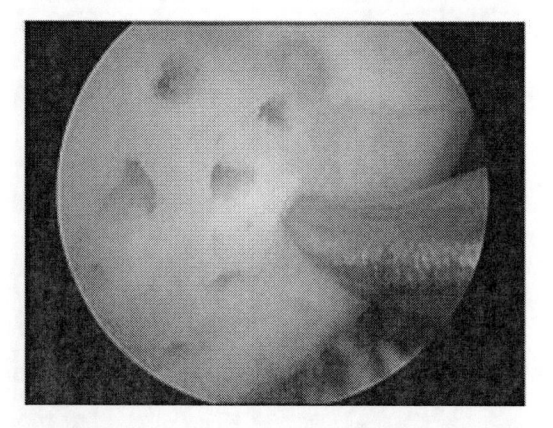

Figure 3. Arthroscopic image illustrating microfracture to femoral condyle articular cartilage lesion.

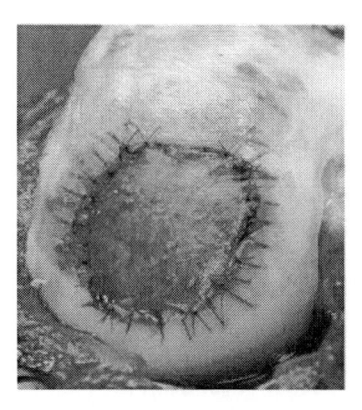

Figure 4. Intra-operative image demonstrating femoral condyle articular cartilage lesion after ACI implantation with patch.

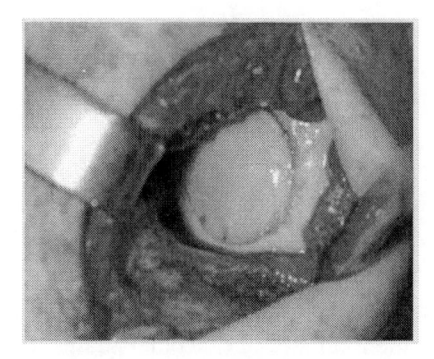

Figure 5. Intra-operative image illustrating OATS to femoral condyle articular cartilage lesion.

Meniscus Pathology

Treatment options for meniscal pathology include debridement, repair, and transplantation. Repair techniques are useful for tears in the peripheral one-third of the meniscus and include outside-in, inside-out, and all-inside techniques. Meniscus allograft transplantation is an invasive technique useful for patients with previous meniscectomies. A variety of transplantation techniques have been described, including the bridge-in-slot technique, bone-plug technique, dovetail technique, and free-end technique.

Role for Combined Procedures

Recent studies have shown that patients with uncorrected varus malalignment do not achieve optimal outcomes with cartilage restorative procedures.[36, 37] For example, HTO performed with a medial meniscus transplant has the potential to both unload the compartment and potentially improve the outcome of a transplant in a varus knee[1, 17, 23, 38-42] Furthermore, biomechanical evidence from Van Thiel *et al*[22] has demonstrated the mechanical benefits of performing HTO with meniscus transplantation. These procedures performed in isolation in the presence of tibiofemoral malalignment may have worse outcomes and higher failure rates due to mechanical overload of the repaired tissue. Alignment correcting procedures such as HTO may unload the damaged compartment enough to allow healing and protect the cartilage and/or meniscal restorative procedure being performed

OUTCOMES

When performed individually for isolated pathology, there are numerous reports of good to excellent outcomes for the procedures mentioned above: osteotomies for malalignment,[3, 43-48] ACL reconstruction for instability,[12, 13, 19, 49, 50] cartilage restoration for chondral disease,[51-53] and meniscus repair/transplantation for meniscal disease.[15-17, 54-57]

In the setting of treatment for combined pathologies, the reported outcomes are not as consistent. As the number of problems in the knee increase, the outcomes are generally diminished irrespective of the treatment employed. Central to the complexity of these clinical challenges is that each of these conditions are essentially interrelated.[58] Chondral disease can be caused by malalignment, which leads to excessive stress on articular cartilage and meniscal pathology.

If the patient has underlying malalignment in the setting of a new cartilage or meniscus injury, it is possible to address the pathology in either a staged fashion or all at once. With regard to instability, however, the clinical situation becomes more complicated. For example, ACL reconstruction does worse if there is concomitant meniscal injury and meniscal repair is not performed or if there is meniscal deficiency in revision settings.

Currently, there are a limited number of outcome studies for combined procedures and it is difficult to draw definitive conclusions based on the short and long-term studies that are available. Gomoll et al[1] reported on seven patients with concomitant meniscus transplantation, chondral repair, and osteotomy. In this clinical study, 6/7 patients returned to unrestricted activities and all experienced significant increases in KOOS, IKDC, and Lysholm scores at 24 months post-operatively. Cameron et al[54] recently reported on 67 patients undergoing meniscus transplantation with/without concomitant procedures in 63 patients. At 31 months post-operatively, 58 (87%) knees had good to excellent results. Of note, in 21 knees with isolated meniscal transplantations, 91% had good to excellent outcomes. In five knees undergoing concomitant ACL reconstruction, 80% had good to excellent outcomes. In 34 knees undergoing concurrent osteotomy, 85% had good to excellent outcomes. Finally, in seven knees undergoing concomitant osteotomy and ACL reconstruction, 86% had good to excellent outcomes. Farr et al[59] reported on 36 patients undergoing concurrent meniscus transplantation and ACI. Of the 29 available for follow-up, 16 had additional concurrent procedures, including tibial tubercle osteotomy, ACL reconstruction, and/or HTO. The authors found significant improvements in outcome surveys, visual analog pain scales, and patient satisfaction with no differences found between subgroups. Within two years post-operatively, the authors reported four failures that went onto revision procedures. Rue et al[18] reported on 31 knees with combined meniscus transplantation and cartilage restoration. Fifty-two percent underwent concomitant ACI while 48% underwent osteochondral allograft. At 3.1 years post-operatively, 76% (80% ACI, 71% osteochondral allograft) were satisfied with their outcomes and showed statistically significant improvements in Lysholm and IKDC scores. There were no significant differences found between groups. Verdonk et al[42] reviewed 27 patients undergiong medial meniscal transplantation and found that patients that also underwent HTO had significantly greater improvements in pain and functional scores compared to those that had isolated transplants. Of note, the 10-year survival rates were 83.3% for the group with a combined transplant and osteotomy versus 74.2% for the medial transplant only group.

CONCLUSION

Treatment of combined knee pathology is a challenging problem. The inter-relationship between malalignment, meniscus pathology, articular cartilage disease, and instability results in complex clinical scenarios. For successful operative management of these patients, proper patient selection is critical. Determining the cause of symptoms (predominantly pain) can be especially difficult in knees with multiple pathologies and treating incidental lesions must be avoided. Current biomechanical and clinical studies suggest a role for combined surgical procedures (either single or staged), but further long-term studies are needed to determine if these results stand over time.

REFERENCES

[1] Gomoll, A. H., Kang, R. W., Chen, A. L., Cole, B. J. Triad of cartilage restoration for unicompartmental arthritis treatment in young patients: meniscus allograft transplantation, cartilage repair and osteotomy. *J. Knee Surg.* Apr. 2009;22(2):137-141.

[2] Anbari, A. Proximal Tibial and Distal Femoral Osteotomy. In: Cole B, Gomoll A, eds. Biologic Joint Reconstruction: Alternatives to Arthroplasty. *Thorofare*: SLACK Inc; 2009.

[3] Wright, J. M., Crockett, H. C., Slawski, D. P., Madsen, M. W., Windsor, RE. . High tibial osteotomy. *J. Am. Acad. Orthop. Surg.* Jul.-Aug. 2005;13(4):279-289.

[4] Morgan, M. C., Gillespie, B., Dedrick, D. Survivorship analysis of total knee arthroplasty. Cumulative rates of survival of 9200 total knee arthroplasties. *J. Bone Joint Surg. Am.* Feb. 1992;74(2):308-309.

[5] Meding, J. B., Wing, J. T., Ritter, M. A. Does high tibial osteotomy affect the success or survival of a total knee replacement? *Clin. Orthop. Relat. Res.* Jul. 2011;469(7):1991-1994.

[6] Lee, S. J., Aadalen, K. J., Malaviya, P., et al. Tibiofemoral contact mechanics after serial medial meniscectomies in the human cadaveric knee. *Am. J. Sports Med.* Aug. 2006;34(8):1334-1344.

[7] McNicholas, M. J., Rowley, D. I., McGurty, D., et al. Total meniscectomy in adolescence. A thirty-year follow-up. *J. Bone Joint Surg. Br.* Mar. 2000;82(2):217-221.

[8] Roos, E. M., Ostenberg, A., Roos, H., Ekdahl, C., Lohmander, L. S. Long-term outcome of meniscectomy: symptoms, function, and performance tests in patients with or without radiographic osteoarthritis compared to matched controls. *Osteoarthritis Cartilage.* May 2001;9(4):316-324.

[9] Roos, H., Lauren, M., Adalberth, T., Roos, E. M., Jonsson, K., Lohmander, L. S. Knee osteoarthritis after meniscectomy: prevalence of radiographic changes after twenty-one years, compared with matched controls. *Arthritis Rheum.* Apr. 1998;41(4):687-693.

[10] Burks, R. T., Metcalf, M. H., Metcalf, R. W. Fifteen-year follow-up of arthroscopic partial meniscectomy. *Arthroscopy.* Dec. 1997;13(6):673-679.

[11] Maletius, W., Messner, K. The effect of partial meniscectomy on the long-term prognosis of knees with localized, severe chondral damage. A twelve- to fifteen-year followup. *Am. J. Sports Med.* May-Jun. 1996;24(3):258-262.

[12] Hart, A. J., Buscombe, J., Malone, A., Dowd, G. S. Assessment of osteoarthritis after reconstruction of the anterior cruciate ligament: a study using single-photon emission computed tomography at ten years. *J. Bone Joint Surg. Br.* Nov. 2005;87(11):1483-1487.

[13] Ruiz, A. L., Kelly, M., Nutton, R. W. Arthroscopic ACL reconstruction: a 5-9 year follow-up. *Knee.* Sep. 2002;9(3):197-200.

[14] Shirazi, R., Shirazi-Adl, A. Analysis of partial meniscectomy and ACL reconstruction in knee joint biomechanics under a combined loading. *Clin. Biomech.* (Bristol, Avon). Nov. 2009;24(9):755-761.

[15] Kang, R. W., Lattermann, C., Cole, B. J. Allograft meniscus transplantation: background, indications, techniques, and outcomes. *J. Knee Surg.* Jul. 2006;19(3):220-230.

[16] Noyes, F. R., Barber-Westin, S. D. Meniscus transplantation: indications, techniques, clinical outcomes. *Instr. Course Lect.* 2005;54:341-353.

[17] Packer, J. D., Rodeo, S. A. Meniscal allograft transplantation. *Clin. Sports Med.* Apr. 2009;28(2):259-283, viii.

[18] Rue, J. P., Yanke, A. B., Busam, M. L., McNickle, A. G., Cole, B. J. Prospective evaluation of concurrent meniscus transplantation and articular cartilage repair: minimum 2-year follow-up. *Am. J. Sports Med.* Sep. 2008;36(9):1770-1778.

[19] Louboutin, H., Debarge, R., Richou, J., et al. Osteoarthritis in patients with anterior cruciate ligament rupture: a review of risk factors. *Knee.* Aug. 2009;16(4):239-244.

[20] Sharma, L., Eckstein, F., Song, J., et al. Relationship of meniscal damage, meniscal extrusion, malalignment, and joint laxity to subsequent cartilage loss in osteoarthritic knees. *Arthritis Rheum.* Jun. 2008;58(6):1716-1726.

[21] Sharma, L., Song, J., Felson, D. T., Cahue, S., Shamiyeh, E., Dunlop, D. D. The role of knee alignment in disease progression and functional decline in knee osteoarthritis. *JAMA.* Jul. 11 2001;286(2):188-195.

[22] Van Thiel, G., Frank, R., Gupta, A., et al. Biomechanical Evaluation of a High Tibial Ostetomy with a Meniscal Transplant. *8th World Congress of the International Cartilage Repair Society.* Miami, FL; 2009.

[23] Verdonk, P. C., Demurie, A., Almqvist, K. F., Veys, E. M., Verbruggen, G., Verdonk, R. Transplantation of viable meniscal allograft. Survivorship analysis and clinical outcome of one hundred cases. *J. Bone Joint Surg. Am.* Apr. 2005;87(4):715-724.

[24] Koshino, T. The treatment of spontaneous osteonecrosis of the knee by high tibial osteotomy with and without bone-grafting or drilling of the lesion. *J. Bone Joint Surg. Am.* Jan. 1982;64(1):47-58.

[25] Cooper, D. Treatment of Combined posterior cruciate ligament and posterolateral injuries of the knee. *Oper. Tech. Sports Med.* 1999;7:135-142.

[26] Fanelli, G., Monahan, T. Complications in posterior cruciate ligament and posterolateral corner surgery. *Oper. Tech. Sports Med.* 2001;9:96-99.

[27] MacGillivray, J., Warren, R. Treatment of acute and chronic injuries to the posterolateral and lateral knee. *Operative Techniques in Orthopaedics.* 1999;9:309-317.

[28] Van Thiel, G. S., Frank, R. M., Gupta, A., et al. Biomechanical evaluation of a high tibial osteotomy with a meniscal transplant. *J. Knee Surg.* Mar. 2011;24(1):45-53.

[29] Verma, N. N., Kolb, E., Cole, B. J., et al. The effects of medial meniscal transplantation techniques on intra-articular contact pressures. *J. Knee Surg.* Jan. 2008;21(1):20-26.

[30] Gallo, R. A., Feeley, B. T. Cartilage defects of the femoral trochlea. *Knee Surg. Sports Traumatol. Arthrosc.* Nov. 2009;17(11):1316-1325.

[31] Sterett, W. I., Steadman, J. R. Chondral resurfacing and high tibial osteotomy in the varus knee. *Am. J. Sports Med.* Jul.-Aug. 2004;32(5):1243-1249.

[32] Willey, M., Wolf, B. R., Kocaglu, B., Amendola, A. Complications associated with realignment osteotomy of the knee performed simultaneously with additional reconstructive procedures. *Iowa Orthop. J.* 2011;30:55-60.

[33] Sterett, W. I., Steadman, J. R., Huang, M. J., Matheny, L. M., Briggs, K. K. Chondral resurfacing and high tibial osteotomy in the varus knee: survivorship analysis. *Am. J. Sports Med.* Jul. 2010;38(7):1420-1424.

[34] Steadman, J. R., Miller, B. S., Karas, S. G., Schlegel, T. F., Briggs, K. K. Hawkins, R. J. The microfracture technique in the treatment of full-thickness chondral lesions of the knee in National Football League players. *J. Knee Surg.* Apr. 2003;16(2):83-86.

[35] Steadman, J. R., Rodkey, W. G., Briggs, K. K. Microfracture to treat full-thickness chondral defects: surgical technique, rehabilitation, and outcomes. *J. Knee Surg.* Summer 2002;15(3):170-176.

[36] Minas, T. The role of cartilage repair techniques, including chondrocyte transplantation, in focal chondral knee damage. *Instr. Course Lect.* 1999;48:629-643.

[37] Minas, T. Autologous chondrocyte implantation in the arthritic knee. *Orthopedics.* Sep. 2003;26(9):945-947.

[38] Garrett, J. C. Meniscal transplantation. *Am. J. Knee Surg.* Winter 1996;9(1):32-34.

[39] Peters, G., Wirth, C. J. The current state of meniscal allograft transplantation and replacement. *Knee.* Mar. 2003;10(1):19-31.

[40] Bonasia, D. E., Amendola, A. Combined medial meniscal transplantation and high tibial osteotomy. *Knee Surg. Sports Traumatol. Arthrosc.* Jul. 2010;18(7):870-873.

[41] Noyes, F. R., Barber-Westin, S. D., Hewett, T. E. High tibial osteotomy and ligament reconstruction for varus angulated anterior cruciate ligament-deficient knees. *Am. J. Sports Med.* May-Jun. 2000;28(3):282-296.

[42] Verdonk, P. C., Verstraete, K. L., Almqvist, K. F., et al. Meniscal allograft transplantation: long-term clinical results with radiological and magnetic resonance imaging correlations. *Knee Surg. Sports Traumatol. Arthrosc.* Aug. 2006;14(8):694-706.

[43] Coventry, M. B. Upper tibial osteotomy for osteoarthritis. *J. Bone Joint Surg. Am.* Sep. 1985;67(7):1136-1140.

[44] Coventry, M. B., Ilstrup, D. M., Wallrichs, S. L. Proximal tibial osteotomy. A critical long-term study of eighty-seven cases. *J. Bone Joint Surg. Am.* Feb. 1993;75(2):196-201.

[45] Gardiner, A., Gutierrez Sevilla, G. R., Steiner, M. E., Richmond, J. C. Osteotomies about the knee for tibiofemoral malalignment in the athletic patient. *Am. J. Sports Med.* May 2010;38(5):1038-1047.

[46] Preston, C. F., Fulkerson, E. W., Meislin, R., Di Cesare, P. E. Osteotomy about the knee: applications, techniques, and results. *J. Knee Surg.* Oct. 2005;18(4):258-272.

[47] Wolcott, M. Osteotomies around the knee for the young athlete with osteoarthritis. *Clin. Sports Med.* Jan. 2005;24(1):153-161.

[48] Wolcott, M., Traub, S., Efird, C. High tibial osteotomies in the young active patient. *Int. Orthop.* Feb. 2010;34(2):161-166.

[49] Asano, H., Muneta, T., Ikeda, H., Yagishita, K., Kurihara, Y., Sekiya, I. Arthroscopic evaluation of the articular cartilage after anterior cruciate ligament reconstruction: a short-term prospective study of 105 patients. *Arthroscopy.* May 2004;20(5):474-481.

[50] Kessler, M. A., Behrend, H., Henz, S., Stutz, G., Rukavina, A., Kuster, M. S. Function, osteoarthritis and activity after ACL-rupture: 11 years follow-up results of conservative versus reconstructive treatment. *Knee Surg. Sports Traumatol. Arthrosc.* May 2008;16(5):442-448.

[51] Alford, J. W., Cole, B. J. Cartilage restoration, part 2: techniques, outcomes, and future directions. *Am. J. Sports Med.* Mar. 2005;33(3):443-460.

[52] Alford, J. W., Cole, B. J. Cartilage restoration, part 1: basic science, historical perspective, patient evaluation, and treatment options. *Am. J. Sports Med.* Feb. 2005;33(2):295-306.

[53] Buckwalter, J. A., Mankin, H. J. Articular cartilage: degeneration and osteoarthritis, repair, regeneration, and transplantation. *Instr. Course Lect.* 1998;47:487-504.

[54] Cameron, J. C., Saha, S. Meniscal allograft transplantation for unicompartmental arthritis of the knee. *Clin. Orthop. Relat. Res.* Apr. 1997(337):164-171.

[55] Cole, B. J., Carter, T. R., Rodeo, S. A. Allograft meniscal transplantation: background, techniques, and results. *Instr. Course Lect.* 2003;52:383-396.

[56] Hergan, D., Thut, D., Sherman, O., Day, M. S. Meniscal Allograft Transplantation. *Arthroscopy.* Sep. 28 2010.

[57] Noyes, F. R., Barber-Westin, S. D., Rankin, M. Meniscal transplantation in symptomatic patients less than fifty years old. *J. Bone Joint Surg. Am.* Jul. 2004;86-A(7):1392-1404.

[58] Cole, B. J., Harner, C. D. Degenerative arthritis of the knee in active patients: evaluation and management. *J. Am. Acad. Orthop. Surg.* Nov.-Dec. 1999;7(6):389-402.

[59] Farr, J., Rawal, A., Marberry, K. M. Concomitant meniscal allograft transplantation and autologous chondrocyte implantation: minimum 2-year follow-up. *Am. J. Sports Med.* Sep. 2007;35(9):1459-1466.

In: The Knee
Editor: Randy Mascarenhas

ISBN: 978-1-61942-268-1
© 2012 Nova Science Publishers, Inc.

Chapter XII

TRANSPHYSEAL ANTERIOR CRUCIATE LIGAMENT RECONSTRUCTION IN THE SKELETALLY IMMATURE ATHLETE

R. Mascarenhas, J. D. Dillon and P. MacDonald

Pan Am Clinic, Section of Orthopaedic Surgery,
University of Manitoba, Winnipeg, Canada

ABSTRACT

Background: The surgical management of ACL rupture in the teenage athlete with open physes remains controversial. The purpose of this study was to evaluate the functional and radiographic outcome of transphyseal ACL reconstruction with medial hamstring autograft in skeletally immature patients with open physes.

Hypothesis: Transphyseal ACL reconstruction with hamstring autograft can yield satisfactory clinical and functional outcomes with a low incidence of clinically significant leg length discrepancy or malalignment.

Study Design: Case Series

Methods: ACL reconstruction involved drilling tunnels through the tibial and femoral physes and placing a hamstring graft. Follow-up evaluation included objective clinical data (ROM and laxity testing), imaging (scanograms to assess for limb length discrepancies and MRI to assess for bony bar formation), and subjective patient-reported data (IKDC and ACL QOL forms).

Results: Seventeen patients were reviewed at an average clinical follow-up of 8.2 years after surgery (range 5-9 years). No patients had significant leg-length discrepancies or bony bar formation. Subjective results showed an average ACL QOL score of 73.2 (range 37-100) and 88.2% of patients had normal or nearly normal knees as per the IKDC survey. Fifteen out of seventeen patients (88.2%) returned to competitive sports after surgery.

Conclusions: Transphyseal ACL reconstruction with semitendinosus/ gracilis autograft was performed successfully in seventeen skeletally immature adolescents with clearly open growth plates with little apparent risk for growth disturbance.

Keywords: Anterior Cruciate Ligament, Skeletally Immature, Athlete, Transphyseal

INTRODUCTION

Anterior Cruciate Ligament (ACL) ruptures in skeletally immature athletes are not uncommon injuries and the management of such injuries remains a topic of debate[1]. The incidence of ACL tears in teens participating in high-risk sports such as soccer, basketball, and football ranges from 1% to 3.4 % [2]. Non-operative treatment has been advocated in the past to avoid growth disturbances, but the outcomes of such treatment have generally been poor [1]. Young athletes tend to continue participation in sport, which leads to recurrent episodes of knee instability in the affected leg and an increased incidence of new meniscal and chondral injury [3]. While ACL reconstruction may prevent the development of further insult to the skeletally immature knee, ideal surgical technique and timing of surgery in patients with open physes remains controversial. Neither extra-articular reconstruction [4] or primary repair of the ACL have been proven to consistently restore knee stability [5].

The purpose of this study was to evaluate patient outcomes following transphyseal ACL reconstruction with medial hamstring autograft in skeletally immature athletes with open physes. This technique offers an anatomic reconstruction with fixation distant from the physis and a graft consisting only of soft tissue traversing the physis. The incidence of growth disturbances in this patient populations was also investigated and we hypothesized that transphyseal ACL reconstruction with hamstring autograft would yield acceptable objective and subjective clinical outcomes with a low incidence of post-operative growth disturbance.

MATERIALS AND METHODS

Inclusion/Exclusion Criteria

Inclusion criteria were patients who had sustained an ACL injury during their main sport of participation and had wide-open physes on radiographs before undergoing tibial and femoral transphsyeal ACL reconstruction with hamstring autograft. Exclusion criteria were previous surgery and/or documented injury to the affected knee. Skeletal maturity was determined by AP and lateral radiographs of the affected knee where wide open physes were defined as complete radiolucency at the distal femur, proximal tibia, and tibial tubercle [6,7].

Pre-Operative Assessment

All patients had undergone a pre-operative history and physical exam that included measurement of active and passive knee ROM and laxity testing. Pre-operative imaging included standing AP, lateral, and patellar view radiographs and magnetic resonance imaging (MRI) to confirm the diagnosis of ACL rupture and identify other associated injuries.

Post-Operative Assessment

All patients were followed up at a minimum of five years post-surgery. Subjective patient reported outcomes were assessed with the International Knee Documentation Committee (IKDC) subjective knee score [8] and ACL Quality of Life (ACL QOL) forms [9]. Objective outcomes were measured via physical exam with Lachman and Pivot Shift testing, as well as range of motion of the affected knee. Post-operative scanograms were obtained to look for limb length discrepancies and magnetic resonance imaging was done to assess for bony bar formation.

Surgical Technique

All surgeries were performed by the senior author. The surgical procedure was performed under general anesthesia with the patient supine on the operating table and a tourniquet around the proximal thigh on the affected leg. A thorough examination under anesthesia was performed before beginning the operation. An incision was made over the proximal medial tibia with dissection carried down through subcutaneous tissue and sartorius fascia until the gracilis and semitendinosus tendons were reached. The tendons were then dissected out distally and cleared of any adhesions proximally before being harvested with a tendon-stripper. The ACL graft was prepared in a standard fashion and placed over an Endobutton (Smith and Nephew Endoscopy, Andover, Massachusetts). Standard arthroscopic anterolateral and anteromedial portal were next utilized to perform a diagnostic arthroscopy of the affected knee. Meniscal and/or chondral injuries were managed if present and requiring treatment. The intercondylar notch was visualized and the stump of the ACL was debrided if still present. The notch width was assessed and a notchplasty performed if necessary. A tibial tunnel was placed in the posterior aspect of the footprint of ACL with use of a tibial guide at 55 degrees and the tibial tunnel was reamed according to the diameter of the graft. A transtibial femoral offset guide was positioned and a guidewire was placed and overreamed to create the femoral tunnel. The depth of the femoral tunnel was measured with a depth gauge, and the guidewire was replaced to allow reaming of the femoral tunnel to the appropriate depth. The graft was then brought through the tibial tunnel across the joint and through the femoral tunnel. The Endobutton (Smith and Nephew Endoscopy, Andover, Massachusetts) was then flipped and tension was applied to the graft to assess its stability after which the knee was extended fully to assess notch impingement. The knee was cycled and the tibial fixation was performed with a bioabsorbable interference screw with tension on the graft with the knee at 30 degrees of flexion. The stability of the graft was then checked prior to the end of the procedure.

Post-Operative Rehabilitation

The patient was allowed to be weight-bearing as tolerated with a hinged knee brace set at 0 to 90 degrees of flexion. Mobilization from full extension to 90 degrees began immediately post-operatively and was progressed to full range of motion after two weeks. If a meniscal repair was performed at the time of ACL reconstruction, toe-touch weight-bearing was allowed for four to six weeks and progression to full range of motion was delayed until six weeks postoperatively. Progressive rehabilitation including range of motion and closed-chain strengthening was then begun and eventually led to jogging and sport specific exercises at three months post-operatively. Return to full activity, including cutting sports, was usually allowed at six months post-operatively. A knee brace was prescribed to all patients to use during cutting and pivoting activities for the first six months after return to sports.

RESULTS

Seventeen patients (eleven females and six males) were available for review. The mean age at the time of surgery was 15.5 years (range 14-16 years). The average interval time from injury to surgery was 5.75 months (0.75-12 months). The average length of follow-up was 8.2 years (range 5-9 years). The primary sports of participation of the patients can be seen in table 1. All patients had complete radiolucency of the distal femoral and proximal tibial physes. A quadruple-stranded hamstring transphyseal technique utilizing semitendinosus and gracilis tendons was used in all cases. Endobutton femoral fixation and tibial fixation with a bioabsorbable screw were used in all cases. Meniscal tears were found in 64.7% of patients (11/17) with seven tears (63.6%) of the medial meniscus, three tears (27.2%) of the lateral meniscus, and one case (9.1%) with bilateral tears. Two out of the twelve tears (both lateral menisci) were deemed stable and no surgical intervention was deemed necessary, while ten tears were repaired at the time of ACL reconstruction.

Changes in pre- and post-operative Lachman and Pivot Shift results are shown in Figures 1 and 2, respectively. Pre-operatively, 88.2% (15/17) of patients had a 2+ Lachman and 11.8% (2/17) had a 1+ Lachman. Similarly, the pre-operative Pivot shift was also 2+ in 88.2% (15/17) of patients and one patient had a 1+ Pivot Shift (11.8%). Post-operatively, 35.3% of patients (6/17) had a 1+ Lachman and the remaining 64.7% of patients (11/17) had a negative Lachman. Post-operatively, 17.6% (3/17) of patients had a 1+ Pivot shift compared to fourteen out of seventeen patients (82.4%) that had a negative Pivot Shift. In terms of range of motion, no significant differences were seen in hyperextension or mean maximum flexion between the ACL-reconstructed knee and the contralateral knee. IKDC scoring revealed 12/17 normal (70.6%), 3/17 near normal (17.6%) and 2/17 (11.8%) abnormal knees. ACL QOL scores averaged 73.2% post-operatively (Range 37-100). A successful return to pre-injury activity levels was achieved by 88.2% (15/17) of patients.

Table 1. Primary Sport at Time of Injury

Sport	Patients
Soccer	5
Basketball	4
Ice Hockey	4
Football	2
Ballet	1
Speed Skating	1

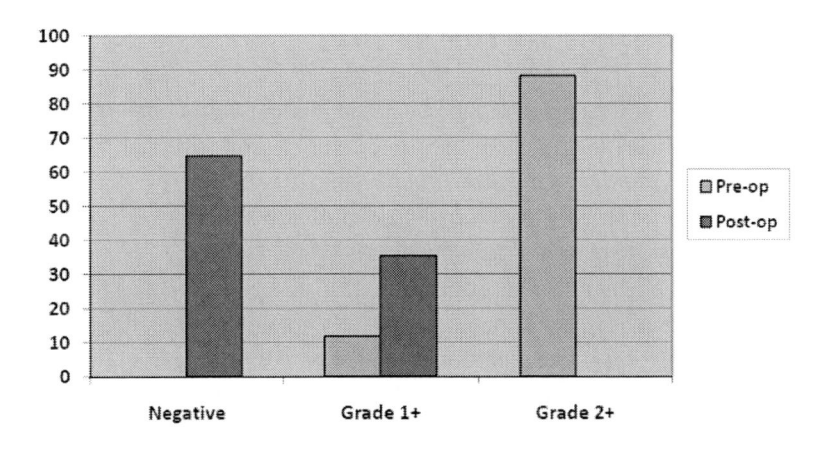

Figure 1. Lachman Laxity Grading Pre- and Post-operatively.

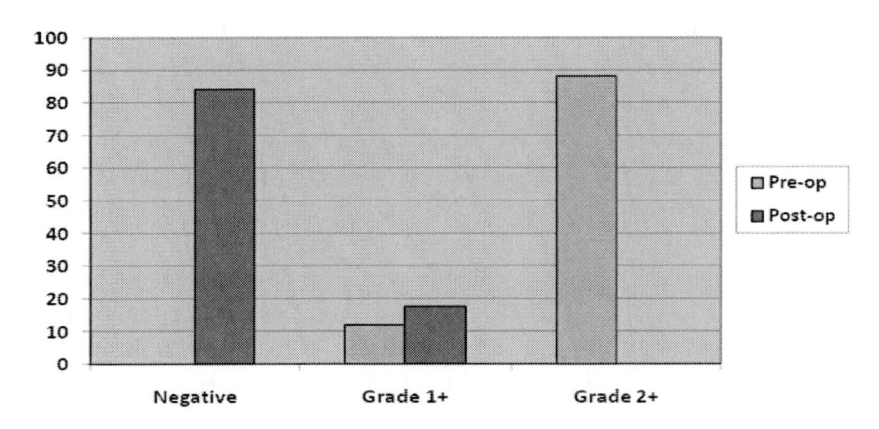

Figure 2. Pivot Shift Grading Pre- and Post-operatively.

Radiographs at final follow-up showed no growth plate disturbances, angular deformities, or joint space narrowing in any of the patients. No significant side-to-side differences were observed on the scanograms on review. Post-operative radiological evaluation revealed that growth plates were closed in all patients at the time of latest follow-up. Post-operative MRI did not show any evidence of bony bar formation.

There were no infections, deep vein thromboses, or neurovascular injuries encountered in this patient population. Additionally, no patients sustained disruption of their ACL graft. Five patients (29.4%) required subsequent surgical procedures to the affected knee. One patient developed arthrofibrosis and required manipulation of the affected knee under anesthesia at three months post-operatively and had no further complications. Another patient required debridement of a Cyclops lesion six years after the initial surgery and also had no further complications. One patient had failure of their medial meniscal repair requiring a repeat repair two years after the initial surgery and suffered no further complications. Two patients who underwent meniscal repair at the time of surgery (one lateral and one medial) required partial meniscectomies six years after the initial surgery. They had no further complications.

DISCUSSION

While transphyseal ACL reconstruction in the patient with open physes has gained significant popularity in the last decade, the topic remains controversial. Some surgeons are still proponents of delaying ligament reconstruction until skeletal maturity to decrease the risk of growth disturbance, attributing most growth disturbances following ACL reconstruction surgery to bone or hardware placed across the physis [10,11].

Non-operative management may be recommended in order to delay reconstruction until skeletal maturity is reached, and may consist of bracing, physiotherapy, and activity modification [12]. This form of treatment may be successful in young children or in patients with partial tears [13], but non-operative management of complete ACL ruptures has been shown to result in poor outcomes due to recurrent instability leading to further meniscal and chondral injury [1,3]. Data from several authors [14,15] has suggested that although skeletally immature patients have a relatively high rate of meniscal injury at the time of ACL disruption, meniscal tears can also occur in the time interval between the initial injury and ACL reconstruction despite patient counseling on activity restrictions [6]. These meniscal injuries and the chondral damage associated with them can have important implications in the long-term prognosis of the knee and the risk of future degenerative joint disease [13].

Surgical procedures used to treat ACL rupture in patients with open growth plates have included primary ligament repair, extra-articular tenodesis, physeal sparing reconstruction, partial transphyseal reconstruction, and transphyseal reconstruction [13]. Primary repair of the ACL [16] and extra-articular tenodesis alone [3,4] have had poor results in both children and adults. A number of physeal sparing procedures have been described to avoid drilling tunnels across open physes [5,15,17], while partial transphyseal reconstructions violate only the proximal tibial physis [18,19]. Finally, transphyseal reconstructions with tunnels that cross both the distal femoral and the proximal tibial physes have been performed with a variety of soft tissue grafts [6,7,13,20,21].

Several animal studies have investigated the risk of growth plate disturbances following drilling and placement of soft tissue grafts across open physes. Stadelmaier et al. [22] showed no relative change in growth plate function after intra-articular ACL reconstruction using a fascia lata autograft in skeletally immature dogs, while Edwards and colleagues [23] found significant valgus deformities of the femur and varus deformities of the tibia using a similar technique in dogs. Additionally, studies by Guzzanti et al. [24] and Houle and colleagues [25] reported growth disturbances after tensioning of a tendon graft in a bone tunnel across rabbit physes. Studies such as these indicate the concern for potential growth plate disturbance with ACL reconstruction, but results in human studies have been encouraging.

Within the last decade, many authors have presented excellent results with no growth disturbances or angular deformities seen after drilling tunnels across both the tibial and femoral physes in patients with open growth plates undergoing ACL reconstruction [6,7,13,20,21]. Our results match these and lend more evidence to the growing body of knowledge that suggests that transphyseal ACL reconstruction is a safe treatment option in the patient with open growth plates.

This investigation has several limitations. The authors recognize the fact that several similar studies are present in the literature, but feel that our study is also important as multiple studies all showing similar positive results are required to lend supporting evidence to proposed surgical interventions. Our study did not have any statistics performed as it was a retrospective observational study, lacking pre-operative outcome scores. The relatively small sample size in this study imparts low statistical power, and its retrospective nature did not allow for standardization of preoperative data collection.

The mean ACL quality of life outcome scores may have been skewed as there was one main outlier with a score of 37/ 100, which was much lower than the remainder of the patient population. This patient had bilateral meniscal tears which were repaired at the time of ACL reconstruction, and was one of the two patients who failed to return to athletic activity. The patient also went on to have a partial meniscectomy six years after the original surgery.

Additionally, skeletal maturity was assessed only with radiographs without assessment of physiologic maturity. While all patients were skeletally immature on radiographs, the average age of our patient population was 15.5 years of age. This suggests that our patient population may have been closer to skeletal maturity than younger patient populations described in other studies. Other weaknesses include the fact that pre-operative leg lengths were not measured and also there was no control group treated with another type of ACL reconstruction technique for comparison.

CONCLUSION

In conclusion, transphyseal ACL reconstruction with semitendinosus/ gracilis autograft was performed successfully in seventeen skeletally immature adolescents with clearly open growth plates with little apparent risk for growth disturbance. On the basis of our findings, we believe that transphyseal reconstruction of the anterior cruciate ligament with use of an autogenous quadrupled hamstrings-tendon graft is a reasonable treatment option for skeletally immature patients with open growth plates.

REFERENCES

[1]   Aichroth, P. M., Patel, D. V., Zorrilla, P. The natural history and treatment of rupture of the anterior cruciate ligament in children and adolescents. A prospective review. *J. Bone Joint Surg. Br.* 2002 Jan.;84(1):38-41.

[2]   Johnston, D. R., Ganley, T. J., Flynn, J. M., Gregg, J. R. Anterior cruciate ligament injuries in skeletally immature patients. *Orthopedics.* 2002 Aug.;25(8):864-71.

[3]   McCarroll, J. R., Rettig, A. C., Shelbourne, K. D. Anterior cruciate ligament injuries in the young athlete with open physes. *Am. J. Sports Med.* 1988 Jan.-Feb.;16(1):44-7.

[4]   Graf, B. K., Lange, R. H., Fujisaki, C. K., Landry, G. L., Saluja, R. K. Anterior cruciate ligament tears in skeletally immature patients: meniscal pathology at presentation and after attempted conservative treatment. *Arthroscopy.* 1992;8(2):229-33.

[5]   DeLee, J. C., Curtis, R. Anterior cruciate ligament insufficiency in children. *Clin. Orthop. Relat. Res.* 1983 Jan.-Feb.;(172):112-8.

[6]   McIntosh, A. L., Dahm, D. L., Stuart, M. J. Anterior cruciate ligament reconstruction in the skeletally immature patient. *Arthroscopy.* 2006 Dec.;22(12):1325-30.

[7] Shelbourne, K. D., Gray, T., Wiley, B. V. Results of transphyseal anterior cruciate ligament reconstruction using patellar tendon autograft in tanner stage 3 or 4 adolescents with clearly open growth plates. *Am. J. Sports Med.* 2004 Jul.-Aug.;32(5):1218-22.

[8] Irrgang, J. J., Anderson, A. F., Boland, A. L., Harner, C. D., Kurosaka, M., Neyret, P., Richmond, J. C., Shelborne, K. D. Development and validation of the international knee documentation committee subjective knee form. *Am. J. Sports. Med.* 2001 Sep.-Oct.;29(5):600-13.

[9] Mohtadi, N. Development and validation of the quality of life outcome measure (questionnaire) for chronic anterior cruciate ligament deficiency. *Am. J. Sports Med.* 1998 May-Jun.;26(3):350-9.

[10] Koman, J. D., Sanders, J. O. Valgus deformity after reconstruction of the anterior cruciate ligament in a skeletally immature patient. A case report. *J. Bone Joint Surg. Am.* 1999 May;81(5):711-5.

[11] Lipscomb, A. B., Anderson, A. F. Tears of the anterior cruciate ligament in adolescents. *J. Bone Joint Surg. Am.* 1986 Jan.;68(1):19-28.

[12] Pressman, A. E., Letts, R. M., Jarvis, J. G. Anterior cruciate ligament tears in children: an analysis of operative versus nonoperative treatment. *J. Pediatr. Orthop.* 1997 Jul.-Aug.;17(4):505-11.

[13] Kocher, M. S., Smith, J. T., Zoric, B. J., Lee, B., Micheli, L. J. Transphyseal anterior cruciate ligament reconstruction in skeletally immature pubescent adolescents. *J. Bone Joint Surg. Am.* 2007 Dec.;89(12):2632-9.

[14] Millett, P. J., Willis, A. A., Warren, R. F. Associated injuries in pediatric and adolescent anterior cruciate ligament tears: does a delay in treatment increase the risk of meniscal tear? *Arthroscopy.* 2002 Nov.-Dec.;18(9):955-9.

[15] Woods, G. W., O'Connor, D. P. Delayed anterior cruciate ligament reconstruction in adolescents with open physes. *Am. J. Sports Med.* 2004 Jan.-Feb.;32(1):201-10.

[16] Clanton, T. O., DeLee, J.C., Sanders, B., Neidre, A. Knee ligament injuries in children. *J. Bone Joint Surg. Am.* 1979 Dec.;61(8):1195-201.

[17] Kim, S. H., Ha, K. I., Ahn, J. H., Chang, D. K. Anterior cruciate ligament reconstruction in the young patient without violation of the epiphyseal plate. *Arthroscopy.* 1999 Oct.;15(7):792-5.

[18] Bisson, L. J., Wickiewicz, T., Levinson, M., Warren, R. ACL reconstruction in children with open physes. *Orthopedics.* 1998 Jun.;21(6):659-63.

[19] Lo, I. K., Kirkley, A., Fowler, P. J., Miniaci, A. The outcome of operatively treated anterior cruciate ligament disruptions in the skeletally immature child. *Arthroscopy.* 1997 Oct.;13(5):627-34.

[20] Aronowitz, E. R., Ganley, T. J., Goode, J. R., Gregg, J. R., Meyer, J. S. Anterior cruciate ligament reconstruction in adolescents with open physes. *Am. J. Sports Med.* 2000 Mar.-Apr.;28(2):168-75.

[21] Matava, M. J., Siegel, M. G. Arthroscopic reconstruction of the ACL with semitendinosus-gracilis autograft in skeletally immature adolescent patients. *Am. J. Knee Surg.* 1997 Spring;10(2):60-9.

[22] Stadelmaier, D. M., Arnoczky, S. P., Dodds, J., Ross, H. The effect of drilling and soft tissue grafting across open growth plates. A histologic study. *Am. J. Sports Med.* 1995 Jul.-Aug.;23(4):431-5.

[23] Edwards, T. B., Greene, C. C., Baratta, R. V., Zieske, A., Willis, R. B. The effect of placing a tensioned graft across open growth plates. A gross and histologic analysis. *J. Bone Joint Surg. Am.* 2001 May;83-A(5):725-34.

[24] Guzzanti, V., Falciglia, F., Gigante, A., Fabbriciani, C. The effect of intra-articular ACL reconstruction on the growth plates of rabbits. *J. Bone Joint Surg. Br.* 1994 Nov;76(6):960-3.

[25] Houle, J. B., Letts, M., Yang, J. Effects of a tensioned tendon graft in a bone tunnel across the rabbit physis. *Clin. Orthop. Relat. Res.* 2001 Oct.;(391):

INDEX

T